Machine Learning in Medicine - a Complete Overview

Ton J. Cleophas • Aeilko H. Zwinderman

Machine Learning in Medicine - a Complete Overview

With the help from HENNY I. CLEOPHAS-ALLERS, BChem

Springer

Ton J. Cleophas
Department Medicine
Albert Schweitzer Hospital
Sliedrecht, The Netherlands

Aeilko H. Zwinderman
Department Biostatistics and Epidemiology
Academic Medical Center
Amsterdam, The Netherlands

Additional material to this book can be downloaded from http://extras.springer.com.

ISBN 978-3-319-38638-6 ISBN 978-3-319-15195-3 (eBook)
DOI 10.1007/978-3-319-15195-3

Springer Cham Heidelberg New York Dordrecht London

Softcover reprint of the hardcover 1st edition 2015

Printed on acid-free paper

Springer International Publishing AG Switzerland is part of Springer Science+Business Media (www.springer.com)

Preface

The amount of data stored in the world's databases doubles every 20 months, as estimated by Usama Fayyad, one of the founders of machine learning and co-author of the book *Advances in Knowledge Discovery and Data Mining* (ed. by the American Association for Artificial Intelligence, Menlo Park, CA, USA, 1996), and clinicians, familiar with traditional statistical methods, are at a loss to analyze them.

Traditional methods have, indeed, difficulty to identify outliers in large datasets, and to find patterns in big data and data with multiple exposure/outcome variables. In addition, analysis-rules for surveys and questionnaires, which are currently common methods of data collection, are, essentially, missing. Fortunately, the new discipline, machine learning, is able to cover all of these limitations.

So far, medical professionals have been rather reluctant to use machine learning. Ravinda Khattree, co-author of the book *Computational Methods in Biomedical Research* (ed. by Chapman & Hall, Baton Rouge, LA, USA, 2007) suggests that there may be historical reasons: technological (doctors are better than computers (?)), legal, cultural (doctors are better trusted). Also, in the field of diagnosis making, few doctors may want a computer checking them, are interested in collaboration with a computer or with computer engineers.

Adequate health and health care will, however, soon be impossible without proper data supervision from modern machine learning methodologies like cluster models, neural networks, and other data mining methodologies. The current book is the first publication of a complete overview of machine learning methodologies for the medical and health sector, and it was written as a training companion, and as a must-read, not only for physicians and students, but also for anyone involved in the process and progress of health and health care.

Some of the 80 chapters have already appeared in Springer's Cookbook Briefs, but they have been rewritten and updated. All of the chapters have two core characteristics. First, they are intended for current usage, and they are, particularly, concerned with improving that usage. Second, they try and tell what readers need to know in order to understand the methods.

In a nonmathematical way, stepwise analyses of the below three most important classes of machine learning methods will be reviewed:

Cluster and classification models (Chaps. 1, 2, 3, 4, 5, 6, 7, 8, 9, 10, 11, 12, 13, 14, 15, 16, 17, and 18),
(Log)linear models (Chaps. 19, 20, 21, 22, 23, 24, 25, 26, 27, 28, 29, 30, 31, 32, 33, 34, 35, 36, 37, 38, 39, 40, 41, 42, 43, 44, 45, 46, 47, 48, and 49),
Rules models (Chaps. 50, 51, 52, 53, 54, 55, 56, 57, 58, 59, 60, 61, 62, 63, 64, 65, 66, 67, 68, 69, 70, 71, 72, 73, 74, 75, 76, 77, 78, 79, and 80).

The book will include basic methodologies like typology of medical data, quantile-quantile plots for making a start with your data, rate analysis and trend analysis as more powerful alternatives to risk analysis and traditional tests, probit models for binary effects on treatment frequencies, higher order polynomes for circadian phenomena, contingency tables and its myriad applications. Particularly, Chaps. 9, 14, 15, 18, 45, 48, 49, 79, and 80 will review these methodologies.

Chapter 7 describes the use of visualization processes instead of calculus methods for data mining. Chapter 8 describes the use of trained clusters, a scientifically more appropriate alternative to traditional cluster analysis. Chapter 69 describes evolutionary operations (evops), and the evop calculators, already widely used for chemical and technical process improvement.

Various automated analyses and simulation models are in Chaps. 4, 29, 31, and 32. Chapters 67, 70, 71 review spectral plots, Bayesian networks, and support vector machines. A first description of several methods already employed by technical and market scientists, and of their suitabilities for clinical research, is given in Chaps. 37, 38, 39, and 56 (ordinal scalings for inconsistent intervals, loglinear models for varying incident risks, and iteration methods for cross-validations).

Modern methodologies like interval censored analyses, exploratory analyses using pivoting trays, repeated measures logistic regression, doubly multivariate analyses for health assessments, and gamma regression for best fit prediction of health parameters are reviewed in Chaps. 10, 11, 12, 13, 16, 17, 42, 46, and 47.

In order for the readers to perform their own analyses, SPSS data files of the examples are given in extras.springer.com, as well as XML (eXtended Markup Language), SPS (Syntax), and ZIP (compressed) files for outcome predictions in future patients. Furthermore, four csv type excel files are available for data analysis in the Konstanz information miner (Knime) and Weka (Waikato University New Zealand) miner, widely approved free machine learning software packages on the internet since 2006. Also a first introduction is given to SPSS modeler (SPSS' data mining workbench, Chaps. 61, 64, 65), and to SPSS Amos, the graphical and non-graphical data analyzer for the identification of cause-effect relationships as principle goal of research (Chaps. 48 and 49). The free Davidwees polynomial grapher is used in Chap. 79.

This book will demonstrate that machine learning performs sometimes better than traditional statistics does. For example, if the data perfectly fit the cut-offs for node splitting, because, e.g., ages > 55 years give an exponential rise in infarctions, then decision trees, optimal binning, and optimal scaling will be better analysis-methods than traditional regression methods with age as continuous predictor. Machine learning may have little options for adjusting confounding and interaction, but you can add propensity scores and interaction variables to almost any machine learning method.

Each chapter will start with purposes and scientific questions. Then, step-by-step analyses, using both real data and simulated data examples, will be given. Finally, a paragraph with conclusion, and references to the corresponding sites of three introductory textbooks previously written by the same authors, is given.

Lyon, France
December 2015

Ton J. Cleophas
Aeilko H. Zwinderman

Contents

Part I Cluster and Classification Models

1 Hierarchical Clustering and K-Means Clustering to Identify Subgroups in Surveys (50 Patients) 3
General Purpose 3
Specific Scientific Question 3
Hierarchical Cluster Analysis 4
K-Means Cluster Analysis 6
Conclusion 7
Note 8

2 Density-Based Clustering to Identify Outlier Groups in Otherwise Homogeneous Data (50 Patients) 9
General Purpose 9
Specific Scientific Question 9
Density-Based Cluster Analysis 10
Conclusion 11
Note 11

3 Two Step Clustering to Identify Subgroups and Predict Subgroup Memberships in Individual Future Patients (120 Patients) 13
General Purpose 13
Specific Scientific Question 13
The Computer Teaches Itself to Make Predictions 14
Conclusion 15
Note 15

4 Nearest Neighbors for Classifying New Medicines (2 New and 25 Old Opioids) 17
General Purpose 17
Specific Scientific Question 17

Example ... 17
Conclusion ... 24
Note ... 24

5 Predicting High-Risk-Bin Memberships (1,445 Families) ... 25
General Purpose ... 25
Specific Scientific Question ... 25
Example ... 25
Optimal Binning ... 26
Conclusion ... 29
Note ... 29

6 Predicting Outlier Memberships (2,000 Patients) ... 31
General Purpose ... 31
Specific Scientific Question ... 31
Example ... 31
Conclusion ... 34
Note ... 34

7 Data Mining for Visualization of Health Processes (150 Patients) ... 35
General Purpose ... 35
Primary Scientific Question ... 35
Example ... 36
Knime Data Miner ... 37
Knime Workflow ... 38
Box and Whiskers Plots ... 39
Lift Chart ... 39
Histogram ... 40
Line Plot ... 41
Matrix of Scatter Plots ... 42
Parallel Coordinates ... 43
Hierarchical Cluster Analysis with SOTA (Self Organizing Tree Algorithm) ... 44
Conclusion ... 45
Note ... 46

8 Trained Decision Trees for a More Meaningful Accuracy (150 Patients) ... 47
General Purpose ... 47
Primary Scientific Question ... 47
Example ... 48
Downloading the Knime Data Miner ... 49
Knime Workflow ... 50
Conclusion ... 52
Note ... 52

9 **Typology of Medical Data (51 Patients)** 53
General Purpose 53
Primary Scientific Question 54
Example 54
Nominal Variable 55
Ordinal Variable 56
Scale Variable 57
Conclusion 59
Note 60

10 **Predictions from Nominal Clinical Data (450 Patients)** 61
General Purpose 61
Primary Scientific Question 61
Example 61
Conclusion 65
Note 65

11 **Predictions from Ordinal Clinical Data (450 Patients)** 67
General Purpose 67
Primary Scientific Question 67
Example 68
Conclusion 70
Note 70

12 **Assessing Relative Health Risks (3,000 Subjects)** 71
General Purpose 71
Primary Scientific Question 71
Example 71
Conclusion 75
Note 75

13 **Measuring Agreement (30 Patients)** 77
General Purpose 77
Primary Scientific Question 77
Example 77
Conclusion 79
Note 79

14 **Column Proportions for Testing Differences Between Outcome Scores (450 Patients)** 81
General Purpose 81
Specific Scientific Question 81
Example 81
Conclusion 85
Note 85

15 Pivoting Trays and Tables for Improved Analysis of Multidimensional Data (450 Patients) 87
General Purpose 87
Primary Scientific Question 87
Example 87
Conclusion 94
Note 94

16 Online Analytical Procedure Cubes, a More Rapid Approach to Analyzing Frequencies (450 Patients) 95
General Purpose 95
Primary Scientific Question 95
Example 95
Conclusion 99
Note 99

17 Restructure Data Wizard for Data Classified the Wrong Way (20 Patients) 101
General Purpose 101
Primary Scientific Question 103
Example 103
Conclusion 104
Note 104

18 Control Charts for Quality Control of Medicines (164 Tablet Desintegration Times) 105
General Purpose 105
Primary Scientific Question 105
Example 106
Conclusion 109
Note 110

Part II (Log) Linear Models

19 Linear, Logistic, and Cox Regression for Outcome Prediction with Unpaired Data (20, 55, and 60 Patients) 113
General Purpose 113
Specific Scientific Question 113
Linear Regression, the Computer Teaches Itself to Make Predictions 114
Conclusion 116
Note 116
Logistic Regression, the Computer Teaches Itself to Make Predictions 116
Conclusion 118
Note 118
Cox Regression, the Computer Teaches Itself to Make Predictions 118
Conclusion 121
Note 121

20 Generalized Linear Models for Outcome Prediction with Paired Data (100 Patients and 139 Physicians) ... 123
General Purpose ... 123
Specific Scientific Question ... 123
Generalized Linear Modeling, the Computer Teaches Itself to Make Predictions ... 123
Conclusion ... 125
Generalized Estimation Equations, the Computer Teaches Itself to Make Predictions ... 126
Conclusion ... 129
Note ... 129

21 Generalized Linear Models Event-Rates (50 Patients) ... 131
General Purpose ... 131
Specific Scientific Question ... 131
Example ... 131
The Computer Teaches Itself to Make Predictions ... 132
Conclusion ... 135
Note ... 135

22 Factor Analysis and Partial Least Squares (PLS) for Complex-Data Reduction (250 Patients) ... 137
General Purpose ... 137
Specific Scientific Question ... 137
Factor Analysis ... 138
Partial Least Squares Analysis (PLS) ... 140
Traditional Linear Regression ... 142
Conclusion ... 142
Note ... 142

23 Optimal Scaling of High-Sensitivity Analysis of Health Predictors (250 Patients) ... 143
General Purpose ... 143
Specific Scientific Question ... 143
Traditional Multiple Linear Regression ... 144
Optimal Scaling Without Regularization ... 145
Optimal Scaling With Ridge Regression ... 146
Optimal Scaling With Lasso Regression ... 147
Optimal Scaling With Elastic Net Regression ... 147
Conclusion ... 148
Note ... 148

24 Discriminant Analysis for Making a Diagnosis from Multiple Outcomes (45 Patients) ... 149
General Purpose ... 149
Specific Scientific Question ... 149
The Computer Teaches Itself to Make Predictions ... 150
Conclusion ... 153
Note ... 153

25 Weighted Least Squares for Adjusting Efficacy Data with Inconsistent Spread (78 Patients) 155
General Purpose 155
Specific Scientific Question 155
Weighted Least Squares 156
Conclusion 158
Note 158

26 Partial Correlations for Removing Interaction Effects from Efficacy Data (64 Patients) 159
General Purpose 159
Specific Scientific Question 159
Partial Correlations 160
Conclusion 162
Note 163

27 Canonical Regression for Overall Statistics of Multivariate Data (250 Patients) 165
General Purpose 165
Specific Scientific Question 165
Canonical Regression 166
Conclusion 169
Note 169

28 Multinomial Regression for Outcome Categories (55 Patients) 171
General Purpose 171
Specific Scientific Question 171
The Computer Teaches Itself to Make Predictions 172
Conclusion 174
Note 174

29 Various Methods for Analyzing Predictor Categories (60 and 30 Patients) 175
General Purpose 175
Specific Scientific Questions 175
Example 1 175
Example 2 179
Conclusion 182
Note 182

30 Random Intercept Models for Both Outcome and Predictor Categories (55 patients) 183
General Purpose 183
Specific Scientific Question 184
Example 184
Conclusion 187
Note 187

31 Automatic Regression for Maximizing Linear Relationships (55 patients) 189
General Purpose 189
Specific Scientific Question 189
Data Example 189
The Computer Teaches Itself to Make Predictions 192
Conclusion 193
Note 194

32 Simulation Models for Varying Predictors (9,000 Patients) 195
General Purpose 195
Specific Scientific Question 195
Instead of Traditional Means and Standard Deviations, Monte Carlo Simulations of the Input and Outcome Variables are Used to Model the Data. This Enhances Precision, Particularly, With non-Normal Data 196
Conclusion 200
Note 201

33 Generalized Linear Mixed Models for Outcome Prediction from Mixed Data (20 Patients) 203
General Purpose 203
Specific Scientific Question 203
Example 203
Conclusion 206
Note 206

34 Two-Stage Least Squares (35 Patients) 207
General Purpose 207
Primary Scientific Question 207
Example 208
Conclusion 210
Note 210

35 Autoregressive Models for Longitudinal Data (120 Mean Monthly Population Records) 211
General Purpose 211
Specific Scientific Question 211
Example 212
Conclusion 216
Note 217

36 Variance Components for Assessing the Magnitude of Random Effects (40 Patients) 219
General Purpose 219
Primary Scientific Question 219
Example 220
Conclusion 222
Note 222

37 Ordinal Scaling for Clinical Scores with Inconsistent Intervals (900 Patients) ... 223
General Purpose ... 223
Primary Scientific Questions ... 223
Example ... 223
Conclusion ... 227
Note ... 227

38 Loglinear Models for Assessing Incident Rates with Varying Incident Risks (12 Populations) ... 229
General Purpose ... 229
Primary Scientific Question ... 230
Example ... 230
Conclusion ... 232
Note ... 232

39 Loglinear Modeling for Outcome Categories (445 Patients) ... 233
General Purpose ... 233
Primary Scientific Question ... 233
Example ... 234
Conclusion ... 239
Note ... 239

40 Heterogeneity in Clinical Research: Mechanisms Responsible (20 Studies) ... 241
General Purpose ... 241
Primary Scientific Question ... 241
Example ... 242
Conclusion ... 244
Note ... 244

41 Performance Evaluation of Novel Diagnostic Tests (650 and 588 Patients) ... 245
General Purpose ... 245
Primary Scientific Question ... 245
Example ... 245
Binary Logistic Regression ... 248
C-Statistics ... 249
Conclusion ... 251
Note ... 251

42 Quantile-Quantile Plots, a Good Start for Looking at Your Medical Data (50 Cholesterol Measurements and 58 Patients) ... 253
General Purpose ... 253
Specific Scientific Question ... 253
Q-Q Plots for Assessing Departures from Normality ... 253

Q-Q Plots as Diagnostics for Fitting Data to Normal (and Other Theoretical) Distributions ... 256
Conclusion ... 258
Note ... 259

43 Rate Analysis of Medical Data Better than Risk Analysis (52 Patients) ... 261
General Purpose ... 261
Specific Scientific Question ... 261
Example ... 261
Conclusion ... 264
Note ... 264

44 Trend Tests Will Be Statistically Significant if Traditional Tests Are Not (30 and 106 Patients) ... 265
General Purpose ... 265
Specific Scientific Questions ... 265
Example 1 ... 265
Example 2 ... 267
Conclusion ... 269
Note ... 269

45 Doubly Multivariate Analysis of Variance for Multiple Observations from Multiple Outcome Variables (16 Patients) ... 271
General Purpose ... 271
Primary Scientific Question ... 271
Example ... 272
Conclusion ... 276
Note ... 276

46 Probit Models for Estimating Effective Pharmacological Treatment Dosages (14 Tests) ... 279
General Purpose ... 279
Primary Scientific Question ... 279
Example ... 279
Simple Probit Regression ... 279
Multiple Probit Regression ... 282
Conclusion ... 286
Note ... 287

47 Interval Censored Data Analysis for Assessing Mean Time to Cancer Relapse (51 Patients) ... 289
General Purpose ... 289
Primary Scientific Question ... 289
Example ... 290
Conclusion ... 292
Note ... 293

48 Structural Equation Modeling (SEM) with SPSS Analysis of Moment Structures (Amos) for Cause Effect Relationships I (35 Patients) 295
General Purpose 295
Primary Scientific Question 296
Example 296
Conclusion 300
Note 300

49 Structural Equation Modeling (SEM) with SPSS Analysis of Moment Structures (Amos) for Cause Effect Relationships in Pharmacodynamic Studies II (35 Patients) 301
General Purpose 301
Primary Scientific Question 302
Example 302
Conclusion 306
Note 306

Part III Rules Models

50 Neural Networks for Assessing Relationships That Are Typically Nonlinear (90 Patients) 309
General Purpose 309
Specific Scientific Question 309
The Computer Teaches Itself to Make Predictions 310
Conclusion 311
Note 312

51 Complex Samples Methodologies for Unbiased Sampling (9,678 Persons) 313
General Purpose 313
Specific Scientific Question 313
The Computer Teaches Itself to Predict Current Health Scores from Previous Health Scores 315
The Computer Teaches Itself to Predict Individual Odds Ratios of Current Health Scores Versus Previous Health Scores 317
Conclusion 318
Note 319

52 Correspondence Analysis for Identifying the Best of Multiple Treatments in Multiple Groups (217 Patients) 321
General Purpose 321
Specific Scientific Question 321
Correspondence Analysis 322
Conclusion 325
Note 325

53 Decision Trees for Decision Analysis (1,004 and 953 Patients) 327
General Purpose 327
Specific Scientific Question 327
Decision Trees with a Binary Outcome 327
Decision Trees with a Continuous Outcome 331
Conclusion 334
Note 334

54 Multidimensional Scaling for Visualizing Experienced Drug Efficacies (14 Pain-Killers and 42 Patients) 335
General Purpose 335
Specific Scientific Question 335
Proximity Scaling 336
Preference Scaling 338
Conclusion 343
Note 344

55 Stochastic Processes for Long Term Predictions from Short Term Observations 345
General Purpose 345
Specific Scientific Questions 345
Example 1 345
Example 2 347
Example 3 349
Conclusion 351
Note 351

56 Optimal Binning for Finding High Risk Cut-offs (1,445 Families) 353
General Purpose 353
Specific Scientific Question 353
Optimal Binning 354
Conclusion 357
Note 357

57 Conjoint Analysis for Determining the Most Appreciated Properties of Medicines to Be Developed (15 Physicians) 359
General Purpose 359
Specific Scientific Question 359
Constructing an Analysis Plan 359
Performing the Final Analysis 361
Conclusion 364
Note 364

58 Item Response Modeling for Analyzing Quality of Life with Better Precision (1,000 Patients) 365
General Purpose 365
Primary Scientific Question 365
Example 365
Conclusion 369
Note 369

59 Survival Studies with Varying Risks of Dying (50 and 60 Patients) 371
General Purpose 371
Primary Scientific Question 371
Examples 371
Cox Regression with a Time-Dependent Predictor 371
Cox Regression with a Segmented Time-Dependent Predictor 373
Conclusion 374
Note 375

60 Fuzzy Logic for Improved Precision of Dose-Response Data (8 Induction Dosages) 377
General Purpose 377
Specific Scientific Question 377
Example 378
Conclusion 381
Note 381

61 Automatic Data Mining for the Best Treatment of a Disease (90 Patients) 383
General Purpose 383
Specific Scientific Question 383
Example 383
Step 1 Open SPSS Modeler 385
Step 2 The Distribution Node 385
Step 3 The Data Audit Node 386
Step 4 The Plot Node 387
Step 5 The Web Node 388
Step 6 The Type and c5.0 Nodes 389
Step 7 The Output Node 390
Conclusion 390
Note 390

62 Pareto Charts for Identifying the Main Factors of Multifactorial Outcomes (2,000 Admissions to Hospital) 391
General Purpose 391
Primary Scientific Question 391
Example 392
Conclusion 396
Note 396

63 Radial Basis Neural Networks for Multidimensional Gaussian Data (90 Persons) 397
General Purpose 397
Specific Scientific Question 397
Example 397
The Computer Teaches Itself to Make Predictions 398
Conclusion 400
Note 400

64 Automatic Modeling of Drug Efficacy Prediction (250 Patients) 401
General Purpose 401
Specific Scientific Question 401
Example 401
Step 1 Open SPSS Modeler (14.2) 402
Step 2 The Statistics File Node 403
Step 3 The Type Node 403
Step 4 The Auto Numeric Node 404
Step 5 The Expert Node 405
Step 6 The Settings Tab 407
Step 7 The Analysis Node 407
Conclusion 408
Note 408

65 Automatic Modeling for Clinical Event Prediction (200 Patients) 409
General Purpose 409
Specific Scientific Question 409
Example 409
Step 1 Open SPSS Modeler (14.2) 410
Step 2 The Statistics File Node 411
Step 3 The Type Node 411
Step 4 The Auto Classifier Node 412
Step 5 The Expert Tab 413
Step 6 The Settings Tab 414
Step 7 The Analysis Node 415
Conclusion 416
Note 416

66 Automatic Newton Modeling in Clinical Pharmacology (15 Alfentanil Dosages, 15 Quinidine Time-Concentration Relationships) 417
General Purpose 417
Specific Scientific Question 418
Examples 418
  Dose-Effectiveness Study 418
  Time-Concentration Study 420
Conclusion 422
Note 422

67 Spectral Plots for High Sensitivity Assessment of Periodicity (6 Years' Monthly C Reactive Protein Levels) 423
General Purpose 423
Specific Scientific Question 423
Example 423
Conclusion 427
Note 428

68 Runs Test for Identifying Best Regression Models (21 Estimates of Quantity and Quality of Patient Care) 429
General Purpose 429
Primary Scientific Question 429
Example 429
Conclusion 433
Note 433

69 Evolutionary Operations for Process Improvement (8 Operation Room Air Condition Settings) 435
General Purpose 435
Specific Scientific Question 435
Example 436
Conclusion 437
Note 438

70 Bayesian Networks for Cause Effect Modeling (600 Patients) 439
General Purpose 439
Primary Scientific Question 439
Example 440
Binary Logistic Regression in SPSS 440
Konstanz Information Miner (Knime) 441
Knime Workflow 442
Conclusion 443
Note 444

71 Support Vector Machines for Imperfect Nonlinear Data (200 Patients with Sepsis) 445
General Purpose 445
Primary Scientific Question 445
Example 446
Knime Data Miner 446
Knime Workflow 447
File Reader Node 447
The Nodes X-Partitioner, svm Learner, svm Predictor, X-Aggregator 448
Error Rates 448
Prediction Table 448
Conclusion 449
Note 449

72 Multiple Response Sets for Visualizing Clinical Data Trends (811 Patient Visits) 451
General Purpose 451
Specific Scientific Question 451
Example 451
Conclusion 457
Note 457

73 Protein and DNA Sequence Mining 459
General Purpose 459
Specific Scientific Question 459
Data Base Systems on the Internet 460
Example 1 461
Example 2 462
Example 3 462
Example 4 463
Conclusion 464
Note 464

74 Iteration Methods for Crossvalidations (150 Patients with Pneumonia) 465
General Purpose 465
Primary Scientific Question 465
Example 465
Downloading the Knime Data Miner 466
Knime Workflow 467
Crossvalidation 467
Conclusion 469
Note 469

75 Testing Parallel-Groups with Different Sample Sizes and Variances (5 Parallel-Group Studies) 471
General Purpose 471
Primary Scientific Question 471
Examples 472
Conclusion 473
Note 473

76 Association Rules Between Exposure and Outcome (50 and 60 Patients) 475
General Purpose 475
Primary Scientific Question 475
Example 475
  Example One 477
  Example Two 478
Conclusion 479
Note 479

77 Confidence Intervals for Proportions and Differences in Proportions (100 and 75 Patients) 481
General Purpose 481
Primary Scientific Question 481
Example 482
Confidence Intervals of Proportions 482
Confidence Intervals of Differences in Proportions 483
Conclusion 484
Note 484

78 Ratio Statistics for Efficacy Analysis of New Drugs (50 Patients) 485
General Purpose 485
Primary Scientific Question 485
Example 485
Conclusion 489
Note 489

79 Fifth Order Polynomes of Circadian Rhythms (1 Patient with Hypertension) 491
General Purpose 491
Primary Scientific Question 492
Example 492
Conclusion 495
Note 496

80 Gamma Distribution for Estimating the Predictors of Medical Outcome Scores (110 Patients) 497
General Purpose 497
Primary Scientific Question 498
Example 498
Conclusion 503
Note 503

Index 505

Part I
Cluster and Classification Models

Chapter 1
Hierarchical Clustering and K-Means Clustering to Identify Subgroups in Surveys (50 Patients)

General Purpose

Clusters are subgroups in a survey estimated by the distances between the values needed to connect the patients, otherwise called cases. It is an important methodology in explorative data mining.

Specific Scientific Question

In a survey of patients with mental depression of different ages and depression scores, how do different clustering methods perform in identifying so far unobserved subgroups.

This chapter was previously published in "Machine learning in medicine-cookbook 1" as Chap. 1, 2013.

T.J. Cleophas, A.H. Zwinderman, *Machine Learning in Medicine - a Complete Overview*, DOI 10.1007/978-3-319-15195-3_1

1	2	3
20,00	8,00	1
21,00	7,00	2
23,00	9,00	3
24,00	10,00	4
25,00	8,00	5
26,00	9,00	6
27,00	7,00	7
28,00	8,00	8
24,00	9,00	9
32,00	9,00	10
30,00	1,00	11
40,00	2,00	12
50,00	3,00	13
60,00	1,00	14
70,00	2,00	15
76,00	3,00	16
65,00	2,00	17
54,00	3,00	18

Var 1 age
Var 2 depression score (0 = very mild, 10 = severest)
Var 3 patient number (called cases here)

Only the first 18 patients are given, the entire data file is entitled "hierk-meansdensity" and is in extras.springer.com.

Hierarchical Cluster Analysis

SPSS 19.0 will be used for data analysis. Start by opening the data file.

Command:

Analyze….Classify….Hierarchical Cluster Analysis….enter variables….Label Case by: case variable with the values 1-50….Plots: mark Dendrogram….Method ….Cluster Method: Between-group linkage….Measure: Squared Euclidean Distance….Save: click Single solution….Number of clusters: enter 3….Continue ….OK.

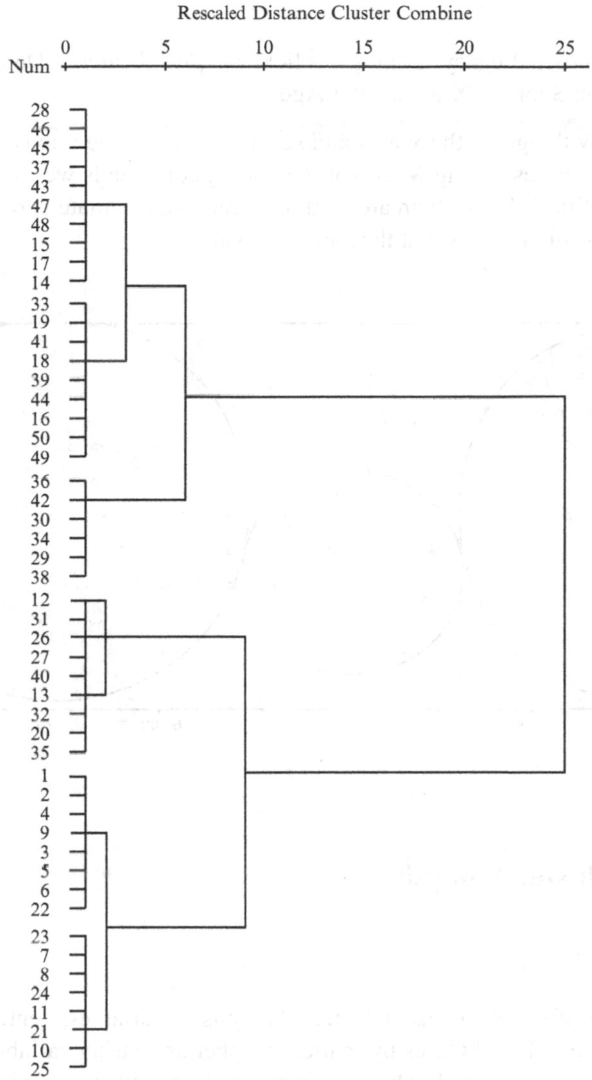

In the output a dendrogram of the results is given. The actual distances between the cases are rescaled to fall into a range of 0–25 units (0 = minimal distance, 25 = maximal distance). The cases no. 1–11, 21–25 are clustered together in cluster 1, the cases 12, 13, 20, 26, 27, 31, 32, 35, 40 in cluster 2, both at a rescaled distance from 0 at approximately 3 units, the remainder of the cases is clustered at approximately 6 units. And so, as requested, three clusters have been identified with cases more similar to one another than to the other clusters. When minimizing the output, the data file comes up and it now shows the cluster membership of each case. We will use SPSS again to draw a Dotter graph of the data.

Command:

Analyze....Graphs....Legacy Dialogs: click Simple Scatter....Define....Y-axis: enter Depression Score....X-axis: enter Age....OK.

The graph (with age on the x-axis and severity score on the y-axis) produced by SPSS shows the cases. Using Microsoft's drawing commands we can encircle the clusters as identified. All of them are oval and even, approximately, round, because variables have similar scales, but they are different in size.

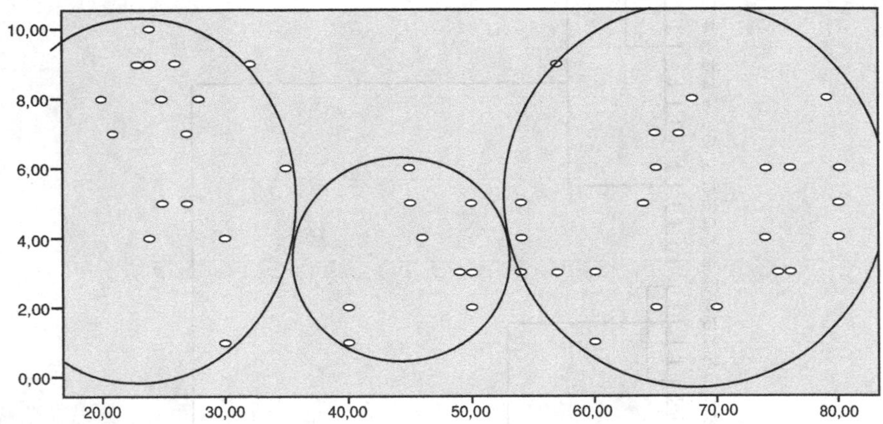

K-Means Cluster Analysis

Command:

Analyze....Classify....K-means Cluster Analysis....Variables: enter Age and Depression score....Label Cases by: patient number as a string variable....Number of clusters: 3 (in our example chosen for comparison with the above method).... click Method: mark Iterate....click Iterate: Maximal Iterations: mark 10.... Convergence criterion: mark 0....click Continue....click Save: mark Cluster Membership....click Continue....click Options: mark Initiate cluster centers.... mark ANOVA table....mark Cluster information for each case....click Continue.... OK.

The output shows that the three clusters identified by the k-means cluster model were significantly different from one another both by testing the y-axis (depression score) and the x-axis variable (age). When minimizing the output sheets, the data file comes up and shows the cluster membership of the three clusters.

ANOVA

	Cluster		Error			
	Mean square	df	Mean square	df	F	Sig.
Age	8712,723	2	31,082	47	280,310	,000
Depression score	39,102	2	4,593	47	8,513	,001

We will use SPSS again to draw a Dotter graph of the data.

Command:

Analyze....Graphs....Legacy Dialogs: click Simple Scatter....Define....Y-axis: enter Depression Score....X-axis: enter Age....OK.

The graph (with age on the x-axis and severity score on the y-axis) produced by SPSS shows the cases. Using Microsoft's drawing commands we can encircle the clusters as identified. All of them are oval and even approximately round because variables have similar scales, and they are approximately equal in size.

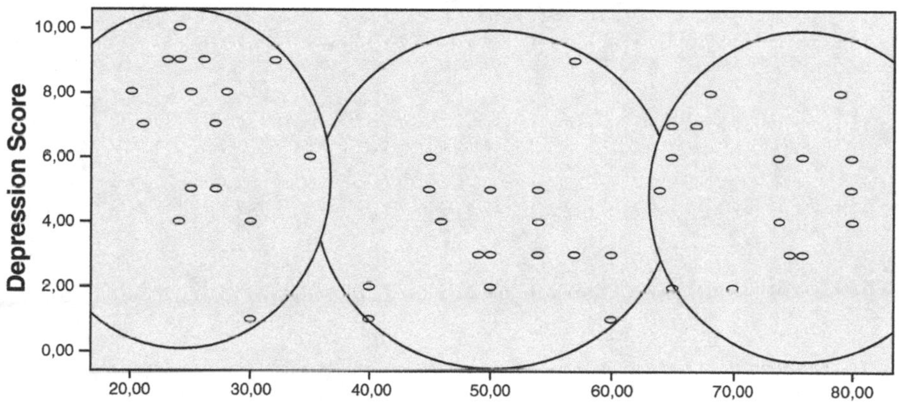

Conclusion

Clusters are estimated by the distances between the values needed to connect the cases. It is an important methodology in explorative data mining. Hierarchical clustering is adequate if subgroups are expected to be different in size, k-means clustering if approximately similar in size. Density-based clustering is more appropriate if small outlier groups between otherwise homogenous populations are expected. The latter method is in Chap. 2.

Note

More background, theoretical and mathematical information of the two methods is given in Machine learning in medicine part two, Chap. 8 Two-dimensional Clustering, pp 65–75, Springer Heidelberg Germany 2013. Density-based clustering will be reviewed in the next chapter.

Chapter 2
Density-Based Clustering to Identify Outlier Groups in Otherwise Homogeneous Data (50 Patients)

General Purpose

Clusters are subgroups in a survey estimated by the distances between the values needed to connect the patients, otherwise called cases. It is an important methodology in explorative data mining. Density-based clustering is used.

Specific Scientific Question

In a survey of patients with mental depression of different ages and depression scores, how does density-based clustering perform in identifying so far unobserved subgroups.

This chapter was previously published in "Machine learning in medicine-cookbook 1" as Chap. 2, 2013.

T.J. Cleophas, A.H. Zwinderman, *Machine Learning in Medicine - a Complete Overview*, DOI 10.1007/978-3-319-15195-3_2

1	2	3
20,00	8,00	1
21,00	7,00	2
23,00	9,00	3
24,00	10,00	4
25,00	8,00	5
26,00	9,00	6
27,00	7,00	7
28,00	8,00	8
24,00	9,00	9
32,00	9,00	10
30,00	1,00	11
40,00	2,00	12
50,00	3,00	13
60,00	1,00	14
70,00	2,00	15
76,00	3,00	16
65,00	2,00	17
54,00	3,00	18

Var 1 age
Var 2 depression score (0 = very mild, 10 = severest)
Var 3 patient number (called cases here)

Only the first 18 patients are given, the entire data file is entitled "hierk-meansdensity" and is in extras.springer.com.

Density-Based Cluster Analysis

The DBSCAN method was used (density based spatial clustering of application with noise). As this method is not available in SPSS, an interactive JAVA Applet freely available at the Internet was used [Data Clustering Applets. http://webdocs.cs.ualberts.ca/~yaling/Cluster/applet]. The DBSCAN connects points that satisfy a density criterion given by a minimum number of patients within a defined radius (radius = Eps; minimum number = Min pts).

Command:

User Define....Choose data set: remove values given....enter you own x and y values....Choose algorithm: select DBSCAN....Eps: mark 25....Min pts: mark 3.... Start....Show.

Three cluster memberships are again shown. We will use SPSS 19.0 again to draw a Dotter graph of the data.

Command:

Analyze....Graphs....Legacy Dialogs: click Simple Scatter....Define....Y-axis: enter Depression Score....X-axis: enter Age....OK.

The graph (with age on the x-axis and severity score on the y-axis) shows the cases. Using Microsoft's drawing commands we can encircle the clusters as identified. Two very small ones, one large one. All of the clusters identified are non-circular and, are, obviously, based on differences in patient-density.

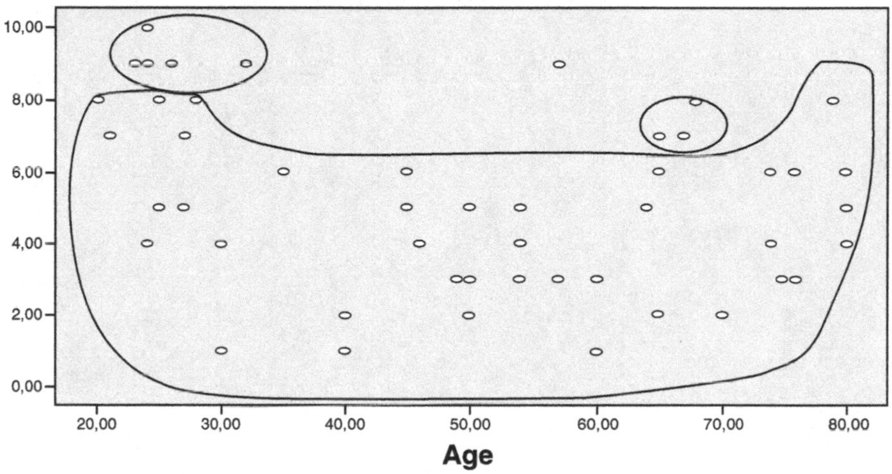

Conclusion

Clusters are estimated by the distances between the values needed to connect the cases. It is an important methodology in explorative data mining. Density-based clustering is suitable if small outlier groups between otherwise homogeneous populations are expected. Hierarchical and k-means clustering are more appropriate if subgroups have Gaussian-like patterns (Chap. 1).

Note

More background, theoretical and mathematical information of the three methods is given in Machine learning in medicine part two, Chap. 8 Two-dimensional clustering, pp 65–75, Springer Heidelberg Germany 2013. Hierarchical and k-means clustering are reviewed in the previous chapter.

Chapter 3
Two Step Clustering to Identify Subgroups and Predict Subgroup Memberships in Individual Future Patients (120 Patients)

General Purpose

To assess whether two step clustering of survey data can be trained to identify subgroups and subgroup membership.

Specific Scientific Question

In patients with mental depression, can the item scores of depression severity be used to classify subgroups and to predict subgroup membership of future patients.

Var 1	Var 2	Var 3	Var 4	Var 5	Var 6	Var 7	Var 8	Var 9
9,00	9,00	9,00	2,00	2,00	2,00	2,00	2,00	2,00
8,00	8,00	6,00	3,00	3,00	3,00	3,00	3,00	3,00
7,00	7,00	7,00	4,00	4,00	4,00	4,00	4,00	4,00
4,00	9,00	9,00	2,00	2,00	6,00	2,00	2,00	2,00
8,00	8,00	8,00	3,00	3,00	3,00	3,00	3,00	3,00
7,00	7,00	7,00	4,00	4,00	4,00	4,00	4,00	4,00
9,00	5,00	9,00	9,00	2,00	2,00	2,00	2,00	2,00
8,00	8,00	8,00	3,00	3,00	3,00	3,00	3,00	3,00
7,00	7,00	7,00	4,00	6,00	4,00	4,00	4,00	4,00
9,00	9,00	9,00	2,00	2,00	2,00	2,00	2,00	2,00
4,00	4,00	4,00	9,00	9,00	9,00	3,00	3,00	3,00
3,00	3,00	3,00	8,00	8,00	8,00	4,00	4,00	4,00

Var 1–9 = depression score 1–9

This chapter was previously published in "Machine learning in medicine-cookbook 1" as Chap. 3, 2013.

T.J. Cleophas, A.H. Zwinderman, *Machine Learning in Medicine - a Complete Overview*, DOI 10.1007/978-3-319-15195-3_3

Only the first 12 patients are given, the entire data file is entitled “twostepclustering” and is in extras.springer.com.

The Computer Teaches Itself to Make Predictions

SPSS 19.0 is used for data analysis. It will use XML (eXtended Markup Language) files to store data. Now start by opening the data file.

Command:

Click Transform....click Random Number Generators....click Set Starting Point ....click Fixed Value (2000000)....click OK....click Analyze....Classify....TwoStep Cluster....Continuous Variables: enter depression 1-9....click Output: in Working Data File click Create cluster membership....in XML Files click Export final model....click Browse....File name: enter "export2step"....click Save....click Continue....click OK.

Returning to the data file we will observe that three subgroups have been identified and for each patient the subgroup membership is given as a novel variable, and the name of this novel variable is TSC (two step cluster). The saved XML file will now be used to compute the predicted subgroup membership in five future patients. For convenience the XML file is given in extras.springer.com.

Var 1	Var 2	Var 3	Var 4	Var 5	Var 6	Var 7	Var 8	Var 9
4,00	5,00	3,00	4,00	6,00	9,00	8,00	7,00	6,00
2,00	2,00	2,00	2,00	2,00	2,00	2,00	2,00	2,00
5,00	4,00	6,00	7,00	6,00	5,00	3,00	4,00	5,00
9,00	8,00	7,00	6,00	5,00	4,00	3,00	2,00	2,00
7,00	7,00	7,00	3,00	3,00	3,00	9,00	9,00	9,00

Var 1–9 = Depression score 1–9

Enter the above data in a new SPSS data file.

Command:

Utilities....click Scoring Wizard....click Browse....click Select....Folder: enter the export2step.xml file....click Select....in Scoring Wizard click Next....click Use value substitution....click Next....click Finish.

The above data file now gives subgroup memberships of the five patients as computed by the two step cluster model with the help of the XML file.

Var 1	Var 2	Var 3	Var 4	Var 5	Var 6	Var 7	Var 8	Var 9	Var 10
4,00	5,00	3,00	4,00	6,00	9,00	8,00	7,00	6,00	2,00
2,00	2,00	2,00	2,00	2,00	2,00	2,00	2,00	2,00	2,00
5,00	4,00	6,00	7,00	6,00	5,00	3,00	4,00	5,00	3,00
9,00	8,00	7,00	6,00	5,00	4,00	3,00	2,00	2,00	1,00
7,00	7,00	7,00	3,00	3,00	3,00	9,00	9,00	9,00	2,00

Var 1–9 Depression score 1–9
Var 10 predicted value

Conclusion

Two step clustering can be readily trained to identify subgroups in patients with mental depression, and, with the help of an XML file, it can, subsequently, be used to identify subgroup memberships in individual future patients.

Note

More background, theoretical and mathematical information of two step and other methods of clustering is available in Machine learning in medicine part two, Chaps. 8 and 9, entitled "Two-dimensional clustering" and "Multidimensional clustering", pp 65–75 and 77–91, Springer Heidelberg Germany 2013.

Chapter 4
Nearest Neighbors for Classifying New Medicines (2 New and 25 Old Opioids)

General Purpose

Nearest neighbor methodology has a long history, and has, initially, been used for data imputation in demographic data files. This chapter is to assess whether it can also been used for classifying new medicines.

Specific Scientific Question

For most diseases a whole class of drugs rather than a single compound is available. Nearest neighbor methods can be used for identifying the place of a new drug within its class.

Example

Two newly developed opioid compounds are assessed for their similarities with the standard opioids in order to determine their potential places in therapeutic regimens. Underneath are the characteristics of 25 standard opioids and two newly developed opioid compounds.

This chapter was previously published in "Machine learning in medicine-cookbook 2" as Chap. 1, 2014.

T.J. Cleophas, A.H. Zwinderman, *Machine Learning in Medicine - a Complete Overview*, DOI 10.1007/978-3-319-15195-3_4

Drugname	analgesia score	antitussive score	constipation score	respiratory score	abuse score	eliminate time	duration time
buprenorphine	7,00	4,00	5,00	7,00	4,00	5,00	9,00
butorphanol	7,00	3,00	4,00	7,00	4,00	2,70	4,00
codeine	5,00	6,00	6,00	5,00	4,00	2,90	7,00
heroine	8,00	6,00	8,00	8,00	10,00	9,00	15,00
hydromorphone	8,00	6,00	6,00	8,00	8,00	2,60	5,00
levorphanol	8,00	6,00	6,00	8,00	8,00	11,00	20,00
mepriridine	7,00	2,00	4,00	8,00	6,00	3,20	14,00
methadone	9,00	6,00	6,00	8,00	6,00	25,00	5,00
morphine	8,00	6,00	8,00	8,00	8,00	3,10	5,00
nalbuphine	7,00	2,00	4,00	7,00	4,00	5,10	4,50
oxycodone	6,00	6,00	6,00	6,00	8,00	5,00	4,00
oxymorphine	8,00	5,00	6,00	8,00	8,00	5,20	3,50
pentazocine	7,00	2,00	4,00	7,00	5,00	2,90	3,00
propoxyphene	5,00	2,00	4,00	5,00	5,00	3,30	2,00
nalorphine	2,00	3,00	6,00	8,00	1,00	1,40	3,20
levallorphan	3,00	2,00	5,00	4,00	1,00	11,00	5,00
cyclazocine	2,00	3,00	6,00	3,00	2,00	1,60	2,80
naloxone	1,00	2,00	5,00	8,00	1,00	1,20	3,00
naltrexon	1,00	3,00	5,00	8,00	,00	9,70	14,00
alfentanil	7,00	6,00	7,00	4,00	6,00	1,60	,50
alphaprodine	6,00	5,00	6,00	3,00	5,00	2,20	2,00
fentanyl	6,00	5,00	7,00	5,00	4,00	3,70	,50
meptazinol	4,00	3,00	5,00	5,00	3,00	1,60	2,00
norpropoxyphene	8,00	6,00	8,00	5,00	7,00	6,00	4,00
sufentanil	7,00	6,00	8,00	6,00	8,00	2,60	5,00
newdrug1	5,00	5,00	4,00	3,00	6,00	5,00	12,00
newdrug2	8,00	6,00	3,00	4,00	5,00	7,00	16,00

Var = variable
Var 1 analgesia score (0–10)
Var 2 antitussive score (0–10)
Var 3 constipation score (0–10)
Var 4 respiratory depression score (1–10)
Var 5 abuse liability score (1–10)
Var 6 elimination time ($t_{1/2}$ in hours)
Var 7 duration time analgesia (hours)

The data file is entitled "nearestneighbor" and is in extras.springer.com.

SPSS statistical software is used for data analysis. Start by opening the data file. The drug names included, eight variables are in the file. A ninth variable entitled "partition" must be added with the value 1 for the opioids 1–25 and 0 for the two new compounds (cases 26 and 27).

Then command:

Analyze....Classify....Nearest Neighbor Analysis....enter the variable "drugsname" in Target....enter the variables "analgesia" to "duration of analgesia" in Features.... click Partitions....click Use variable to assign cases....enter the variable "Partition"....click OK.

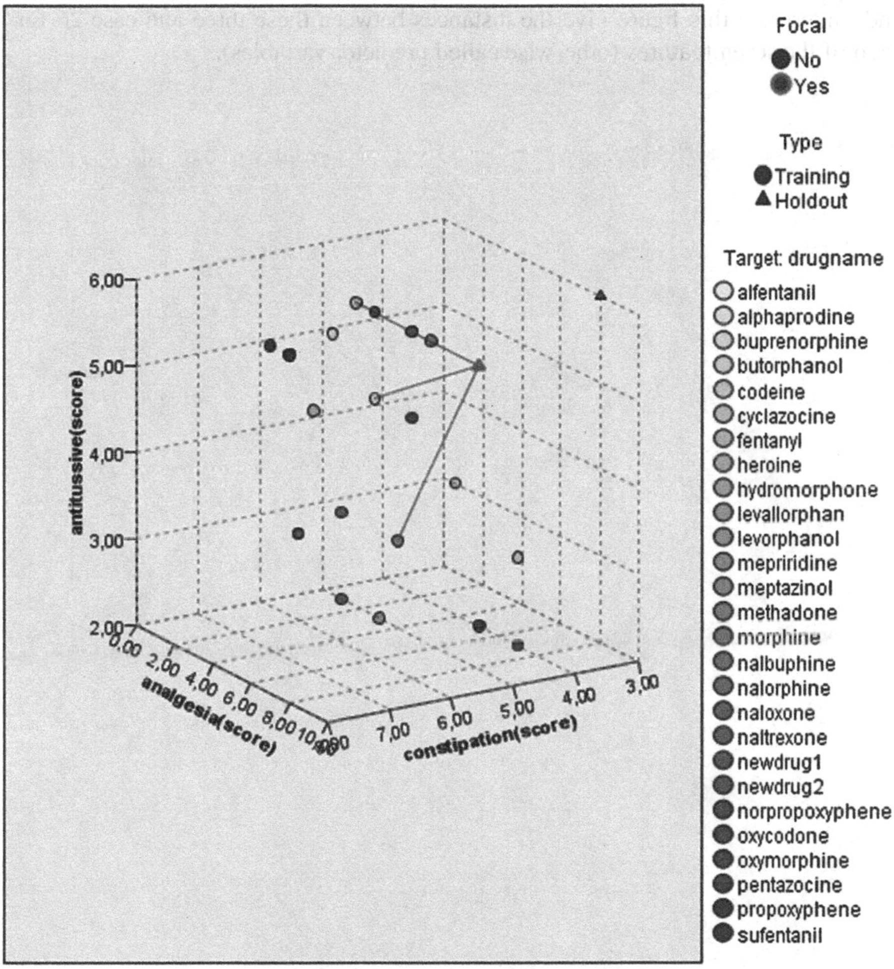

Select points to use as focal records

This chart is a lower-dimensional projection of the predictor space, which contains a total of 7 predictors.

The above figure shows as an example the place of the two new compounds (the small triangles) as compared with those of the standard opioids. Lines connect them to their 3 nearest neighbors. In SPSS' original output sheets the graph can by double-clicking be placed in the "model viewer", and, then, (after again clicking on it) be interactively rotated in order to improve the view of the distances. SPSS uses 3 nearest neighbors by default, but you can change this number if you like. The names of the compounds are given in alphabetical order. Only three of seven variables are given in the initial figure, but if you click on one of the small triangles in this figure, an auxiliary view comes up right from the main view. Here are all the details of the analysis. The upper left graph of it shows that the opioids 21, 3, and 23 have the best average nearest neighbor records for case 26 (new drug 1). The seven figures alongside and underneath this figure give the distances between these three and case 26 for each of the seven features (otherwise called predictor variables).

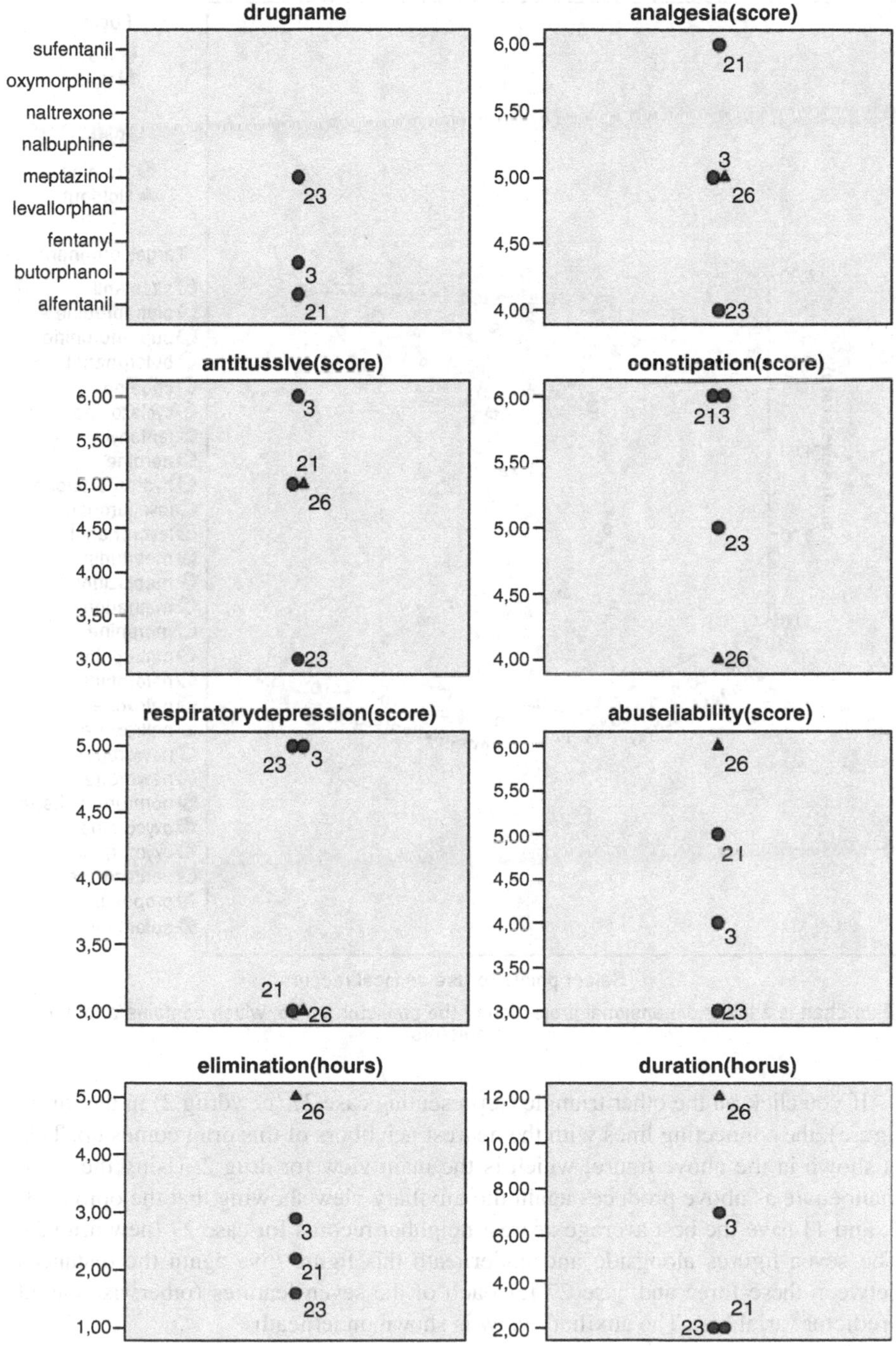
drugname
sufentanil
oxymorphine
naltrexone
nalbuphine
meptazinol
levallorphan
fentanyl
butorphanol
alfentanil
23
3
21
analgesia(score)
6,00
5,50
5,00
4,50
4,00
21
3
26
23
antitussive(score)
6,00
5,50
5,00
4,50
4,00
3,50
3,00
3
21
26
23
constipation(score)
6,00
5,50
5,00
4,50
4,00
213
23
26
respiratorydepression(score)
5,00
4,50
4,00
3,50
3,00
23
3
21
26
abuseliability(score)
6,00
5,50
5,00
4,50
4,00
3,50
3,00
26
21
3
23
elimination(hours)
5,00
4,00
3,00
2,00
1,00
26
3
21
23
duration(horus)
12,00
10,00
8,00
6,00
4,00
2,00
26
3
21
23

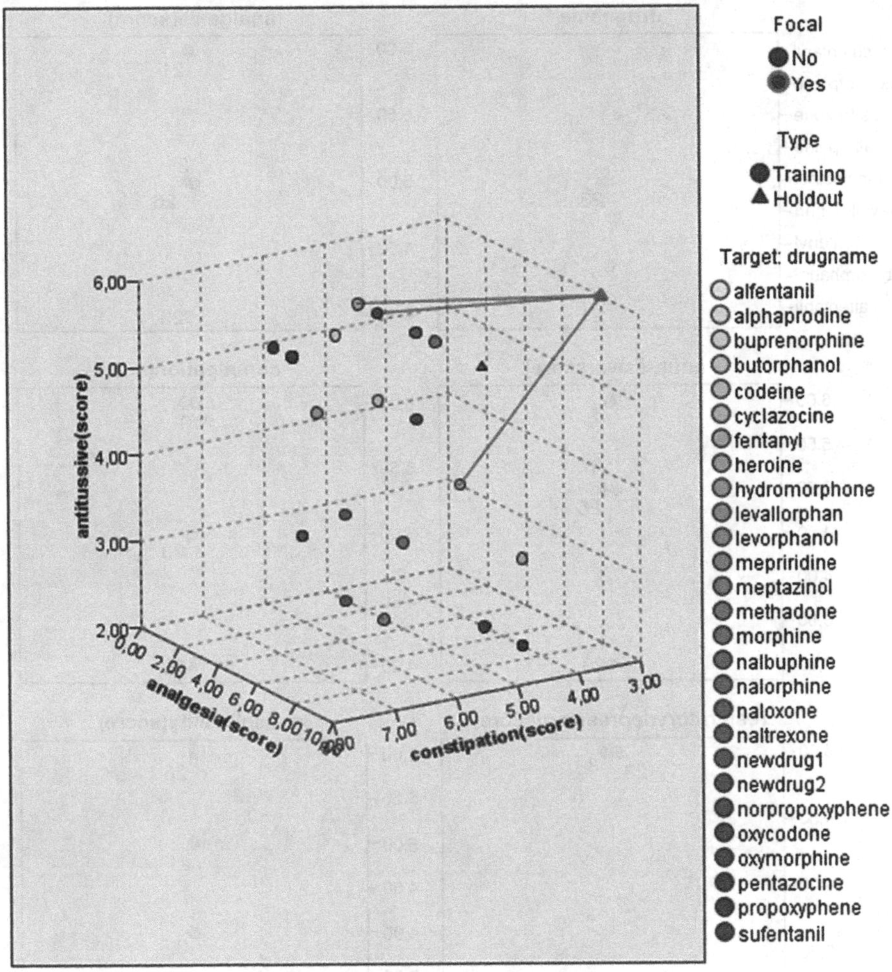

Select points to use as focal records

This chart is a lower-dimensional projection of the predictor space, which contains a total of 7 predictors.

If you click on the other triangle (representing case 27 (newdrug 2) in the initial figure), the connecting lines with the nearest neighbors of this drug comes up. This is shown in the above figure, which is the main view for drug 2. Using the same manoeuvre as above produces again the auxiliary view showing that the opioids 3, 1, and 11 have the best average nearest neighbor records for case 27 (new drug 2). The seven figures alongside and underneath this figure give again the distances between these three and case 27 for each of the seven features (otherwise called predictor variables). The auxiliary view is shown underneath.

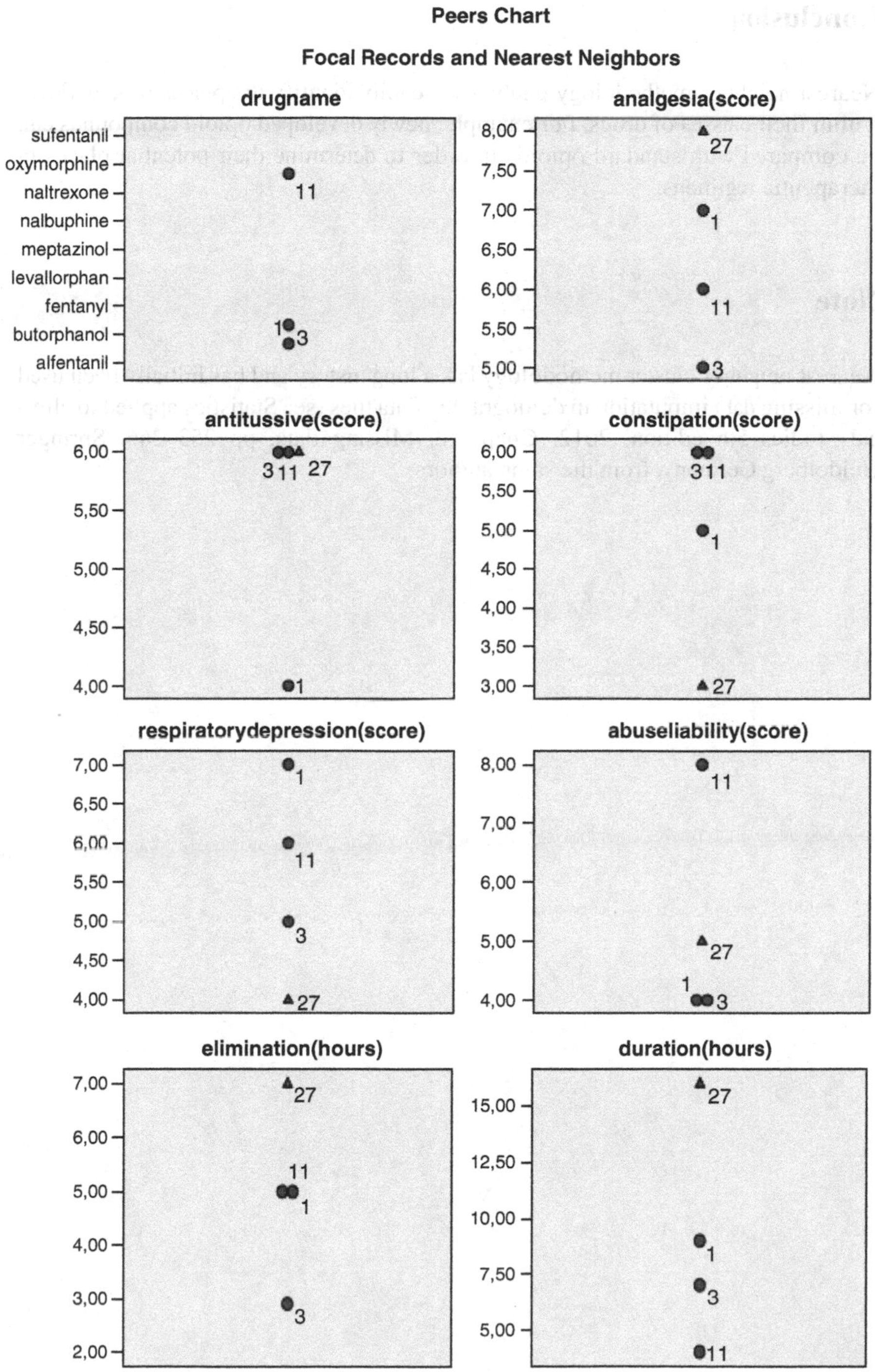
Peers Chart
Focal Records and Nearest Neighbors
drugname
sufentanil
oxymorphine
naltrexone
nalbuphine
meptazinol
levallorphan
fentanyl
butorphanol
alfentanil
11
1
3
analgesia(score)
8,00
7,50
7,00
6,50
6,00
5,50
5,00
27
1
11
3
antitussive(score)
6,00
5,50
5,00
4,50
4,00
3 11 27
1
constipation(score)
6,00
5,50
5,00
4,50
4,00
3,50
3,00
3 11
1
27
respiratorydepression(score)
7,00
6,50
6,00
5,50
5,00
4,50
4,00
1
11
3
27
abuseliability(score)
8,00
7,00
6,00
5,00
4,00
11
27
1
3
elimination(hours)
7,00
6,00
5,00
4,00
3,00
2,00
27
11
1
3
duration(hours)
15,00
12,50
10,00
7,50
5,00
27
1
3
11

Conclusion

Nearest neighbor methodology enables to readily identify the places of new drugs within their classes of drugs. For example, newly developed opioid compounds can be compared with standard opioids in order to determine their potential places in therapeutic regimens.

Note

Nearest neighbor cluster methodology has a long history and has initially been used for missing data imputation in demographic data files (see Statistics applied to clinical studies 5th edition, 2012, Chap. 22, Missing data, pp 253–266, Springer Heidelberg Germany, from the same authors).

Chapter 5
Predicting High-Risk-Bin Memberships (1,445 Families)

General Purpose

Optimal bins describe continuous predictor variables in the form of best fit categories for making predictions, e.g., about families at high risk of bank loan defaults. In addition, it can be used for, e.g., predicting health risk cut-offs about individual future families, based on their characteristics (Chap. 56).

Specific Scientific Question

Can optimal binning also be applied for other medical purposes, e.g., for finding high risk cut-offs for overweight children in particular families?

Example

A data file of 1,445 families was assessed for learning the best fit cut-off values of unhealthy lifestyle estimators to maximize the difference between low and high risk of overweight children. These cut-off values were, subsequently, used to determine the risk profiles (the characteristics) in individual future families.

This chapter was previously published in "Machine learning in medicine-cookbook 2" as Chap. 2, 2014.

T.J. Cleophas, A.H. Zwinderman, *Machine Learning in Medicine - a Complete Overview*, DOI 10.1007/978-3-319-15195-3_5

Var 1	Var 2	Var 3	Var 4	Var 5
0	11	1	8	0
0	7	1	9	0
1	25	7	0	1
0	11	4	5	0
1	5	1	8	1
0	10	2	8	0
0	11	1	6	0
0	7	1	8	0
0	7	0	9	0
0	15	3	0	0

Var = variable
Var 1 fruitvegetables (times per week)
Var 2 unhealthysnacks (times per week)
Var 3 fastfoodmeal (times per week)
Var 4 physicalactivities (times per week)
Var 5 overweightchildren (0 = no, 1 = yes)

Only the first 10 families of the original learning data file are given, the entire data file is entitled "optimalbinning1" and is in extras.springer.com.

Optimal Binning

SPSS 19.0 is used for analysis. Start by opening the data file.

Command:

Transform….Optimal Binning….Variables into Bins: enter fruitvegetables, unhealthysnacks, fastfoodmeal, physicalactivities….Optimize Bins with Respect to: enter "overweightchildren"….click Output….Display: mark Endpoints….mark Descriptive statistics….mark Model Entropy….click Save: mark Create variables that contain binned data….Save Binning Rules in a Syntax file: click Browse…. open appropriate folder….File name: enter, e.g., "exportoptimalbinning"….click Save….click OK.

fruitvegetables/wk

Bin	End point		Number of cases by level of overweight children		
	Lower	Upper	No	Yes	Total
1	a	14	802	340	1142
2	14	a	274	29	303
Total			1076	369	1445

unhealthysnacks/wk

Bin	End point		Number of cases by level of overweight children		
	Lower	Upper	No	Yes	Total
1	[a]	12	830	143	973
2	12	19	188	126	314
3	19	[a]	58	100	158
Total			1076	369	1445

fastfoodmeal/wk

Bin	End point		Number of cases by level of overweight children		
	Lower	Upper	No	Yes	Total
1	[a]	2	896	229	1125
2	2	[a]	180	140	320
Total			1076	369	1445

physicalactivities/wk

Bin	End point		Number of cases by level of overweight children		
	Lower	Upper	No	Yes	Total
1	[a]	8	469	221	690
2	8	[a]	607	148	755
Total			1076	369	1445

Each bin is computed as Lower <= physicalactivities/wk <Upper

a. Unbounded

In the output sheets the above table is given. It shows the high risk cut-offs for overweight children of the four predicting factors. E.g., in 1,142 families scoring under 14 units of (1) fruit/vegetable per week, are put into bin 1 and 303 scoring over 14 units per week, are put into bin 2. The proportion of overweight children in bin 1 is much larger than it is in bin 2: 340/1,142 = 0.298 (30 %) and 29/303 = 0.096 (10 %). Similarly high risk cut-offs are found for (2) unhealthy snacks less than 12, 12–19, and over 19 per week, (3) fastfood meals less than 2, and over 2 per week, (4) physical activities less than 8 and over 8 per week. These cut-offs will be used as meaningful recommendation limits to 11 future families.

fruit	snacks	fastfood	physical
13	11	4	5
2	5	3	9
12	23	9	0
17	9	6	5
2	3	3	3
10	8	4	3
15	9	3	6
9	5	3	8
2	5	2	7
9	13	5	0
28	3	3	9

Var 1 fruitvegetables (times per week)
Var 2 unhealthysnacks (times per week)
Var 3 fastfoodmeal (times per week)
Var 4 physicalactivities (times per week)

The saved syntax file entitled "exportoptimalbinning.sps" will now be used to compute the predicted bins of some future families. Enter the above values in a new data file, entitled, e.g., "optimalbinning2", and save in the appropriate folder in your computer. Then open up the data file "exportoptimalbinning.sps"….subsequently click File….click Open….click Data….Find the data file entitled "optimalbinning2"….click Open….click "exportoptimalbinning.sps" from the file palette at the bottom of the screen….click Run….click All.

When returning to the Data View of "optimalbinning2", we will find the underneath overview of all of the bins selected for our 11 future families.

fruit	snacks	fastfood	physical	fruit _bin	snacks _bin	fastfood _bin	physical _bin
13	11	4	5	1	1	2	1
2	5	3	9	1	1	2	2
12	23	9	0	1	3	2	1
17	9	6	5	2	1	2	1
2	3	3	3	1	1	2	1
10	8	4	3	1	1	2	1
15	9	3	6	2	1	2	1
9	5	3	8	1	1	2	2
2	5	2	7	1	1	2	1
9	13	5	0	1	2	2	1
28	3	3	9	2	1	2	2

This overview is relevant, since families in high risk bins would particularly qualify for counseling.

Conclusion

Optimal bins describe continuous predictor variables in the form of best fit categories for making predictions, and SPSS statistical software can be used to generate a syntax file, called SPS file, for predicting risk cut-offs in future families. In this way families highly at risk for overweight can be readily identified. The nodes of decision trees can be used for similar purposes (Machine learning in medicine Cookbook One, Chap. 16, Decision trees for decision analysis, pp 97–104, Springer Heidelberg Germany, 2014), but it has subgroups of cases, rather than multiple bins for a single case.

Note

More background, theoretical and mathematical information of optimal binning is given in Machine Learning in Medicine Part Three, Chap. 5, Optimal binning, pp 37–48, Springer Heidelberg Germany 2013, and Machine learning in medicine Cookbook One, Optimal binning, Chap. 19, pp 101–106, Springer Heidelberg Germany, 2014, both from the same authors.

Chapter 6
Predicting Outlier Memberships (2,000 Patients)

General Purpose

With large data files outlier recognition requires a more sophisticated approach than the traditional data plots and regression lines. This chapter is to examine whether BIRCH (balanced iterative reducing and clustering using hierarchies) clustering is able to predict outliers in future patients from a known population.

Specific Scientific Question

Is the XML (eXtended Markup Language) file from a 2,000 patient sample capable of making predictions about cluster memberships and outlierships in future patients from the target population.

Example

In a 2,000 patient study of hospital admissions 576 possibly iatrogenic admissions were identified. Based on age and numbers of co-medications a two step BIRCH cluster analysis will be performed. SPSS version 19 and up can be used for the purpose. Only the first 10 patients' data are shown underneath. The entire data file is in extras.springer.com, and is entitled "outlierdetection".

This chapter was previously published in "Machine learning in medicine-cookbook 2" as Chap. 3, 2014.

T.J. Cleophas, A.H. Zwinderman, *Machine Learning in Medicine - a Complete Overview*, DOI 10.1007/978-3-319-15195-3_6

age	gender	admis	duration	mort	iatro	comorb	comed
1939,00	2,00	7,00	,00	,00	1,00	2,00	1,00
1939,00	2,00	7,00	2,00	1,00	1,00	2,00	1,00
1943,00	2,00	11,00	1,00	,00	1,00	,00	,00
1921,00	2,00	9,00	17,00	,00	1,00	3,00	3,00
1944,00	2,00	21,00	30,00	,00	1,00	3,00	3,00
1977,00	2,00	4,00	1,00	,00	1,00	1,00	1,00
1930,00	1,00	20,00	7,00	,00	1,00	2,00	2,00
1932,00	1,00	3,00	2,00	,00	1,00	4,00	4,00
1927,00	1,00	9,00	13,00	1,00	1,00	1,00	2,00
1920,00	2,00	23,00	8,00	,00	1,00	3,00	3,00

admis = admission indication code
duration = days of admission
mort = mortality
iatro = iatrogenic admission
comorb = number of comorbidities
comed = number of comedications

Start by opening the file.

Then command:

click Transform….click Random Number Generators….click Set Starting Point…. click Fixed Value (2000000)….click OK….click Analyze…. Classify….Two Step Cluster Analysis ….Continuous Variables: enter age and co-medications….Distance Measure: mark Euclidean….Clustering Criterion: mark Schwarz's Bayesian Criterion….click Options: mark Use noise handling….percentage: enter 25…. Assumed Standardized: enter age and co-medications….click Continue….mark Pivot tables….mark Charts and tables in Model Viewer….Working Data File: mark Create Cluster membership variable….XML Files: mark Export final model…. click Browse….select the appropriate folder in your computer….File Name: enter, e.g., "exportanomalydetection"….click Save….click Continue….click OK.

In the output sheets the underneath distribution of clusters is given.

Cluster distribution

		N	% of combined	% of total
Cluster	1	181	31,4 %	9,1 %
	2	152	26,4 %	7,6 %
	3	69	12,0 %	3,5 %
	Outlier (−1)	174	30,2 %	8,7 %
	Combined	576	100,0 %	28,8 %
Excluded cases		1,424		71,2 %
Total		2,000		100,0 %

Additional details are given in Machine learning in medicine Part Two, Chap. 10, Anomaly detection, pp 93–103, Springer Heidelberg Germany, 2013. The large outlier category consisted mainly of patients of all ages and extremely many co-medications. When returning to the Data View screen, we will observe that SPSS has created a novel variable entitled "TSC_5980" containing the patients' cluster memberships. The patients given the value −1 are the outliers.

With Scoring Wizard and the exported XML (eXtended Markup Language) file entitled "exportanomalydetection" we can now try and predict from age and number of co-medications of future patients the best fit cluster membership according to the computed XML model.

age	comed
1954,00	1,00
1938,00	7,00
1929,00	8,00
1967,00	1,00
1945,00	2,00
1936,00	3,00
1928,00	4,00

comed = number of co-medications

Enter the above data in a novel data file and command:

Utilities….click Scoring Wizard….click Browse….Open the appropriate folder with the XML file entitled "exportanomalydetection"….click on the latter and click Select….in Scoring Wizard double-click Next….mark Predicted Value….click Finish.

age	comed	PredictedValue
1954,00	1,00	3,00
1938,00	7,00	−1,00
1929,00	8,00	−1,00
1967,00	1,00	3,00
1945,00	2,00	−1,00
1936,00	3,00	1,00
1928,00	4,00	−1,00

PredictedValue = predicted cluster membership

In the above novel data file SPSS has provided the new variable as requested. One patient is in cluster 1, two are in cluster 3, and 4 patients are in the outlier cluster.

Conclusion

An XML (eXtended Markup Language) file from a 2,000 patient sample is capable of making predictions about cluster memberships and outlierships in future patients from the same target population.

Note

More background theoretical and mathematical information of outlier detection.

Is available Machine learning in medicine part two, Chap. 10, Anomaly detection, pp 93–103, Springer Heidelberg Germany, 2013, from the same authors.

Chapter 7
Data Mining for Visualization of Health Processes (150 Patients)

General Purpose

Computer files of clinical data are often complex and multi-dimensional, and they are, frequently, hard to statistically test. Instead, visualization processes can be successfully used as an alternative approach to traditional statistical data analysis.

For example, Knime (Konstanz information miner) software has been developed by computer scientists from Silicon Valley in collaboration with technicians from Konstanz University at the Bodensee in Switzerland, and it pays particular attention to visual data analysis. It is used since 2006 as a freely available package through the Internet. So far, it is mainly used by chemists and pharmacists, but not by clinical investigators. This chapter is to assess, whether visual processing of clinical data may, sometimes, perform better than traditional statistical analysis.

Primary Scientific Question

Can visualization processes of clinical data provide insights that remained hidden with traditional statistical tests?

This chapter was previously published in "Machine learning in medicine-cookbook 3" as Chap. 1, 2014.

T.J. Cleophas, A.H. Zwinderman, *Machine Learning in Medicine - a Complete Overview*, DOI 10.1007/978-3-319-15195-3_7

Example

Four inflammatory markers (CRP (C-reactive protein), ESR (erythrocyte sedimentation rate), leucocyte count (leucos), and fibrinogen) were measured in 150 patients with pneumonia. Based on x-ray chest clinical severity was classified as A (mild infection), B (medium severity), C (severe infection). One scientific question was to assess whether the markers could adequately predict the severity of infection.

CRP	leucos	fibrinogen	ESR	x-ray severity
120,00	5,00	11,00	60,00	A
100,00	5,00	11,00	56,00	A
94,00	4,00	11,00	60,00	A
92,00	5,00	11,00	58,00	A
100,00	5,00	11,00	52,00	A
108,00	6,00	17,00	48,00	A
92,00	5,00	14,00	48,00	A
100,00	5,00	11,00	54,00	A
88,00	5,00	11,00	54,00	A
98,00	5,00	8,00	60,00	A
108,00	5,00	11,00	68,00	A
96,00	5,00	11,00	62,00	A
96,00	5,00	8,00	46,00	A
86,00	4,00	8,00	60,00	A
116,00	4,00	11,00	50,00	A
114,00	5,00	17,00	52,00	A

CRP = C-reactive protein (mg/l)
leucos = leucyte count (*10^9/l)
fibrinogen = fibrinogen level (mg/l)
ESR = erythrocyte sedimentation rate (mm)
x-ray severity = x-chest severity pneumonia score (A–C = mild to severe)

The data file is entitled "decisiontree", and is available in extras.springer.com. Data analysis of these data in SPSS is rather limited. Start by opening the data file in SPSS statistical software.

Command:

click Graphs….Legacy Dialogs….Bar Charts….click Simple….click Define…. Category Axis: enter "severity score"….Variable: enter CRP….mark Other statistics….click OK.

After performing the same procedure for the other variables four graphs are produced as shown underneath. The mean levels of all of the inflammatory markers consistently tended to rise with increasing severities of infection. Univariate multinomial logistic regression with severity as outcome gives a significant effect of all of the markers. However, this effect is largely lost in the multiple multinomial logistic regression, probably due to interactions.

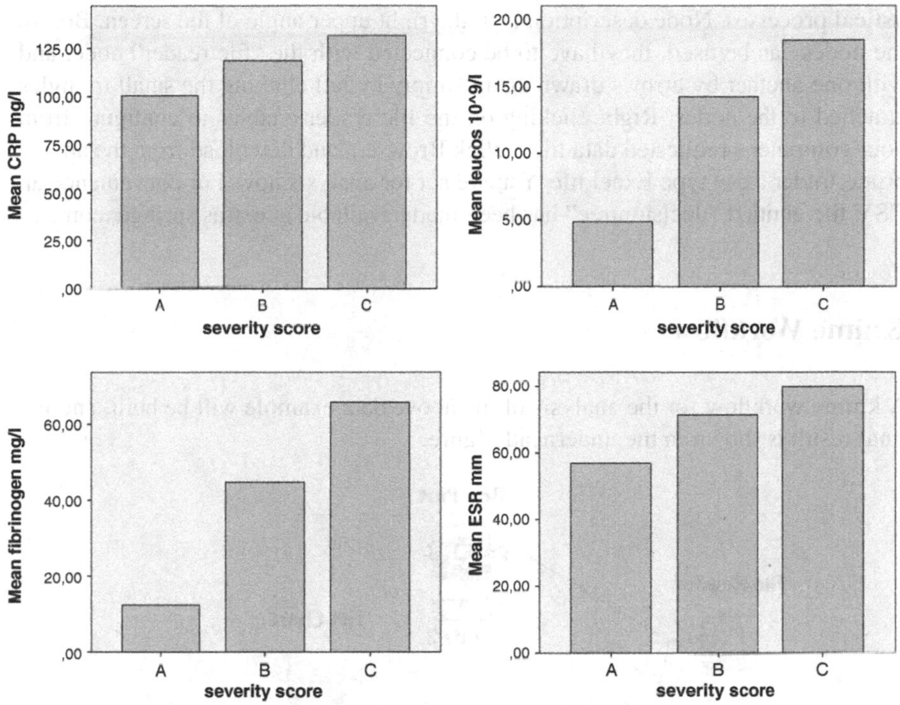

We are interested to explore these results for additional effects, for example, hidden data effects, like different predictive effects and frequency distributions for different subgroups. For that purpose Knime data miner will be applied. SPSS data files can not be downloaded directly in the Knime software, but excel files can, and SPSS data can be saved as an excel file (the csv file type available in your computer must be used).

Command in SPSS:

click File....click Save as....in "Save as" type: enter Comma Delimited (*.csv).... click Save.

Knime Data Miner

In Google enter the term "knime". Click Download and follow instructions. After completing the pretty easy download procedure, open the knime workbench by clicking the knime welcome screen. The center of the screen displays the workflow editor like the canvas in SPSS modeler. It is empty, and can be used to build a stream of nodes, called workflow in knime. The node repository is in the left lower angle of the screen, and the nodes can be dragged to the workflow editor simply by left-clicking. The nodes are computer tools for data analysis like visualization and statistical processes. Node description is in the right upper angle of the screen. Before the nodes can be used, they have to be connected with the "file reader" node, and with one another by arrows drawn again simply by left clicking the small triangles attached to the nodes. Right clicking on the file reader enables to configure from your computer a requested data file....click Browse....and download from the appropriate folder a csv type Excel file. You are set for analysis now. For convenience an CSV file entitled "decisiontree" has been made available at extras.springer.com.

Knime Workflow

A knime workflow for the analysis of the above data example will be built, and the final result is shown in the underneath figure.

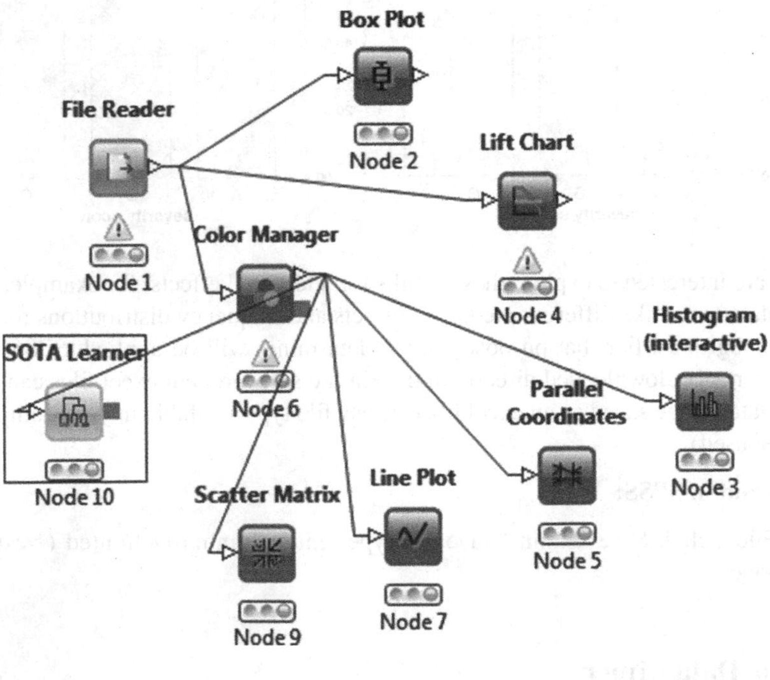

Box and Whiskers Plots

In the node repository find the node Box Plot. First click the IO option (import/export option nodes). Then click "Read", then the File Reader node is displayed, and can be dragged by left clicking to the workflow editor. Enter the requested data file as described above. A Node dialog is displayed underneath the node entitled Node 1. Its light is orange at this stage, and should turn green before it can be applied. If you right click the node's center, and then left click File Table a preview of the data is supplied.

Now, in the search box of the node repository find and click Data Views....then "Box plot"....drag to workflow editor....connect with arrow to File reader....right click File reader....right click execute....right click Box Plot node....right click Configurate....right click Execute and open view....

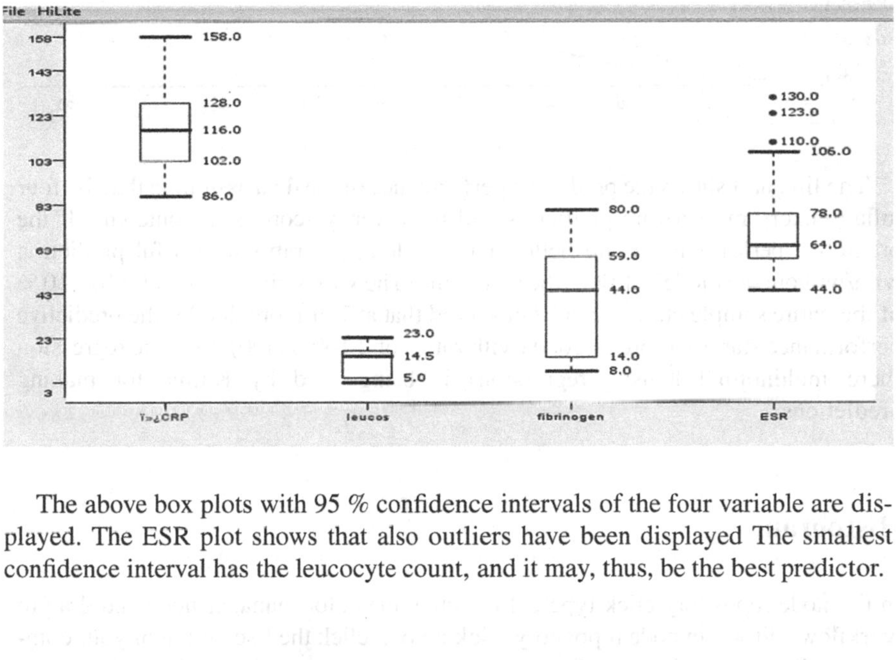

The above box plots with 95 % confidence intervals of the four variable are displayed. The ESR plot shows that also outliers have been displayed The smallest confidence interval has the leucocyte count, and it may, thus, be the best predictor.

Lift Chart

In the node repository....click Lift Chart and drag to workflow editor.... connect with arrow to File reader....right click execute Lift Chart node....right click Configurate.... right click Execute and open view....

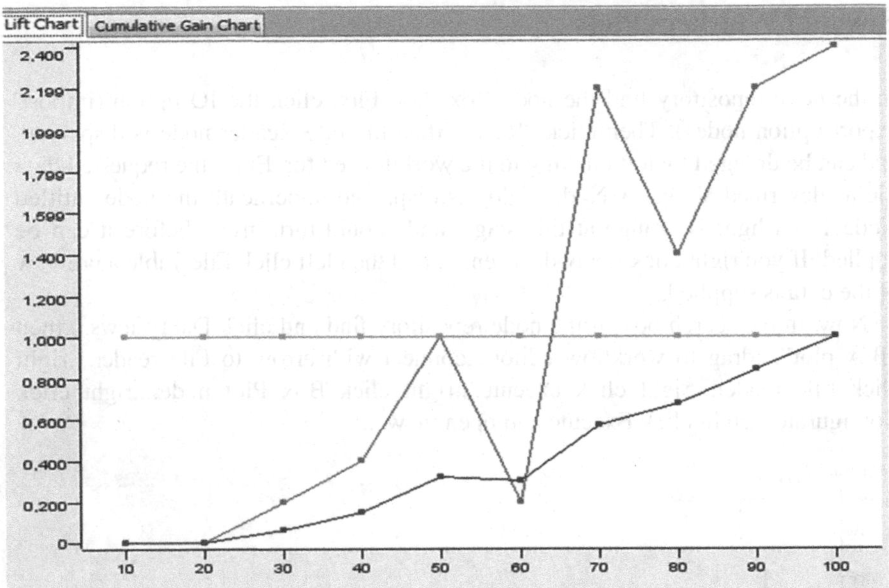

The lift chart shows the predictive performance of the data assuming that the four inflammatory markers are predictors and the severity score is the outcome. If the predictive performance is no better than random, the ratio successful prediction with/without the model = 1.000 (the green line) The x-axis give dociles (1 = 10 = 10 % of the entire sample etc.). It can be observed that at 7 or more dociles the predictive performance start to be pretty good (with ratios of 2.100–2.400). Logistic regression (here multinomial logistic regression) is being used by Knime for making predictions.

Histogram

In the node repository click type color....click the color manager node and drag to workflow editor....in node repository click color....click the Esc button of your computer....click Data Views....select interactive histogram and transfer to workflow editor....connect color manager node with File Reader…connect color manager with "interactive histogram node"....right click Configurate....right click Execute and open view....

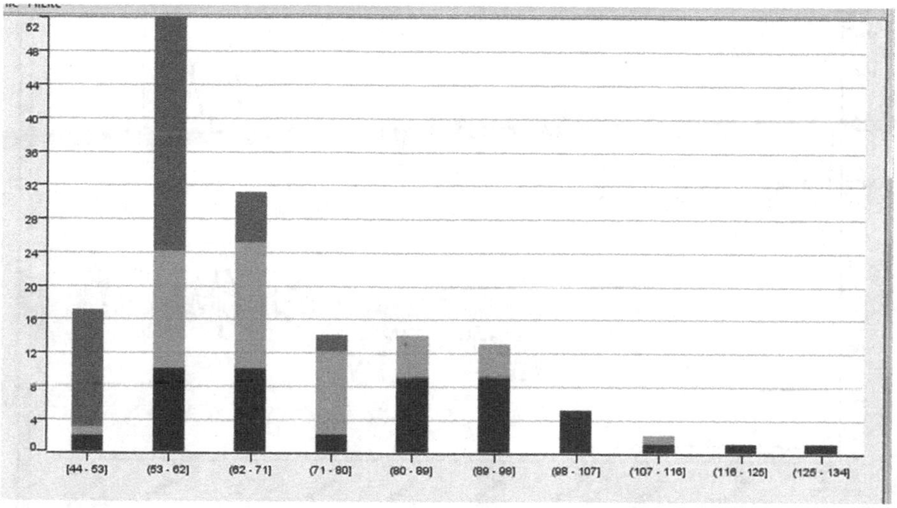

Interactive histograms with bins of ESR values are given. The colors provide the proportions of cases with mild severity (A, red), medium severity (B, green), and severe pneumonias (C, blue). It can be observed that many mild cases (red) are in the ESR 44–71 mm cut-off. Above ESR of 80 mm blue (severe pneumonia) is increasingly present. The software program has selected only the ESR values 44–134. Instead of histograms with ESR, those with other predictor variables can be made.

Line Plot

In the node repository click Data Views....select the node Line plots and transfer to workflow editor....connect color manager with "Line plots"....right click Configurate....right click Execute and open view....

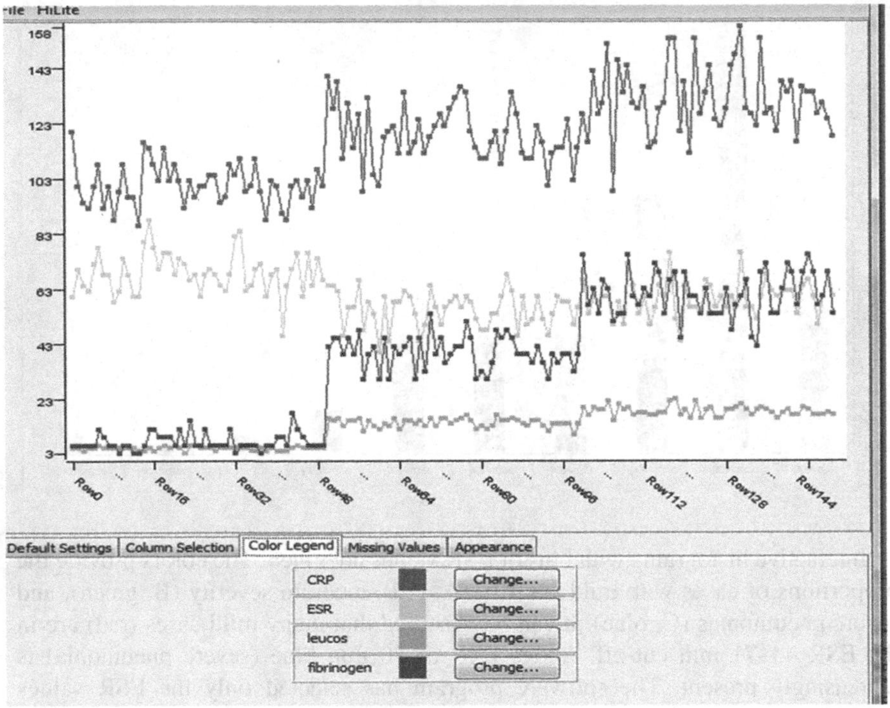

The line plot gives the values of all cases along the x-axis. The upper curve are the CRP values, The middle one the ESR values. The lower part are the leucos and fibrinogen values. The rows 0–50 are the cases with mild pneumonia, the rows 51–100 the medium severity cases, and the rows 101–150 the severe cases. It can be observed that particularly the CRP-, fibrinogen-, and leucos levels increase with increased severity of infection. This is not observed with the ESR levels.

Matrix of Scatter Plots

In the node repository click Data Views....select "Matrix of scatter plots" and transfer to workflow editor....connect color manager with "Matrix of scatter plots" .... right click Configurate....right click Execute and open view....

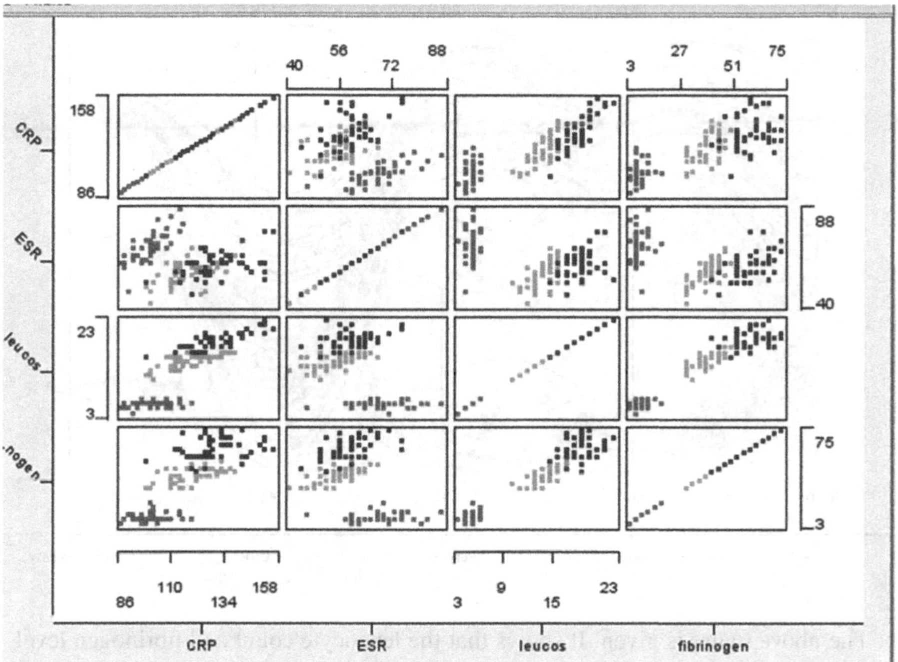

The above figure gives the results. The four predictors variables are plotted against one another. by the colors (blue for severest, red for mildest pneumonias) the fields show that the severest pneumonias are predominantly in the right upper quadrant, the mildest in the left lower quadrant.

Parallel Coordinates

In the node repository click Data Views....select "Parallel coordinates" and transfer to workflow editor....connect color manager with "Parallel coordinates" ....right click Configurate....right click Execute and open view....click Appearance....click Draw (spline) Curves instead of lines....

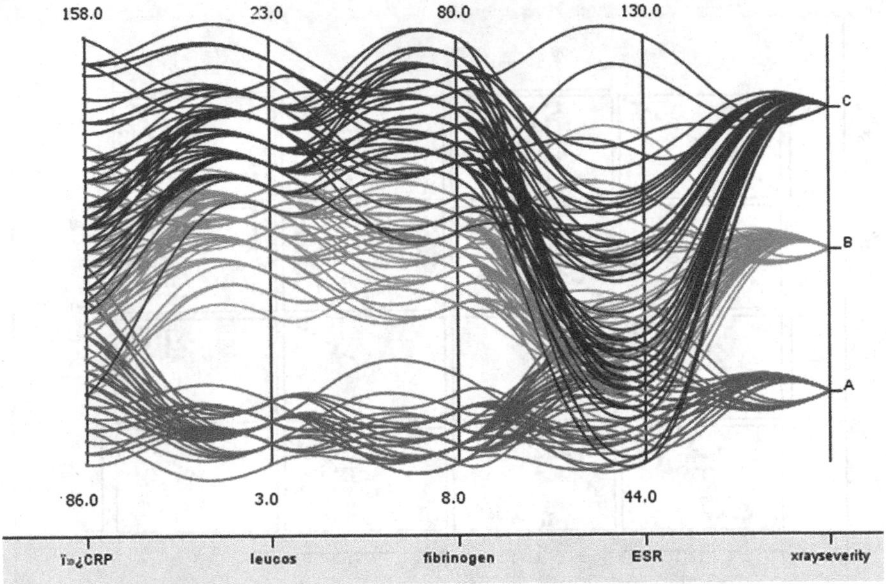

The above figure is given. It shows that the leucocyte count and fibrinogen level are excellent predictors of infection severities. CRP and ESR are also adequate predictors of infections with mild and medium severities, however, poor predictors of levels of severe infections.

Hierarchical Cluster Analysis with SOTA (Self Organizing Tree Algorithm)

In the node repository click Mining....select the node SOTA (Self Organizing tree Algorithm) Learner and transfer to workflow editor....connect color manager with "SOTA learner"....right click Configurate....right click Execute and open view....

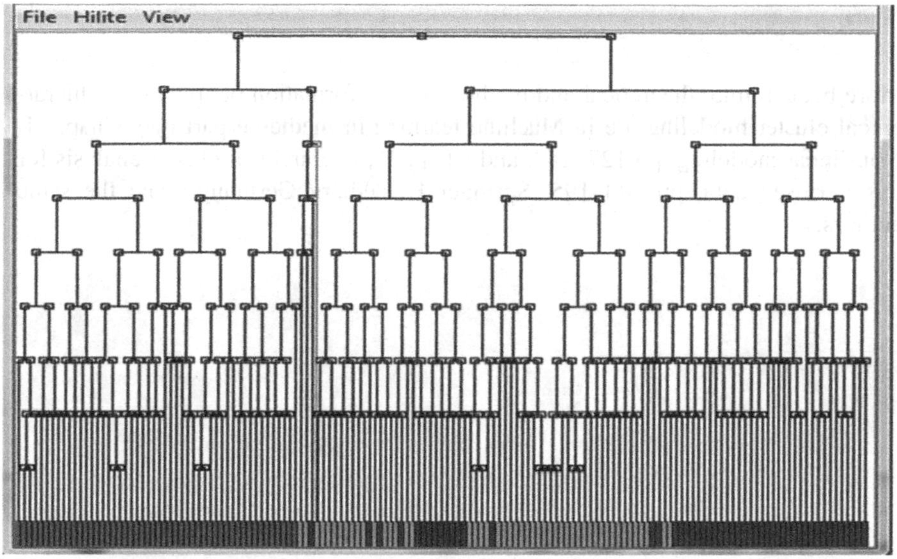

SOTA learning is a modified hierarchical cluster analysis, and it uses in this example the between-case distances of fibrinogen as variable. On the y-axis the standardized distances of the cluster combinations. Clicking the small squares interactively demonstrates the row numbers of the individual cases. It can be observed at the bottom of the figure that the severity classes very well cluster, with the mild cases (red) left, medium severity (green) in the middle, and severe cases (blue) right.

Conclusion

Clinical computer files are complex, and hard to statistically test. Instead, visualization processes can be successfully used as an alternative approach to traditional statistical data analysis. For example, Knime (Konstanz information miner) software developed by computer scientists at Konstanz University Technical Department at the Bodensee, although mainly used by chemists and pharmacists, is able to visualize multidimensional clinical data, and this approach may, sometimes, perform better than traditional statistical testing. In the current example it was able to demonstrate the clustering of inflammatory markers to identify different classes of pneumonia severity. Also to demonstrate that leucocyte count and fibrinogen were the best markers, and that ESR was a poor marker. In all of the markers the best predictive performance was obtained in the severest cases of disease. All of these observations were unobserved in the traditional statistical analysis in SPSS.

Note

More background, theoretical and mathematical information of splines and hierarchical cluster modeling are in Machine learning in medicine part one, Chap. 11, Non-linear modeling, pp 127–143, and Chap. 15, Hierarchical cluster analysis for unsupervised data, pp 183–195, Springer Heidelberg Germany, from the same authors.

Chapter 8
Trained Decision Trees for a More Meaningful Accuracy (150 Patients)

General Purpose

Traditionally, decision trees are used for finding the best predictors of health risks and improvements (Chap. 53). However, this method is not entirely appropriate, because a decision tree is built from a data file, and, subsequently, the same data file is applied once more for computing the health risk probabilities from the built tree. Obviously, the accuracy must be close to 100 %, because the test sample is 100 % identical to the sample used for building the tree, and, therefore, this accuracy does not mean too much. With neural networks this problem of duplicate usage of the same data is solved by randomly splitting the data into two samples, a training sample and a test sample (Chap. 12 in Machine learning in medicine part one, pp 145–156, Artificial intelligence, multilayer perceptron modeling, Springer Heidelberg Germany, 2013, from the same authors). The current chapter is to assess whether the splitting methodology, otherwise called partitioning, is also feasible for decision trees, and to assess its level of accuracy. Decision trees are both appropriate for data with categorical and continuous outcome (Chap. 53).

Primary Scientific Question

Can inflammatory markers adequately predict pneumonia severities wit the help of a decision tree. Can partitioning of the data improve the methodology and is sufficient accuracy of the methodology maintained.

This chapter was previously published in "Machine learning in medicine-cookbook 3" as Chap. 2, 2014.

T.J. Cleophas, A.H. Zwinderman, *Machine Learning in Medicine - a Complete Overview*, DOI 10.1007/978-3-319-15195-3_8

Example

Four inflammatory markers (CRP (C-reactive protein), ESR (erythrocyte sedimentation rate), leucocyte count (leucos), and fibrinogen) were measured in 150 patients. Based on x-ray chest clinical severity was classified as A (mild infection), B (medium severity), C (severe infection). A major scientific question was to assess what markers were the best predictors of the severity of infection.

CRP	leucos	fibrinogen	ESR	x-ray severity
120,00	5,00	11,00	60,00	A
100,00	5,00	11,00	56,00	A
94,00	4,00	11,00	60,00	A
92,00	5,00	11,00	58,00	A
100,00	5,00	11,00	52,00	A
108,00	6,00	17,00	48,00	A
92,00	5,00	14,00	48,00	A
100,00	5,00	11,00	54,00	A
88,00	5,00	11,00	54,00	A
98,00	5,00	8,00	60,00	A
108,00	5,00	11,00	68,00	A
96,00	5,00	11,00	62,00	A
96,00	5,00	8,00	46,00	A
86,00	4,00	8,00	60,00	A
116,00	4,00	11,00	50,00	A
114,00	5,00	17,00	52,00	A

CRP = C-reactive protein (mg/l)
leucos = leucyte count ($*10^9$/l)
fibrinogen = fibrinogen level (mg/l)
ESR = erythrocyte sedimentation rate (mm)
x-ray severity = x-chest severity pneumonia score (A–C = mild to severe)

The first 16 patients are in the above table, the entire data file is in "decisiontree" and can be obtained from "extras.springer.com" on the internet. We will start by opening the data file in SPSS.

Command:

click Classify….Tree….Dependent Variable: enter severity score….Independent Variables: enter CRP, Leucos, fibrinogen, ESR….Growing Method: select CHAID….click Output: mark Tree in table format….Criteria: Parent Node type 50, Child Node type 15….click Continue…. ….click OK.

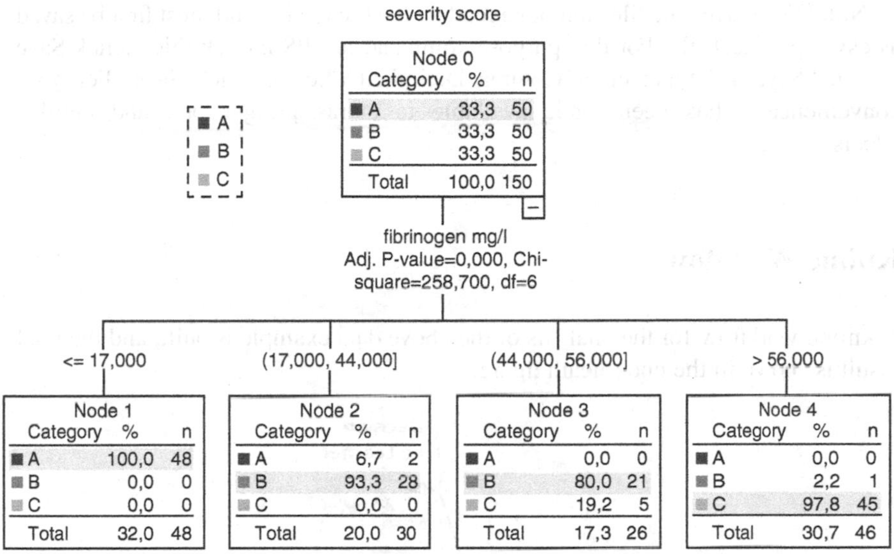

The above decision tree is displayed. A fibrinogen level <17 is 100 % predictor of severity score A (mild disease). Fibrinogen 17–44 gives 93 % chance of severity B, fibrinogen 44–56 gives 81 % chance of severity B, and fibrinogen >56 gives 98 % chance of severity score C. The output also shows that the overall accuracy of the model is 94.7 %, but we have to account that this model is somewhat flawed, because all of the data are used twice, one, for building the tree, and, second, for using the tree for making predictions.

Downloading the Knime Data Miner

In Google enter the term "knime". Click Download and follow instructions. After completing the pretty easy download procedure, open the knime workbench by clicking the knime welcome screen. The center of the screen displays the workflow editor. Like the canvas in SPSS Modeler, it is empty., and can be used to build a stream of nodes, called workflow in knime. The node repository is in the left lower angle of the screen, and the nodes can be dragged to the workflow editor simply by left-clicking. The nodes are computer tools for data analysis like visualization and statistical processes. Node description is in the right upper angle of the screen. Before the nodes can be used, they have to be connected with the "file reader" node, and with one another by arrows, drawn, again, simply by left clicking the small triangles attached to the nodes. Right clicking on the file reader enables to configure from your computer a requested data file....click Browse....and download from the appropriate folder a csv type Excel file. You are set for analysis now.

Note: the above data file cannot be read by the file reader, and must first be saved as csv type Excel file. For that purpose command in SPSS: click File....click Save as....in "Save as" type: enter Comma Delimited (*.csv)....click Save. For your convenience it has been made available in extras.springer.com, and entitled "decisiontree".

Knime Workflow

A knime workflow for the analysis of the above data example is built, and the final result is shown in the underneath figure.

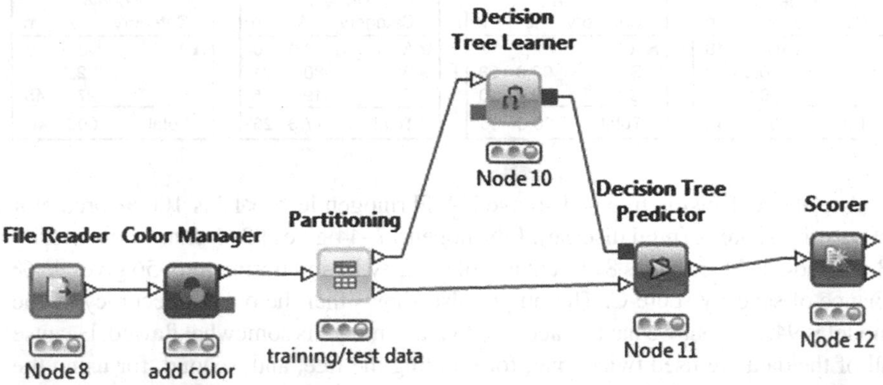

In the node repository click and type color....click the color manager node and drag to workflow editor....in node repository click again color....click the Esc button of your computer....in the node repository click again and type partitioning....the partitioning node is displayed....drag it to the workflow editor....perform the same actions and type respectively Decision Tree Learner, Decision Tree Predictor, and Scorer....Connect, by left clicking, all of the nodes with arrows as indicated above.... Configurate and execute all of the nodes by right clicking the nodes and then the texts "Configurate" and "Execute"....the red lights will successively turn orange and then green....right click the Decision Tree Predictor again....right click the text "View: Decision Tree View".

The underneath decision tree comes up. It is pretty much similar to the above SPSS tree, although it does not use 150 cases but only 45 cases (the test sample from which 100 were resampled). Fibrinogen is again the best predictor. A level <29 mg/l gives you 100 % chance of severity score A. A level 29–57.5 gives 92.1 % chance of Severity B, and a level over 57.5 gives 100 % chance of severity C.

Right clicking the scorer node gives you the accuracy statistics, and shows that the sensitivity of A, B, an C are respectively 100, 93.3, and 90.5 %, and that the overall accuracy is 94 %, slightly less than that of the SPSS tree (94.7 %), but still pretty good. In addition, the current analysis is appropriate, and does not use identical data twice.

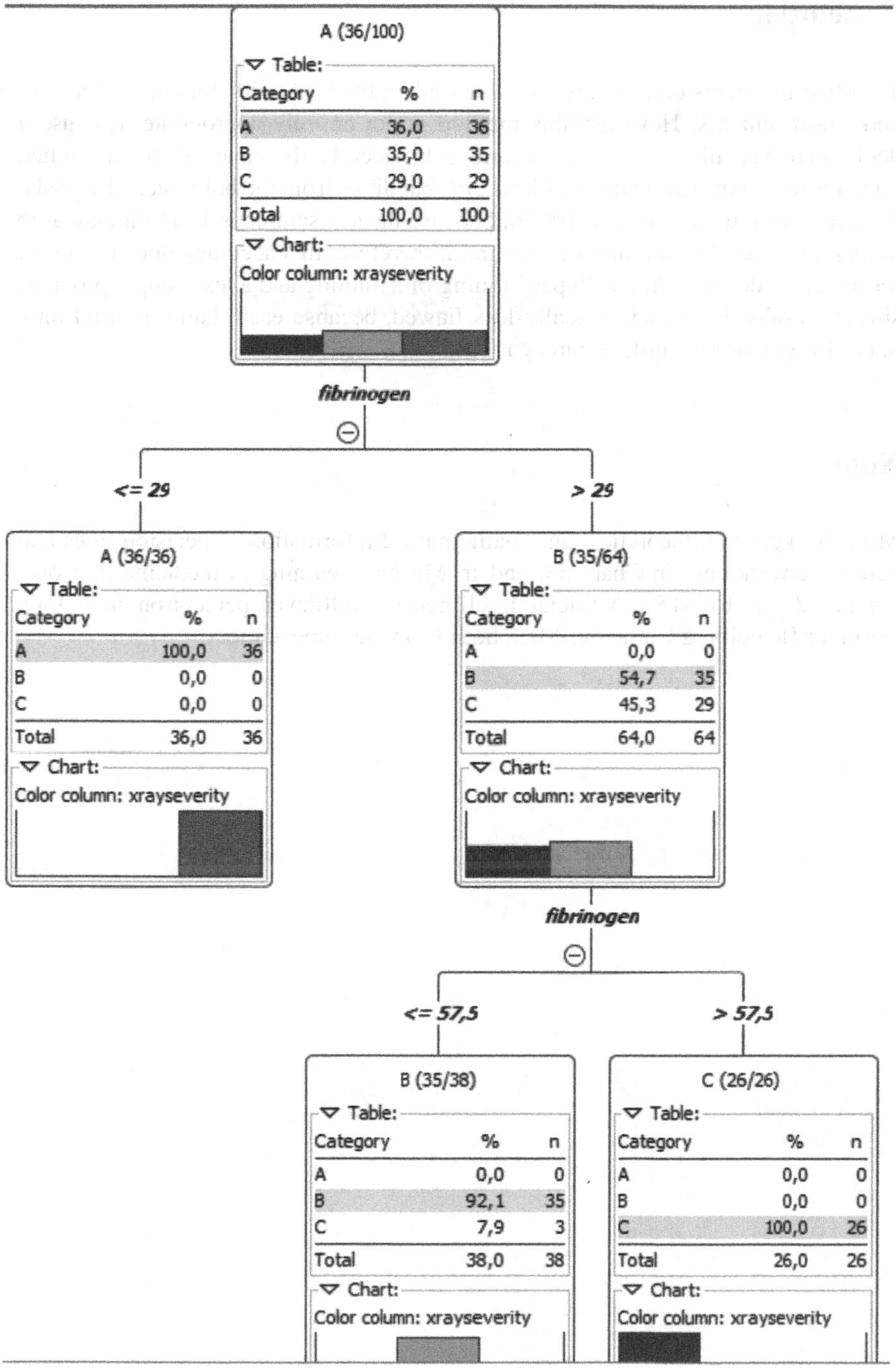
A (36/100)
Table:
Category % n
A 36,0 36
B 35,0 35
C 29,0 29
Total 100,0 100
Chart:
Color column: xrayseverity
fibrinogen
<= 29
> 29
A (36/36)
Table:
Category % n
A 100,0 36
B 0,0 0
C 0,0 0
Total 36,0 36
Chart:
Color column: xrayseverity
B (35/64)
Table:
Category % n
A 0,0 0
B 54,7 35
C 45,3 29
Total 64,0 64
Chart:
Color column: xrayseverity
fibrinogen
<= 57,5
> 57,5
B (35/38)
Table:
Category % n
A 0,0 0
B 92,1 35
C 7,9 3
Total 38,0 38
Chart:
Color column: xrayseverity
C (26/26)
Table:
Category % n
A 0,0 0
B 0,0 0
C 100,0 26
Total 26,0 26
Chart:
Color column: xrayseverity

Conclusion

Traditionally, decision trees are used for finding the best predictors of health risks and improvements. However, this method is not entirely appropriate, because a decision tree is built from a data file, and, subsequently, the same data file is applied once more for computing the health risk probabilities from the built tree. Obviously, the accuracy must be close to 100 %, because the test sample is 100 % identical to the sample used for building the tree, and, therefore, this accuracy does not mean too much. A decision tree with partitioning of a training and a test sample provides similar results, but is scientifically less flawed, because each datum is used only once. In spite of this, little accuracy is lost.

Note

More background, theoretical and mathematical information of decision trees and neural networks are in Chap. 53, and in Machine learning in medicine part one, Chap. 12, pp 145–156, Artificial intelligence, multilayer perceptron modeling, Springer Heidelberg Germany, 2013, both from the same authors.

Chapter 9
Typology of Medical Data (51 Patients)

General Purpose

Apart from histograms (see Chap. 1, Statistics applied to clinical studies 5th edition, "Hypotheses, data, stratification". pp 1–14, Springer Heidelberg Germany, 2012), and Q-Q plots (Chap. 42 of current work), the typology of data and frequency procedures (to be reviewed in the Chaps. 10, and 11 of the current work) are a good way to start looking at your data. First, we will address the typology of the data.

Nominal Data

Nominal data are discrete data without a stepping pattern, like genders, age classes, family names. They can be assessed with pie charts, frequency tables and bar charts.

Ordinal Data

Ordinal data are also discrete data, however, with a stepping pattern, like severity scores, intelligence levels, physical strength scores. They are usually assessed with frequency tables and bar charts.

Scale Data

Scale data also have a stepping pattern, but, unlike ordinal data, they have steps with equal intervals. With small steps they are called continuous data. They are sometimes called quantitative data, while nominal and ordinal data are traditionally called qualitative data. The scale data are assessed with summary tables and histograms.

The typology of the data values become particularly important when it comes to statistical analyses. E.g., means and standard deviations makes no sense with nominal data. The problem with ordinal data is that the steps are usually not equal, like with scale data. With ordinal data you will usually have a mix-up of larger and smaller steps. This biases the outcome if you use a scale data test for their analysis.

T.J. Cleophas, A.H. Zwinderman, *Machine Learning in Medicine - a Complete Overview*, DOI 10.1007/978-3-319-15195-3_9

The Chap. 37 of the current book, entitled "Ordinal scaling for clinical scores with inconsistent intervals", shows how this problem can mathematically be largely solved by complementary log-log transformations.

Primary Scientific Question

In econometrics and marketing research (Foroni, Econometric models for mixed-frequency data, edited by European University of Economics, Florence, 2012), frequency procedures are routinely used for the assessment of nominal, ordinal and scale data. Can they also be adequately applied for assessing medical data?

Example

The patients of an internist's outpatient clinic are reviewed.

nominal variable	ordinal variable	scale variable
agegroup	severity	time
2,00	2,00	2,50
2,00	1,00	6,00
2,00	1,00	2,50
1,00	3,00	2,00
1,00	1,00	5,00
2,00	1,00	4,00
2,00	3,00	,50
1,00	1,00	2,50
2,00	3,00	4,00
2,00	2,00	1,50

agegroup: 1 = senior, 2 = adult, 3 = adolescent, 4 = child
severity: complaint severity scores 1–4
time: consulting time (minutes)

The first 10 patients are in the above table. The entire file (51 patients) is entitled "frequencies", and is available at extras.springer.com. We will start by opening the file in SPSS statistical software.

Nominal Variable

Command:

click Analyze....Descriptive Statistics....Frequencies....Variable(s): enter agegroups.... mark Display frequency tables....click Charts....click Pie charts....click OK.

The underneath pie chart shows that seniors and adults predominate and that children are just a small portion of the outpatient clinic population.

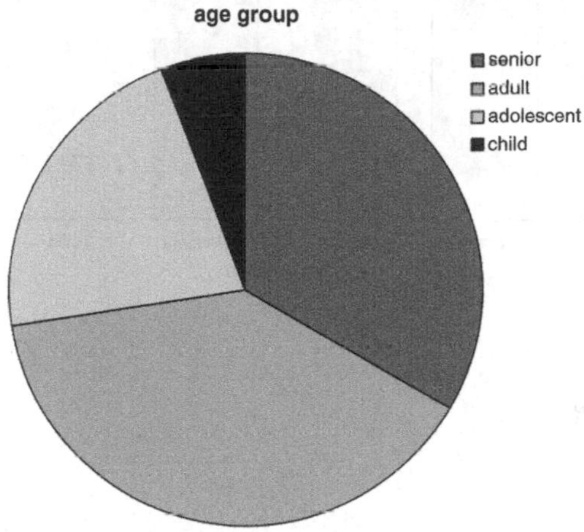

The frequency table shows precise frequencies of the nominal categories.

Age group

		Frequency	Percent	Valid percent	Cumulative percent
Valid	Senior	17	33,3	33,3	33,3
	Adult	20	39,2	39,2	72,5
	Adolescent	11	21,6	21,6	94,1
	Child	3	5,9	5,9	100,0
	Total	51	100,0	100,0	

If you wish, you could present your data in the form of descending or ascending frequencies.

Command:

click Analyze....Descriptive Statistics....Frequencies....Variable(s): enter agegroups ....mark Display frequency tables....click Charts....click Bar charts....click Continue ....click Format....click Descending counts....click Continue.......click OK.

The underneath graph is in the output sheet. It shows an ordered bar chart with adults as largest category.

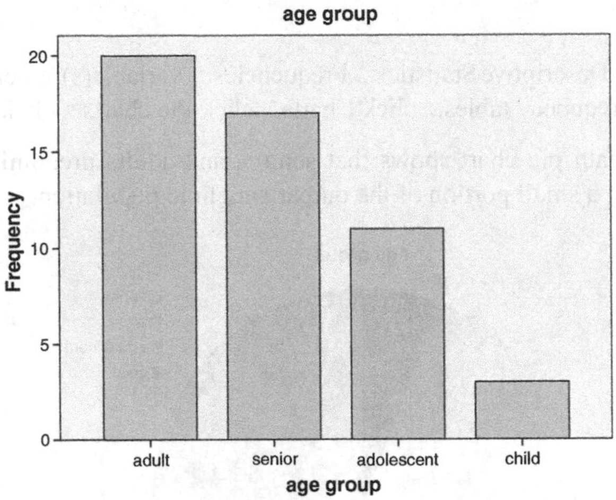

Ordinal Variable

Command:

click Analyze....Descriptive Statistics....Frequencies....Variable(s): enter severity .... mark Display frequency tables....click Charts....click Bar charts....click Continue .... click Format....click Ascending counts....click Continue.......click OK.

According to the severity score count the underneath graph shows the percentages of patients. Most of them are in the score one category, least of them in the score five category.

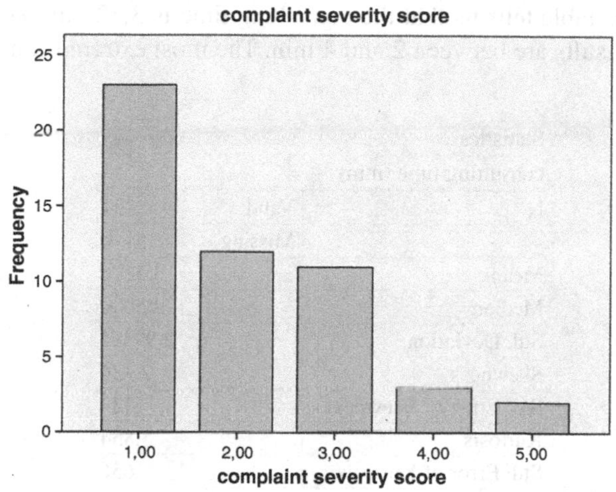

The table gives the precise numbers of patients in each category as well as the percentages. If we have missing values, the valid percent column will give the adjusted percentages, while the cumulative percentage gives the categories one and two, one and two and three etc. percentages.

Complaint severity score

		Frequency	Percent	Valid percent	Cumulative percent
Valid	1,00	23	45,1	45,1	45,1
	2,00	12	23,5	23,5	68,6
	3,00	11	21,6	21,6	90,2
	4,00	3	5,9	5,9	96,1
	5,00	2	3,9	3,9	100,0
	Total	51	100,0	100,0	

Scale Variable

Command:

click Analyze....Descriptive Statistics....Frequencies....Variable(s): enter time .... remove mark from "Display frequency tables"....click Statistics....mark Quartiles.... Std.deviations....Minimum....Maximum.... Mean....Median .... Skewness.... Kurtosis....click Continue....then click Charts....Histograms...mark Show normal curve on histogram....click Continue....click OK.

The statistics table tells us that the consulting time is 3,42 min on average, and 50 % of the consults are between 2 and 4 min. The most extreme consults took 0,5 and 15,0 min.

Statistics		
consulting time (min)		
N	Valid	51
	Missing	0
Mean		3,4216
Median		2,5000
Std. Deviation		2,99395
Skewness		2,326
Std. Error of Skewness		,333
Kurtosis		5,854
Std. Error of Kurtosis		,656
Minimum		,50
Maximum		15,00
Percentiles	25	2,0000
	50	2,5000
	75	4,0000

The histogram shows the frequency distribution of the data and suggests skewness to the right. Most of the consults took as little as less than 5 min but some took no less than 5–15 min. This means that the data are not very symmetric and means, and that standard deviation are not very accurate to summarize these data.

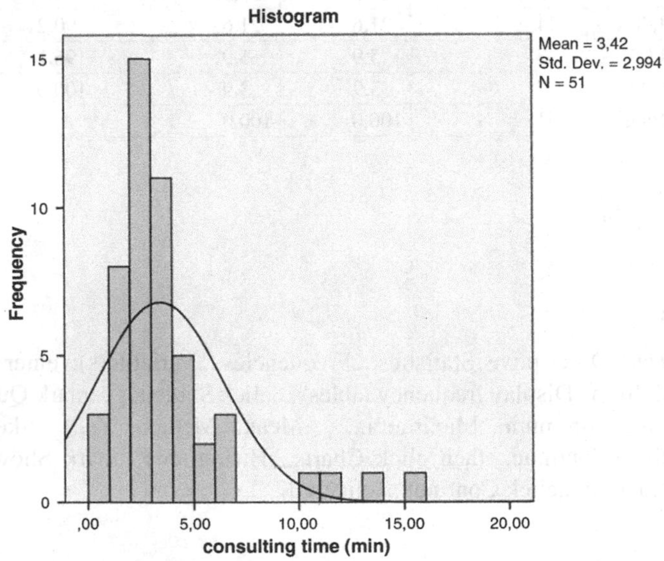

Indeed, a significant level of skewness to the right is in the data, because 2,326/0,333 = 6,985 is much larger than 1,96 (see the above table). We will try and use a logarithmic transformation of these skewed data. because this often "normalizes" the skewness.

Command:

click Transform....Compute Variable....type logtime in Target Variable....type ln(time) in Numeric Expression....click OK.

In the main screen it can be observed that SPSS now has produced a novel variable entitled "logtime". We will perform the scale variable analysis again, and replace the variable "time" with "logtime".

Command:

click Analyze....Descriptive Statistics....Frequencies....Variable(s): enter logtime.... click Charts....Histograms...mark Show normal curve on histogram....click Continue....click OK.

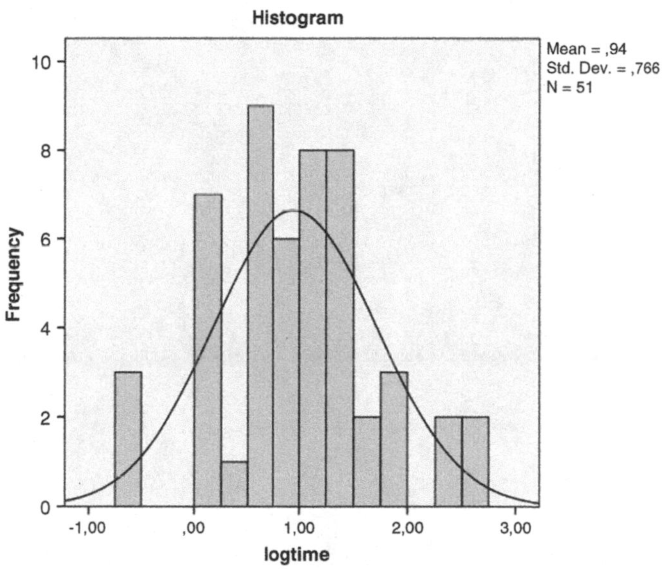

In the output sheets the underneath graph is shown. The data distribution looks less skewed and much closer to a normal distribution now. The logtime data can now be used for data analysis using normal statistical tests.

Conclusion

Data can be classified as nominal, ordinal and scale. For each type frequencies and frequency distributions can readily be calculated, and they enable an unbiased view of their patterns. Nominal data have no mean value. Ordinal data are tricky, because, although they have a stepping pattern, they offer a mix-up of larger and smaller steps. Ordinal regression can largely adjust this irregularity. Skewed scale data often benefit from log-data transformations.

Note

More background, theoretical and mathematical information of ordinal data is given in Chap. 37 of the current book, entitled "Ordinal scaling for clinical scores with inconsistent intervals".

Chapter 10
Predictions from Nominal Clinical Data (450 Patients)

General Purpose

In Chap. 9 the typology of medical data was reviewed. Nominal data are discrete data without a stepping function like genders, age classes, family names. They can be assessed with pie charts, frequency tables and bar charts. Statistical testing is not of much interest. Statistical testing becomes, however, interesting, if we want to know whether two nominal variables like treatment modality and treatment outcome are differently distributed between one another. An interaction matrix of these two nominal variables could, then, be used to test, whether one treatment performs better than the other.

Primary Scientific Question

This chapter assesses the relationship between four treatment modalities, and, as outcome, five levels of quality of life (qol). Can an interaction matrix, otherwise called contingency table or crosstab, be used to assess whether some treatment modalities are associated with a better qol score than others, and to assess the directions of the differences in distribution of the variables.

Example

In 450 patients with coronary artery disease four complementary treatment modalities, including cardiac fitness, physiotherapy, wellness, and hydrotherapy, were assessed for quality of life scores. The first 10 patients are in the table underneath.

T.J. Cleophas, A.H. Zwinderman, *Machine Learning in Medicine - a Complete Overview*, DOI 10.1007/978-3-319-15195-3_10

The entire data file is entitled "Qol.sav", and is in extras.springer.com. The example is also used in the Chap. 11. SPSS is applied for analysis.

treatment	counseling	qol	sat doctor
3	1	4	4
4	0	2	1
2	1	5	4
3	0	4	4
2	1	2	1
2	0	1	4
4	0	4	1
3	0	4	1
4	1	4	4
2	1	3	4

treatment = treatment modality (1 = cardiac fitness, 2 = physiotherapy, 3 = wellness, 4 = hydrotherapy, 5 = nothing)
counseling = counseling given (0 = no, 1 = yes)
qol = quality of life score (1 = very low, 5 = vey high)
sat doctor = satisfaction with doctor (1 = very low, 5 = very high)

Start by opening the data file in SPSS statistical software.

Command

Analyze....Descriptive Statistics....Crosstabs....Rows: enter "treatment".... Columns: enter "qol score"....click Statistics....mark Chi-square....click Continue....click OK.

In the output sheets the underneath tables are given.

Treatment * qol score crosstabulation

Count

		Qol score					
		Very low	Low	Medium	High	Very high	Total
Treatment	Cardiac fitness	21	21	16	24	36	118
	Physiotherapy	22	20	18	20	20	100
	Wellness	23	14	12	30	25	104
	Hydrotherapy	20	18	25	35	30	128
Total		86	73	71	109	111	450

Both hydrotherapy and cardiac fitness produce highest qol scores.

Chi-Square tests			
	Value	df	Asymp. Sig. (2-sided)
Pearson Chi-Square	12,288[a]	12	,423
Likelihood ratio	12,291	12	,423
Linear-by-Linear Association	,170	1	,680
N of valid cases	450		

[a]0 cells (,0 %) have expected countless than 5. The minimum expected count is 15,78

However, the cells are not significantly different from one another, and so the result is due to chance. We have clinical arguments that counseling may support the beneficial effects of treatments, and, therefore, perform an analysis with two layers, one in the patients with and one in those without counseling.

Command

Analyze….Descriptive Statistics….Crosstabs….Rows: enter "treatment"…. Columns: enter "qol score"….Layer 1 of 1: enter "counseling"….click Statistics ….mark Chi-square….mark Contingency coefficient….mark Phi and Cramer's V….mark Lambda….mark Uncertainty coefficient….click Continue….click OK.

The underneath tables are in the output sheets.

Treatment * qol score * counseling crosstabulation								
Count								
			Qol score					
Counseling			Very low	Low	Medium	High	Very high	Total
No	Treatment	Cardiac fitness	19	16	8	8	14	65
		Physiotherapy	8	8	7	7	15	45
		Wellness	23	8	6	15	9	61
		Hydrotherapy	15	14	9	10	11	59
	Total		65	46	30	40	49	230
Yes	Treatment	Cardiac fitness	2	5	8	16	22	53
		Physiotherapy	14	12	11	13	5	55
		Wellness	0	6	6	15	16	43
		Hydrotherapy	5	4	16	25	19	69
	Total		21	27	41	69	62	220

Chi-Square tests				
Counseling		Value	df	Asymp. Sig. (2-sided)
No	Pearson Chi-Square	14,831	12	,251
	Likelihood ratio	14,688	12	,259
	Linear-by-Linear Association	,093	1	,760
	N of valid cases	230		

(continued)

Chi-Square tests				
Counseling		Value	df	Asymp. Sig. (2-sided)
Yes	Pearson Chi-Square	42,961	12	,000
	Likelihood ratio	44,981	12	,000
	Linear-by-Linear Association	,517	1	,472
	N of valid cases	220		

Obviously, if we assess the subjects who received counseling, then the high scores appear to appear very significantly more often in the hydrotherapy and cardiac fitness patients than in the physiotherapy and wellness groups.

Symmetric measures				
Counseling			Value	Approx. Sig.
No	Nominal by nominal	Phi	,254	,251
		Cramer's V	,147	,251
		Contingency coefficient	,246	,251
	N of Valid Cases		230	
Yes	Nominal by nominal	Phi	,442	,000
		Cramer's V	,255	,000
		Contingency coefficient	,404	,000
	N of valid cases		220	

Also the phi value, which is the ratio of the computed Pearson chi-square value and the number of observations, are statistically significant. They support that the differences observed in the yes-counseling group are real findings, not chance findings. Cramer's V and contingency coefficient are rescaled phi values, and furthermore support this conclusion.

Directional measures							
Counseling				Value	Asymp. Std. Error	Approx T	Approx Sig.
No	Nominal by nominal	Lambda	Symmetric	,061	,038	1,570	,116
			Treatment dependent	,079	,061	1,238	,216
			Qol score dependent	,042	,028	1,466	,143
		Goodman and Kruskal tau	Treatment dependent	,021	,011		,277
			Qol score dependent	,018	,009		,182
		Uncertainty coefficient	Symmetric	,022	,011	1,933	,259
			Treatment dependent	,023	,012	1,933	,259
			Qol score dependent	,020	,010	1,933	,259

(continued)

Directional measures							
Counseling				Value	Asymp. Std. Error	Approx T	Approx Sig.
Yes	Nominal by nominal	Lambda	Symmetric	,093	,050	1,806	,071
			Treatment dependent	,132	,054	2,322	,020
			Qol score dependent	,053	,063	,818	,414
		Goodman and Kruskal tau	Treatment dependent	,065	,019		,000
			Qol score dependent	,042	,013		,000
		Uncertainty coefficient	Symmetric	,071	,018	3,839	,000
			Treatment dependent	,074	,019	3,839	,000
			Qol score dependent	,067	,017	3,839	,000

The lambda value is also given. It shows the percentages of misclassifications in the row if you would know the column values, is also statistically significant in the yes-counseling subgroup at p=0.020. The value of 0.132 would mean 1.32 % reduction of misclassification, which is, however, not very much. Goodman and uncertainty coefficients serve similar purpose and are also statistically significant.

Conclusion

In conclusion, many high qol levels are in the hydrotherapy and physiotherapy groups, and, correspondingly, very few low qol levels are a major factor for the overall result of this study assessing the effects of treatment modalities on qol scores. The interaction matrix can be used to assess whether some treatment modalities are associated with a better qol score than others, and to assess the directions of the differences in distribution of the variables.

Note

More background, theoretical and mathematical information of crosstabs is given in Statistics applied to clinical studies 5th edition, Chap. 3, The analysis of safety data, pp 41–59, Edited by Springer Heidelberg Germany, 2012, from the same authors.

Chapter 11
Predictions from Ordinal Clinical Data (450 Patients)

General Purpose

In Chap. 9 the typology of medical data was reviewed. Ordinal data are, like nominal data (Chap. 10), discrete data, however, with a stepping pattern, like severity scores, intelligence levels, physical strength scores. They are usually assessed with frequency tables and bar charts. Unlike scale data, that also have a stepping pattern, they do not necessarily have to have steps with equal intervals. Statistical testing is not of much interest. Statistical testing becomes, however, interesting, if we want to know whether two ordinal variables like levels of satisfaction with treatment and treatment outcome are differently distributed between one another. An interaction matrix of these two ordinal variables could then be used to test whether one treatment level performs better than the other. We should add that sometimes an ordinal variable can very well be analyzed as a nominal one (e.g., treatment outcome in the current Chap. and in Chap. 10).

Primary Scientific Question

This chapter assesses the relationship between five levels of satisfaction with the treating doctor, and, as outcome, five levels of quality of life (qol). Can an interaction matrix, otherwise called contingency table or crosstab, be used to assess whether some "satisfaction-with-treating-doctor" levels are associated with a better qol score than others, and to assess the directions of the differences in distribution of the variables.

T.J. Cleophas, A.H. Zwinderman, *Machine Learning in Medicine - a Complete Overview*, DOI 10.1007/978-3-319-15195-3_11

Example

In 450 patients with coronary artery disease the satisfaction level of patients with their doctor was assumed to be an important predictor of patient qol (quality of life).

treatment	counseling	qol	sat doctor
3	1	4	4
4	0	2	1
2	1	5	4
3	0	4	4
2	1	2	1
2	0	1	4
4	0	4	1
3	0	4	1
4	1	4	4
2	1	3	4

Treatment = treatment modality (1 = cardiac fitness, 2 = physiotherapy, 3 = wellness, 4 = hydrotherapy, 5 = nothing)
counseling = counseling given (0 = no, 1 = yes)
qol = quality of life score (1 = very low, 5 = vey high)
sat doctor = satisfaction with doctor (1 = very low, 5 = very high)

The above table gives the first 10 patients of a 450 patients study of the effects of doctors' satisfaction level and qol. The data are also used in the Chap. 16. The entire data file is in extras.springer.com and is entitled "qol.sav".

SPSS is used for analysis.

Command

Analyze….Descriptive Statistics….Crosstabs….Rows: enter "sat doctor"…. Columns: enter "qol score"….click Statistics….mark Gamma, Somer's d, Kendall's tau-b, Kendall's tau-c….click Continue….click OK.

Sat with doctor * qol score crosstabulation

Count

		Qol score					
		Very low	Low	Medium	High	Very high	Total
Sat with doctor	Very low	11	12	12	11	4	50
	Low	24	16	23	28	15	106
	Medium	21	23	17	22	27	110
	High	18	16	15	32	36	117
	Very high	12	6	4	16	29	67
Total		86	73	71	109	111	450

The above matrix of observed counts is shown in the output sheets. Very high qol was frequently observed in patients who were very satisfied with their doctor, while few patients with very high qol (only 4) had a very low satisfaction with their doctor. We wish to assess whether this association is chance or statistically significant.

"Ordinal x ordinal crosstabs" work differently from "nominal x nominal crosstabs" (Chap. 16). The latter compares the magnitude of the cells, the former compares the magnitude of the concordant and those of the discordant cells, whereby the concordant cells are, e.g., "very low versus very low", "low versus low", etc.

Directional measures

			Value	Asymp. Std. Error[a]	Approx T[b]	Approx Sig.
Ordinal by ordinal	Somers' d	Symmetric	,178	,037	4,817	,000
		Sat with doctor dependent	,177	,037	4,817	,000
		Qol score dependent	,179	,037	4,817	,000

[a]Not assuming the null hypothesis
[b]Using the asymptotic standard error assuming the null hypothesis

Symmetric measures

		Value	Asymp. Std. Error[a]	Approx. T[b]	Approx Sig.
Ordinal by ordinal	Kendall's tau-b	,178	,037	4,817	,000
	Kendall's tau-c	,175	,036	4,817	,000
	Gamma	,225	,046	4,817	,000
N of valid cases		450			

[a]Not assuming the null hypothesis
[b]Using the asymptotic standard error assuming the null hypothesis

The above tables are also in the output. The gamma value equals $\text{probability}_{\text{concordance}} - \text{probability}_{\text{discordance}}$, whereby the tied cells are excluded (the cells that have the same order of both variables). Somer's d measures the same but includes the ties. The measures demonstrate that the association of the two variables is closer than could happen by chance. A positive value means a positive correlation, the higher the order in one variable, the higher it will be in the other one. Tau b and c have similar meanings, but are more appropriate for data where numbers of categories between the two variables are different. Both directional and symmetry measures are statistically very significant. This means that high satisfaction levels with the treating doctors are strongly associated with high qol levels, and that low satisfaction levels are strongly associated with low qol levels.

Conclusion

We can conclude from this analysis that there is a statistically significant positive association between the qol score levels and the levels of satisfaction with the patients' doctors, can make predictions from the levels of satisfaction with the doctor about the expected quality of life in future patients, and could consider to recommend doctors to try and perform better to that aim. An interaction matrix, otherwise called contingency table or crosstab, can be used to assess whether treatment levels are associated with a better outcome score than others, and to assess the directions of the differences in distribution of the variables.

Note

More background, theoretical and mathematical information of crosstabs is given in Statistics applied to clinical studies 5th edition, Chap. 3, The analysis of safety data, pp 41–59, Edited by Springer Heidelberg Germany, 2012, from the same authors.

Chapter 12
Assessing Relative Health Risks (3,000 Subjects)

General Purpose

This chapter is to assess whether interaction matrices, otherwise called contingency tables or simply crosstabs, can be used to test the effect of personal characteristics like gender, age, married status etc. on a person's health risks.

Primary Scientific Question

Can marital status affect a person's health risks.

Example

In 3,000 subjects the effect of married status on being healthy was assessed.

T.J. Cleophas, A.H. Zwinderman, *Machine Learning in Medicine - a Complete Overview*, DOI 10.1007/978-3-319-15195-3_12

ageclass	married	healthy
4,00	1	0
3,00	0	0
2,00	1	0
1,00	1	0
4,00	1	0
3,00	0	0
2,00	1	0
1,00	0	0
4,00	1	0
3,00	1	0

ageclass 1 = 30–40, 2 = 40–50, 3 = 50–60, 4 = 60–70
married 0 = no, 1 = yes
healthy 0 = no, 1 = yes

In the above table the first 10 patients are given. The entire data file is entitled "healthrisk.sav" and is in extras.springer.com. We will start the analysis by opening the data file in SPSS.

Command

Analyze....Descriptive Statistics....Crosstabs....Row(s): enter married....Column(s): enter health....Statistics: mark Observed....mark Rows....click Continue....click OK.

Married * healthy crosstabulation

			Healthy		
			No	Yes	Total
Married	No	Count	192	1,104	1,296
		% within married	14,8 %	85,2 %	100,0 %
	Yes	Count	167	1,537	1,704
		% within married	9,8 %	90,2 %	100,0 %

The crosstab is in the output sheets. It shows that 14.8 % of the unmarried subjects were unhealthy, leaving 85,2 % being healthy. In contrast, 9.8% of the married subjects were unhealthy, 90.2% being healthy. And so, the risk of being unhealthy in this population was 14.8 % in the unmarried and 9.8% in the married subjects. The relative risk of being unhealthy in unmarried versus married subjects was, thus, 14.8/9.8 = 1.512. Similarly, the relative risk of being healthy in unmarried versus married subjects was 85.2/90.2 = 0.944.

Risk estimate

		95% Confidence interval	
	Value	Lower	Upper
Odds ratio for married (no/yes)	1,601	1,283	1,997
For cohort healthy = no	1,512	1,245	1,836
For cohort healthy = yes	,944	,919	,971
N of valid cases	3,000		

The odds of being unhealthy in unmarried subjects was 192/1,104 = 0.1739.

The odds of being unhealthy in married subjects was 167/1,537 = 0.1087.

The ratio of the two, the odds ratio was thus 0.1739/0.1087 = 1.601, as shown in the above table. It is easy to see that this odds ratio is equal to

$$= \frac{\text{the relative risk of being unhealthy in the unmarried versus married subjects}}{\text{the relative risk of being healthy in the unmarried versus married subjects}}$$

$$= 1.512 / 0.944 = 1.601.$$

In order to assess whether this finding is robust, we will add age classes as a layer variable, and test whether different age classes have similar odds ratios.

Command

Analyze....Descriptive Statistics....Crosstabs....Row(s): enter married....Column(s): enter health....Layer 1 of 1: enter ageclass....Statistics: mark Observed....mark Rows ....mark Cochran and Mantel Haenszel Statistics....click Continue....click OK.

Married * healthy * ageclass crosstabulation

				Healthy		
Ageclass				No	Yes	Total
30–40	Married	No	Count	52	138	190
			% within married	27,4 %	72,6 %	100,0 %
		Yes	Count	53	327	380
			% within married	13,9 %	86,1 %	100,0 %
	Total		Count	105	465	570
			% within married	18,4 %	81,6 %	100,0 %
40–50	Married	No	Count	69	352	421
			% within married	16,4 %	83,6 %	100,0 %
		Yes	Count	67	593	660
			% within married	10,2 %	89,8 %	100,0 %
	Total		Count	136	945	1,081
			% within married	12,6 %	87,4 %	100,0 %
50–60	married	No	Count	28	201	229
			% within married	12,2 %	87,8 %	100,0 %
		Yes	Count	17	287	304
			% within married	5,6 %	94,4 %	100,0 %
	Total		Count	45	488	533
			% within married	8,4 %	91,6 %	100,0 %
60–70	Married	No	Count	43	413	456
			% within married	9,4 %	90,6 %	100,0 %
		Yes	Count	30	330	360
			% within married	8,3 %	91,7 %	100,0 %
	Total		Count	73	743	816
			% within married	8,9 %	91,1 %	100,0 %

* Symbol of multiplication

Risk estimate				
			95% Confidence interval	
Ageclass		Value	Lower	Upper
30–40	Odds ratio for married (no/yes)	2,325	1,511	3,578
	For cohort healthy = no	1,962	1,396	2,759
	For cohort healthy = yes	,844	,767	,929
	N of valid cases	570		
40–50	Odds ratio for married (no/yes)	1,735	1,209	2,490
	For cohort healthy = no	1,614	1,180	2,208
	For cohort healthy = yes	,931	,886	,978
	N of valid cases	1,081		
50–60	Odds ratio for married (no/yes)	2,352	1,254	4,411
	For cohort healthy = no	2,186	1,227	3,896
	For cohort healthy = yes	,930	,879	,983
	N of valid cases	533		
60–70	Odds ratio for married (no/yes)	1,145	,703	1,866
	For cohort healthy = no	1,132	,725	1,766
	For cohort healthy = yes	,988	,946	1,031
	N of valid cases	816		

In the output are the crosstabs the odds ratios of the four ageclasses. The odds ratios are pretty heterogeneous, between 1.145 and 2.352, but 95 % confidence intervals were pretty wide. Yet, it is tested whether these odds ratios are significantly different from one another.

Tests of homogeneity of the odds ratio			
	Chi-Squared	df	Asymp. Sig. (2-sided)
Breslow-Day	5,428	3	,143
Tarone's	5,422	3	,143

The above Breslow and the Tarone's tests are the heterogeneity tests. They were insignificant. The differences could, thus, be ascribed to chance findings, rather than real effects. It seems appropriate, therefore, to say that an overall odds ratio of these data adjusted for age classes is meaningful. For that purpose a Mantel Haenszel (MH) odds ratio (OR) will be calculated.

		healthy	
		no	yes
unmarried	no	a	b
	yes	c	d

Having 4 odds ratios with the above structure, it is calculated as follows (n = a + b + c + d):

$$\text{Odds Ratio}_{MH} = \frac{\Sigma\, ad / n}{\Sigma\, cd / n}$$

Tests of conditional independence			
	Chi-Squared	df	Asymp. Sig. (2-sided)
Cochran's	26,125	1	,000
Mantel-Haenszel	25,500	1	,000

Under the conditional independence assumption, Cochran's statistic is asymptotically distributed as a 1 df chi-squared distribution, only if the number of strata is fixed, while the Mantel-Haenszel statistic is always asymptotically distributed as a 1 df chi-squared distribution. Note that the continuity correction is removed from the Mantel-Haenszel statistic when the sum of the differences between the observed and the expected is 0

Mantel-Haenszel common odds ratio estimate			
Estimate			1,781
In(Estimate)			,577
Std. Error of In(Estimate)			,115
Asymp. Sig. (2-sided)			,000
Asymp. 95% confidence interval	Common odds ratio	Lower bound	1,422
		Upper bound	2,230
	In(Common odds ratio)	Lower bound	,352
		Upper bound	,802

The Mantel-Haenszel common odds ratio estimate is asymptotically normally distributed under the common odds ratio of 1,000 assumption. So is the natural log of the estimate

The Cochran's and Mantel Haenszel tests assess whether married status remains an independent predictor of health after adjustment for ageclasses. They are significantly larger than an odds ratio (OR) of 0 at $p<0.0001$. The lower graph gives the OR_{MH} is thus 1.781. This OR is adjusted, and, therefore, more adequate than the unadjusted OR of page 1 of this chapter.

Conclusion

Interaction matrices, otherwise called contingency tables or simply crosstabs, can be used to test the effect of personal characteristics like gender, age, married status etc. on a person's health risks. Results can be adjusted for concomitant effects like the effect of age classes on the relationship between married status and health status. Prior to assessment the homogeneity of the concomitant factors have to tested.

Note

More background, theoretical and mathematical information of relative risk assessments are in Statistics applied to clinical studies, Chap. 3, The analysis of safety data, pp 41–59, Edited by Springer Heidelberg Germany, 2012, from the same authors.

Chapter 13
Measuring Agreement (30 Patients)

General Purpose

Interaction matrices have myriad applications. In the Chap. 12 it can be observed that they perform well for assessing relative health risks, making predictions from nominal and ordinal clinical data (Chap. 9–11), and statistical testing of outcome scores. In this chapter we will assess, if they also can be applied to measure agreement. Agreement, otherwise called reproducibility or reliability, of duplicate observations is the fundament of diagnostic procedures, and, therefore, also the fundament of much of scientific research.

Primary Scientific Question

Can a 2×2 interaction matrix also be used to demonstrate the level of agreement between duplicate observations of the effect of antihypertensive treatment.

Example

In 30 patients with hypertension the effect of an antihypertensive treatment was measured with normotension as outcome. Each patients was tested twice in order to assess the reproducibility of the procedure. the example was used before (Chap. 19, Reliability assessment of qualitative diagnostic tests, in: SPSS for starters part 1, pp 69–70, Springer Heidelberg Germany, 2010, from the same authors as the current work).

T.J. Cleophas, A.H. Zwinderman, *Machine Learning in Medicine - a Complete Overview*, DOI 10.1007/978-3-319-15195-3_13

Variables	
1	2
1,00	1,00
1,00	1,00
1,00	1,00
1,00	1,00
1,00	1,00
1,00	1,00
1,00	1,00
1,00	1,00
1,00	1,00
1,00	1,00
1,00	,00

Variable 1 = responder after first test
(0 = non responder, 1 = responder)
Variable 2 = responder after second test

The above table shows the results of first 11 patients. The entire data file is entitled agreement, and is in extras.springer.com. We will start by opening the file in SPSS.

Command

Analyze....Descriptive Statistics....Crosstabs....Row(s): enter Variable 1....Column(s): enter Variable 2....click Statistics....Mark: kappa....click Continue....click Cells..... mark Observed....click continue....click OK.

VAR00001 * VAR00002 crosstabulation

Count

		VAR00002		
		,00	1,00	Total
VAR00001	,00	11	4	15
	1,00	5	10	15
Total		16	14	30

In the output sheets a interaction matrix of the data is shown. If agreement is 100 %, then the cells b and c would be empty, and the cells a and d would contain 30 patients.

		variable 2	
		0	1
variable 1	0	a	b
	1	c	d

However, the cells a and d contain only 21 patients.

If agreement would be 0 %, then the cells a and d would contain 15 patients. However, 21 is more than 15, and so, this may indicate that agreement is better than 0 %, although less than 100 %. Cohen's Kappa is computed by SPSS to estimate the exact level of agreement.

Symmetric measures

		Value	Asymp. Std. Error[a]	Approx. T[b]	Approx. Sig.
Measure of agreement	Kappa	,400	,167	2,196	,028
N of valid cases		30			

[a]Not assuming the null hypothesis
[b]Using the asymptotic standard error assuming the null hypothesis

The above table shows that the kappa-value equals 0.400. A kappa-value of 0 means poor reproducibility or agreement, a kappa-value of 1 means excellent. This result of 0.400 is moderate. This result is significantly different from an agreement of 0 at $p=0.028$.

Conclusion

In this chapter it is assessed if interaction matrices can be applied to measure agreement. Agreement, otherwise called reproducibility or reliability, of duplicate observations is the fundament of diagnostic procedures, and, therefore, also the fundament of much of scientific research.

A 2×2 interaction matrix can be used to demonstrate the level of agreement between duplicate observations of the effect of antihypertensive treatment. We should add that kappa-values can also be computed from larger interaction matrices, like 3×3, 4×4 contingency tables, etc.

Note

More background, theoretical and mathematical information of correct and incorrect methods for assessing reproducibility or agreement are given in Chap. 45, Testing reproducibility, pp 499–508, in: Statistics applied to clinical studies 5th edition, Springer Heidelberg Germany, 2012, from the same authors.

Chapter 14
Column Proportions for Testing Differences Between Outcome Scores (450 Patients)

General Purpose

In the Chap. 10 the relationship between treatment modality and quality of life (qol) score levels were assessed using a chi-square test of the interaction matrix. Many high qol scores were in the hydrotherapy and physiotherapy treatments, and in the subgroup that received counseling the overall differences from other treatments were statistically significant at $p < 0.0001$. In this chapter, using the same data, we will try and test what levels of qol scores were significantly different from one another, and, thus, provide a more detailed about differences in effects.

Specific Scientific Question

Can the effects of different treatment modalities on outcome score levels previously assessed with a chi-square test of the interaction matrix, be assessed with better precision applying column proportion comparisons using Bonferroni-adjusted z-tests?

Example

A parallel group study of 450 patients assessed the effect of different complementary treatment modalities on qol score levels. The first 11 patients of the data file is underneath. The entire data file is entitled "qol.sav", and is in extras.springer.com.

T.J. Cleophas, A.H. Zwinderman, *Machine Learning in Medicine - a Complete Overview*, DOI 10.1007/978-3-319-15195-3_14

treatment	counseling	qol	satdoctor
3	1	4	4
4	0	2	1
2	1	5	4
3	0	4	4
2	1	2	1
2	0	1	4
4	0	4	1
3	0	4	1
4	1	4	4
2	1	3	4
4	1	5	5

treatment = treatment modality (1 = cardiac fitness, 2 = physiotherapy, 3 = wellness, 4 = hydrotherapy)
counseling = counseling given (0 = no, 1 = yes)
qol = quality of life scores (1 = very low, 5 = very high)
satdoctor = satisfaction with treating doctor (1 = very low, 5 = very high)

We will start by opening the data file in SPSS.

Command:

Analyze....Descriptive Statistics....Crosstabs....Row(s): enter treatment....Column(s): enter qol....click Cells....mark Observed....mark Columns....mark: Compare column properties....mark: Adjusted p-values (Bonferroni method)....click Continue....click OK.

Treatment * qol score crosstabulation

			Qol score					Total
			Very low	Low	Medium	High	Very high	
Treatment	Cardiac fitness	Count	21_a	21_a		24_a	36_a	118
		% within qol score	24,4 %	28,8 %	22,5 %	22,0 %	32,4 %	26,2 %
	Physiotherapy	Count	22^a	20_a	18_a	20_a	20_a	100
		% within qol score	25,6 %	27,4 %	25,4 %	18,3 %	18,0 %	22,2 %

(continued)

Treatment * qol score crosstabulation								
			Qol score					Total
			Very low	Low	Medium	High	Very high	
	Wellness	Count	22_a	14_a	12_a	30_a	25_a	104
		% within qol score	26,7 %	19,2 %	16,9 %	27,5 %	22,5 %	23,1 %
	Hydrotherapy	Count	20_a	18_a	25_a	35_a	30_a	128
		% within qol score	23,3 %	24,7 %	35,2 %	32,1 %	27,0 %	28,4 %
Total		Count	86	73	71	109	111	450
		% within qol score	100,0 %	100,0 %	100,0 %	100,0 %	100,0 %	100,0 %

* Symbol of multiplication
Each subscript letter denotes a subset of qol score categories whose column proportions do not differ significantly from each other at the ,05 level

The above table is in the output sheets. All of the counts in the cells are given with the subscript letter a.

The interpretation of the subscript letters are pretty obvious:

looking in a single row	
a vs a	$p>0.10$
a vs a,b	$0.05<p<0.10$
a vs b	$p<0.05$
a vs c	$p<0.01$
a vs d	$p<0.001$
b vs a,b	$0.05<p<0.10$

This means, that, in the above table, none of the counts is significantly different from one another. This is consistent with the insignificant chi-square test of Chap. 16. We have clinical arguments that counseling may support the beneficial effects of treatments, and, therefore, perform an analysis with two layers, one in the patients with and one in those without counseling.

Command:

Analyze....Descriptive Statistics....Crosstabs....Row(s): enter treatment.... Column(s): enter qol....Layer 1 of 1: enter counseling....click Cells....mark Observed....mark Columns....mark: Compare column properties....mark: Adjusted p-values (Bonferroni method)....click Continue....click OK.

Treatment * qol score * counseling crosstabulation									
				Qol score					
Counseling				Very low	Low	Medium	High	Very high	Total
No	Treatment	Cardiac fitness	Count	19	16	8	8	14	65
			% within qol score	292 %	34,8 %	26,7 %	20,0 %	28,6 %	28,3 %
		Phototherapy	Count	8	8	7	7	15b	45
			% within qol score	12,3 %	17,4 %	23,3 %	17,5 %	30,6 %	19,6 %
		Wellness	Count	23	8	6	15	9	61
			% within qol score	35,4 %	17,4 %	20,0 %	37,5 %	18,4 %	26,5 %
		Hydrotherapy	Count	15	14	9	10	11	59
			% within qol score	23,1 %	30,4 %	30,0 %	25,0 %	22,4 %	25,7 %
	Total		Count	65	46	30	40	49	230
			% within qol score	100,0 %	100,0 %	100,0 %	100,0 %	100,0 %	100,0 %
Yes	Treatment	Cardiac fitness	Count	2	5	8	16	22	53
			% within qol score	9,5 %	18,5 %	19,5 %	23,2 %	35,5 %	24,1 %
		Physiotherapy	Count	14	12	11	13	5	55
			% within qol score	66,7 %	44,4 %	26,8 %	18,8 %	8,1 %	25,0 %
		Wellness	Count	0	6	6	15	16	43
			% within qol score	,0 %	22,2 %	14,6 %	21,7 %	25,8 %	19,5 %
		Hydrotherapy	Count	5	4	16	25	19	69
			% within qol score	23,8 %	14,8 %	39,0 %	36,2 %	30,6 %	31,4 %
	Total		Count	21	27	41	69	62	220
			% within qol score	100,0 %	100,0 %	100,0 %	100,0 %	100,0 %	100,0 %

* Symbol of multiplication

The above table is now shown. It gives the computations for the patients previously counseled separately. Now differences particularly in the patients counseled were larger.

In the cardiac fitness row the very low and very high qol cells the percentages of patients present are 9.5 and 23.2 % (significantly different at $p<0.05$ Bonferroni adjusted), and "very low" versus the three scores in between have a trend to significance $0.05<p<0.10$. The same is true with "very high" versus (vs) the three scores in between. In the physiotherapy row differences were even larger. In the physiotherapy row we have:

1. both 14 vs 11 and 11 vs 5 significantly different at $p<0.05$
2. 14 vs 12, 12 vs 11, 11 vs 13, 13 vs 5 with a trend to significantly different at $0.05<p<0.10$.

Similarly, in the wellness and hydrotherapy rows significant differences and trends to significance were observed.

In the no-counseling patients differences were smaller, but some trends, and two significant differences at $p < 0.05$ (a vs b) were, nonetheless, observed.

In conclusion, only in the physiotherapy row the low qol fraction is large, in the other three the high qol fractions are large. And so, with respect to qol physiotherapy does not perform very well, and may better be skipped from the program.

Note: Bonferroni adjustment for multiple testing works as follows. In order for p-values to be significant, with two tests they need to be smaller than 0.025, with four tests smaller than 0.0125, with ten tests smaller than 0.005, etc.

Conclusion

When assessing the outcome effects of different treatments, column proportions comparisons of interaction matrices can be applied to precisely find what outcome scores are significantly different from one another. This may provide relevant information about some treatment modalities, and may give cause for some treatment modalities to be skipped.

Note

More background, theoretical and mathematical information of interaction matrices is given in Statistics applied to clinical studies 5th edition, Chap. 3, The analysis of safety data, pp 41–59, Springer Heidelberg Germany, 2012, from the same authors, and in the Chaps. 10–13 of this work.

Chapter 15
Pivoting Trays and Tables for Improved Analysis of Multidimensional Data (450 Patients)

General Purpose

Pivot tables can visualize multiple variables data with the help of interactive displays of multiple dimensions. They have been in SPSS statistical software for a long time (from version 7.0), and, gradually, they take over in most modules. They are helpful for improving the analysis by visualizing interaction patterns you so far did not notice.

Primary Scientific Question

Are pivot tables able to visualize interaction pattern in your clinical data that so far were unnoticed?

Example

We will use as example the data also used in the Chaps. 10–14. A parallel group study of 450 patients assessed the effect of different complementary treatment modalities on qol score levels. The first 11 patients of the data file is underneath. The entire data file is entitled "qol.sav", and is in extras.springer.com.

T.J. Cleophas, A.H. Zwinderman, *Machine Learning in Medicine - a Complete Overview*, DOI 10.1007/978-3-319-15195-3_15

treatment	counseling	qol	satdoctor
3	1	4	4
4	0	2	1
2	1	5	4
3	0	4	4
2	1	2	1
2	0	1	4
4	0	4	1
3	0	4	1
4	1	4	4
2	1	3	4
4	1	5	5

treatment = treatment modality (1 = cardiac fitness, 2 = physiotherapy, 3 = wellness, 4 = hydrotherapy)
counseling = counseling given (0 = no, 1 = yes)
qol = quality of life scores (1 = very low, 5 = very high)
satdoctor = satisfaction with treating doctor (1 = very low, 5 = very high)

We will start by opening the data file in SPSS.

Command:

Analyze....Descriptive Statistics....Crosstabs....Row(s): enter treatment....Column(s): enter qol....click Cells....mark Observed....mark Columns....click Continue....click OK.

The underneath table is shown in the output sheets.

Treatment * qol score * counseling crosstabulation

				Qol score					
Counseling				Very low	Low	Medium	High	Very high	Total
No	Treatment	Cardiac fitness	Count	19	16	8	8	14	65
			% within qol score	29,2 %	34,8 %	26,7 %	20,0 %	28,6 %	28,3 %
		Physiotherapy	Count	8	8	7	7	15	45
			% within qol score	12,3 %	17,4 %	23,3 %	17,5 %	30,6 %	19,6 %
		Wellness	Count	23	8	6	15	9	61
			% within qol score	35,4 %	17,4 %	20,0 %	37,5 %	18,4 %	26,5 %
		Hydrotherapy	Count	15	14	9	10	11	59
			% within qol score	23,1 %	30,4 %	30,0 %	25,0 %	22,4 %	25,7 %
	Total		Count	65	46	30	40	49	230
			% within qol score	100,0 %	100,0 %	100,0 %	100,0 %	100,0 %	100,0 %

(continued)

Treatment * qol score * counseling crosstabulation									
				Qol score					Total
Counseling				Very low	Low	Medium	High	Very high	
Yes	Treatment	Cardiac fitness	Count	2	5	8	16	22	53
			% within qol score	9,5 %	18,5 %	19,5 %	23,2 %	35,5 %	24,1 %
		Physiotherapy	Count	14	12	11	13	5	55
			% within qol score	66,7 %	44,4 %	26,8 %	18,8 %	8,1 %	25,0 %
		Wellness	Count	0	6	6	15	16	43
			% within qol score	,0 %	22,2 %	14,6 %	21,7 %	25,8 %	19,5 %
		Hydrotherapy	Count	5	4	16	25	19	69
			% within qol score	23,8 %	14,8 %	39,0 %	36,2 %	30,6 %	31,4 %
	Total		Count	21	27	41	69	62	220
			% within qol score	100,0 %	100,0 %	100,0 %	100,0 %	100,0 %	100,0 %
Total	treatment	Cardiac fitness	Count	21	21	16	24	36	118
			% within qol score	24,4 %	28,8 %	22,5 %	22,0 %	32,4 %	26,2 %
		Physiotherapy	Count	22	20	18	20	20	100
			% within qol score	25,6 %	27,4 %	25,4 %	18,3 %	18,0 %	22,2 %
		Wellness	Count	23	14	12	30	25	104
			% within qol score	26,7 %	19,2 %	16,9 %	27,5 %	22,5 %	23,1 %
		Hydrotherapy	Count	20	18	25	35	30	128
			% within qol score	23,3 %	24,7 %	35,2 %	32,1 %	27,0 %	28,4 %
	Total		Count	86	73	71	109	111	450
			% within qol score	100,0 %	100,0 %	100,0 %	100,0 %	100,0 %	100,0 %

* Symbol of multiplication

We will apply this table for pivoting the data, using the "user interface for pivot tables", otherwise called the pivoting tray.

Command:

Double-click the above table....the term Pivot is added to the menu bar....click Pivot in the menu bar....the underneath Pivoting Tray consisting of all of the variables appears....qol score is a column variables....counseling, treatment, and statistics are row variables....left click the counseling icon and drag it to the column variables.... similarly have statistics dragged to the layer dimension....close the Pivoting Tray.

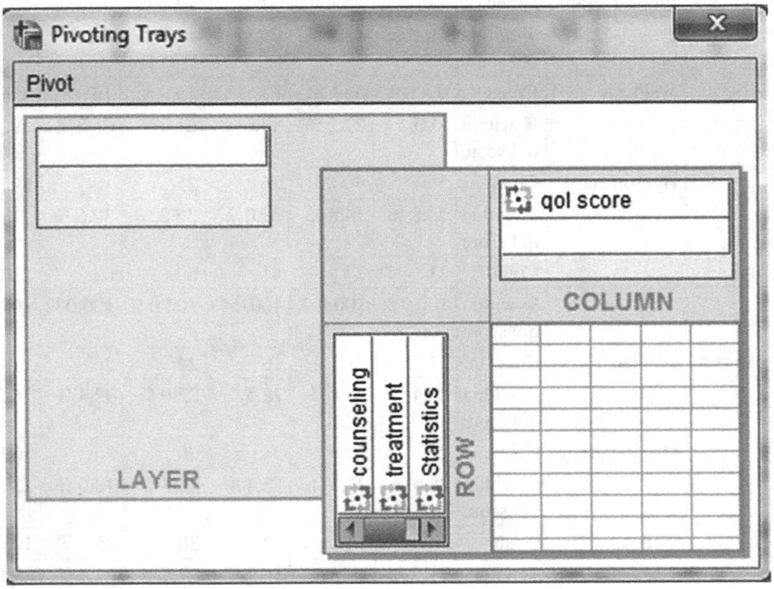

A new table is shown in the output.

Treatment * qol score * counseling crosstabulation

Statistics: % within qol score

		Qol score														
		Very low			Low			Medium			High			Very high		
		Counseling			Counseling			Counseling			Counseling			Counseling		
		No	Yes	Total	No	Yes	Total	No	Yes	Total	No	Yes	Total	No	Yes	Total
Treatment	Cardiac fitness	292 %	9,5 %	24,4 %	348 %	16,5 %	268 %	26,7 %	19,5 %	223 %	20,0 %	23,2 %	228 %	28,6 %	35,5 %	32,4 %
	Physiotherapy	123 %	66,7 %	25,6 %	17,4 %	44,4 %	27,4 %	233 %	26,6 %	25,4 %	17,5 %	18,6 %	183 %	30,6 %	8,1 %	18,0 %
	Wellness	35,4 %	,0 %	26,7 %	17,4 %	222 %	192 %	20,0 %	14,6 %	163 %	378 %	21,7 %	273 %	18,4 %	25,8 %	223 %
	Hydrotherapy	23,1 %	23,8 %	23,3 %	30,4 %	14,6 %	24,7 %	30,0 %	39,0 %	352 %	25,0 %	36,2 %	32,1 %	22,4 %	30,6 %	27,0 %
Total		100,0 %	100,0 %	100,0 %	100,0 %	100,0 %	1008 %	100,0 %	100,0 %	1002 %	100,0 %	100,0 %	1002 %	100,0 %	100,0 %	100,0 %

*Symbol of multiplication

In it click Statistics and click "% within qol score" in the drop box of the table next to Statistics. In the now upcoming table the cell counts have disappeared. They are not relevant, anyway, only the percentages are so. From the Chaps. 2 and 6 we already know, that there is an overall difference between the cells of the yes-counseling matrix, and that the 67 % very low qol is significantly different from the 5 % very high qol in the physical therapy treatment groups. What more can the above pivoted table teach us? It underscores the finding from the Chaps. 2 and 6 by showing next to each other the no-counseling and yes-counseling percentages; very low qol with physiotherapy is observed in respectively 12.3 and 66.7 %, low qol in 17.4 and 44.4 %, and, in contrast, very high qol in respectively 30.6 and 8.1 %.

Restarting with the above unpivoted table once more, give the commands:

Double-click the table....the term Pivot is added to the menu bar....click Pivot in the menu bar....the Pivoting Tray consisting of all of the variables appears....qol score is a column variables....counseling, treatment, and statistics are row variables....drag treatment to the layer dimension....similarly have statistics dragged to the layer dimension....the Pivoting Tray now looks like shown underneath....close it.

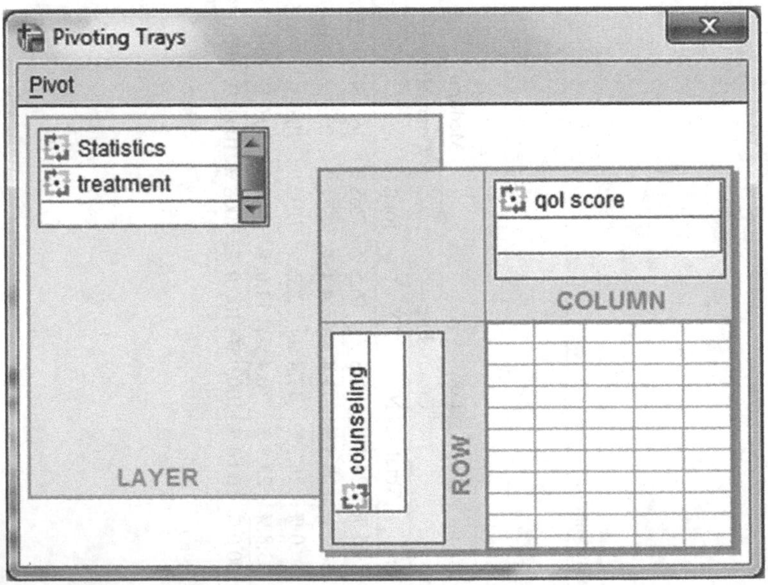

A new pivot table is given in the output. In the left upper angle of it, it has a Statistics and a treatment drop box. Statistics: click Count and select "% within qol score", treatment: select, subsequently, all of the four treatments given. The four underneath tables are produced.

Treatment * qol score * counseling crosstabulation						
Statistics: % within qol score, treatment: treatment cardiac fitness						
	Qol score					
Counseling	Very low	Low	Medium	High	Very high	Total
No	29,2 %	34,8 %	26,7 %	20,0 %	28,6 %	28,3 %
Yes	9,5 %	18,5 %	19,5 %	23,2 %	35,5 %	24,1 %
Total	24,4 %	28,8 %	22,5 %	22,0 %	32,4 %	26,2 %

* Symbol of multiplication

Treatment * qol score * counseling crosstabulation						
Statistics: % within qol score, treatment: treatment physiotherapy						
	Qol score					
Counseling	Very low	Low	Medium	High	Very high	Total
No	12,3 %	17,4 %	23,3 %	17,5 %	30,6 %	19,6 %
Yes	66,7 %	44,4 %	26,8 %	18,8 %	8,1 %	25,0 %
Total	25,6 %	27,4 %	25,4 %	18,3 %	18,0 %	22,2 %

* Symbol of multiplication

Treatment * qol score * counseling crosstabulation						
Statistics: % within qol score, treatment: treatment wellness						
	Qol score					
Counseling	Very low	Low	Medium	High	Very high	Total
No	35,4 %	17,4 %	20,0 %	37,5 %	18,4 %	26,5 %
Yes	,0 %	22,2 %	14,6 %	21,7 %	25,8 %	19,5 %
Total	26,7 %	19,2 %	16,9 %	27,5 %	22,5 %	23,1 %

* Symbol of multiplication

Treatment * qol score * counseling crosstabulation						
Statistics: % within qol score, treatment: treatment hydrotherapy						
	Qol score					
Counseling	Very low	Low	Medium	High	Very high	Total
No	23,1 %	30,4 %	30,0 %	25,0 %	22,4 %	25,7 %
Yes	23,8 %	14,8 %	39,0 %	36,2 %	30,6 %	31,4 %
Total	23,3 %	24,7 %	35,2 %	32,1 %	27,0 %	28,4 %

* Symbol of multiplication

They visualize a big downward trend of percentages from very low to very high qol for the treatments cardiac fitness, wellness and hydrotherapy, and an upward trend for the treatment physiotherapy. Although this is in agreement with the findings from the Chaps. 2 and 6, the patterns are relevant, because they give you an additional idea about how patients experience their treatments.

Conclusion

The interactive pivot tables are not only a way of showing the same in another perspective, but they are also more than that, because they help you better notice what is going on at difference levels of the analysis, and, so, they, actually, can improve the analysis by visualizing data patterns you did not notice before.

Note

Pivot tables are widely applied not only in SPSS and most of the larger statistical software programs, but also in spreadsheets programs like Excel. In SPSS they are being applied with Anova (analysis of variance), Correlations, Crosstabs, Descriptives, Examine, Frequencies, General Linear Models, Nonparametric Tests, Regression, T-tests. In the current book pivot tables were applied in many more Chaps., e.g., the Chaps. 6, 16, and 29.

Chapter 16
Online Analytical Procedure Cubes, a More Rapid Approach to Analyzing Frequencies (450 Patients)

General Purpose

OLAP means online analytical procedures. Cubes is a term used to indicate multidimensional datasets. OLAP cubes were first used in 1970, by SQL Express a software package for storing business data, like financial data, in an electronic warehouse, and, at the same time, turning raw data into meaningful information (business intelligence), and was initially called layered reports. Generally, financial data or production data are being summarized, and from these summaries subsummaries are computed like productions by time-periods, cities, and other subgroups. Instead of quantities of business data, quantities of health outcomes could, similarly, be analyzed. However, to date no such analyses have been performed. This chapter is to assess whether online analytical procedures can also be applied on health outcomes instead of business outcomes.

Primary Scientific Question

Can online analytical processing (OLAP) using summaries and subsummaries of clinical outcome data support traditional crosstab analyses?

Example

We will use as example the data also used in the Chaps. 10 and 11. A parallel group study of 450 patients assessed the effect of different complementary treatment modalities on qol score levels. The first 11 patients of the data file is underneath. The entire data file is entitled "qol.sav", and is in extras.springer.com.

T.J. Cleophas, A.H. Zwinderman, *Machine Learning in Medicine - a Complete Overview*, DOI 10.1007/978-3-319-15195-3_16

treatment	counseling	qol	satdoctor
3	1	4	4
4	0	2	1
2	1	5	4
3	0	4	4
2	1	2	1
2	0	1	4
4	0	4	1
3	0	4	1
4	1	4	4
2	1	3	4
4	1	5	5

treatment = treatment modality (1 = cardiac fitness, 2 = physiotherapy, 3 = wellness, 4 = hydrotherapy)
counseling = counseling given (0 = no, 1 = yes)
qol = quality of life scores (1 = very low, 5 = very high)
satdoctor = satisfaction with treating doctor (1 = very low, 5 = very high)

We will start by opening the data file in SPSS.

Command:

Analyze....Reports....OLAP Cubes....Summary Variable(s): enter qol score.... Grouping Variable(s): enter treatment, counseling....click OK.

Case processing summary

	Cases					
	Included		Excluded		Total	
	N	Percent	N	Percent	N	Percent
Qol score * treatment * counseling	450	100,0 %	0	,0 %	450	100,0 %

* Symbol of multiplication

OLAP cubes

Treatment:Total

Counseling:Total

	Sum	N	Mean	Std. Deviation	% of Total Sum	% of Total N
Qol score	1,436	450	3,19	1,457	100,0 %	100,0 %

The above tables are in the output sheets. The add-up sum of all scores are given (1436), and the overall mean score of the 450 patients (3.19). Next we can slice these results into subgroups, and calculate mean scores by treatment modality. A pivoting tray is used for that purpose.

Command:

Double-click the above table....the term Pivot is added to the menu bar....click Pivot in the menu bar....the underneath Pivoting Tray consisting of all of the variables appears....close the Pivoting Tray.

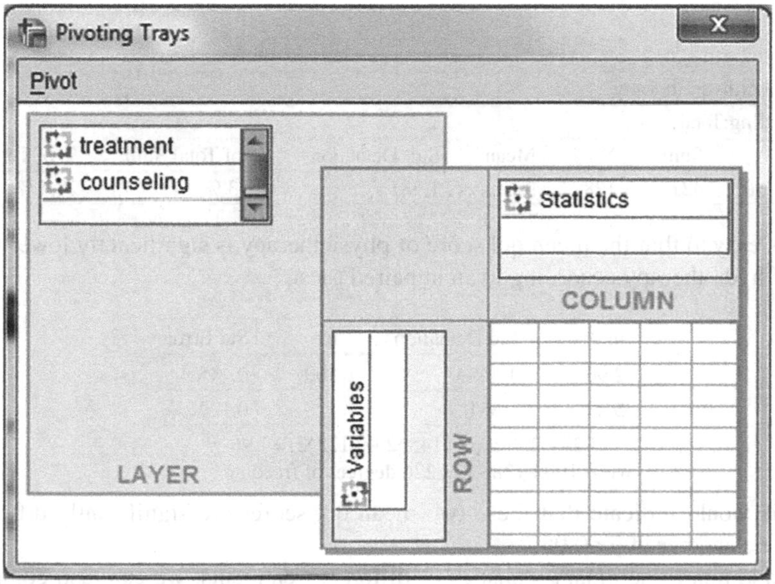

The above table now has in the upper right corner two drop boxes: treatment, and counseling. Treatment: click Total (in blue), and produce the underneath four tables with summary statistics of the four treatment modalities.

OLAP cubes						
Treatment:cardiac fitness						
Counseling:Total						
	Sum	N	Mean	Std. Deviation	% of Total Sum	% of Total N
Qol score	387	118	3,28	1,501	26,9 %	26,2 %

OLAP cubes						
Treatment:physiotherapy						
Counseling:Total						
	Sum	N	Mean	Std. Deviation	% of Total Sum	% of Total N
Qol score	296	100	2,96	1,449	20,6 %	22,2 %

OLAP cubes						
Treatment:wellness						
Counseling:Total						
	Sum	N	Mean	Std. Deviation	% of Total Sum	% of Total N
Qol score	332	104	3,19	1,501	23,1 %	23,1 %

OLAP cubes						
Treatment:hydrotherapy						
Counseling:Total						
	Sum	N	Mean	Std. Deviation	% of Total Sum	% of Total N
Qol score	421	128	3,29	1,381	29,3 %	28,4 %

It is easy to that the mean qol score of physiotherapy is significantly lower than that of hydrotherapy according to an unpaired t-test:

mean	Std Deviation	n	Std Error
2.96	1.449	100	0.145
3.29	1.381	128	0.122

$t=(3.29-2.96)/\sqrt{}(0.145\hat{}2+0.122\hat{}2)=1.96$
with $(100+128-2)=226$ degrees of freedom

This would indicate that these two mean qol scores are significantly different from one another at $p<0.05$.

In addition to summary statistics of different treatments, we can also compute summary statistics of qol scores by counseling yes or no.

Command:

click the treatment drop box....select Total....next click the counseling drop box… first select counseling no....then select counseling yes.

The underneath tables are given.

OLAP cubes						
Treatment:Total						
Counseling:Total						
	Sum	N	Mean	Std. Deviation	% of Total Sum	% of Total N
Qol score	1,436	450	3,19	1,457	100,0 %	100,0 %

OLAP cubes						
Treatment:Total						
Counseling:No						
	Sum	N	Mean	Std. Deviation	% of Total Sum	% of Total N
Qol score	652	230	2,83	1,530	45,4 %	51,1 %

OLAP cubes						
Treatment:Total						
Counseling:Yes						
	Sum	N	Mean	Std. Deviation	% of Total Sum	% of Total N
Qol score	784	220	3,56	1,279	54,6 %	48,9 %

It is again easy to test whether the mean qol score of no-counseling is significantly lower than that of yes-counseling according to an unpaired t-test:

mean	Std Deviation	n	Std Error
2.83	1.530	230	0.101
3.56	1.279	220	0.086

$t=(3.56-2.83)/\sqrt{(0.101^2+0.086^2)}=5.49$
with $(230+220-2)=448$ degrees of freedom

This would indicate that the two means are significantly different from one another at $p<0.0001$.

Conclusion

In the current example the individual qol levels were estimated as 5 scores on a 5-points linear scale. In the Chaps. 2, 6 and 7 analyses took place by comparing frequencies of different qol scores with one another. In the OLAP cubes analysis a different approach is applied. Instead of working with frequencies of different qol scores, it works with mean scores and standard deviations. Other summary measure is also possible like sums of qol scores, medians, ranges or variances etc. Unpaired t-test can be used to test the significance of difference between various subsummaries.

Although we have to admit that the crosstab analyses and OLAP cube lead to essentially the same results, the OLAP cube procedure is faster, and few simple table are enough to tell you what is going on. Also additional statistical testing with the t-test is simple.

Note

More background, theoretical and mathematical information about the analyses of interaction matrices of frequencies are in the Chaps. 9–11. The OLAP cube is another approach with similar results, but it works more rapidly than the other methods.

Chapter 17
Restructure Data Wizard for Data Classified the Wrong Way (20 Patients)

General Purpose

Underneath the opening page of the Restructure Data Wizard in SPSS is given. In the current chapter this tool will be applied for restructuring multiple variables in a single case to multiple cases with a single variables.

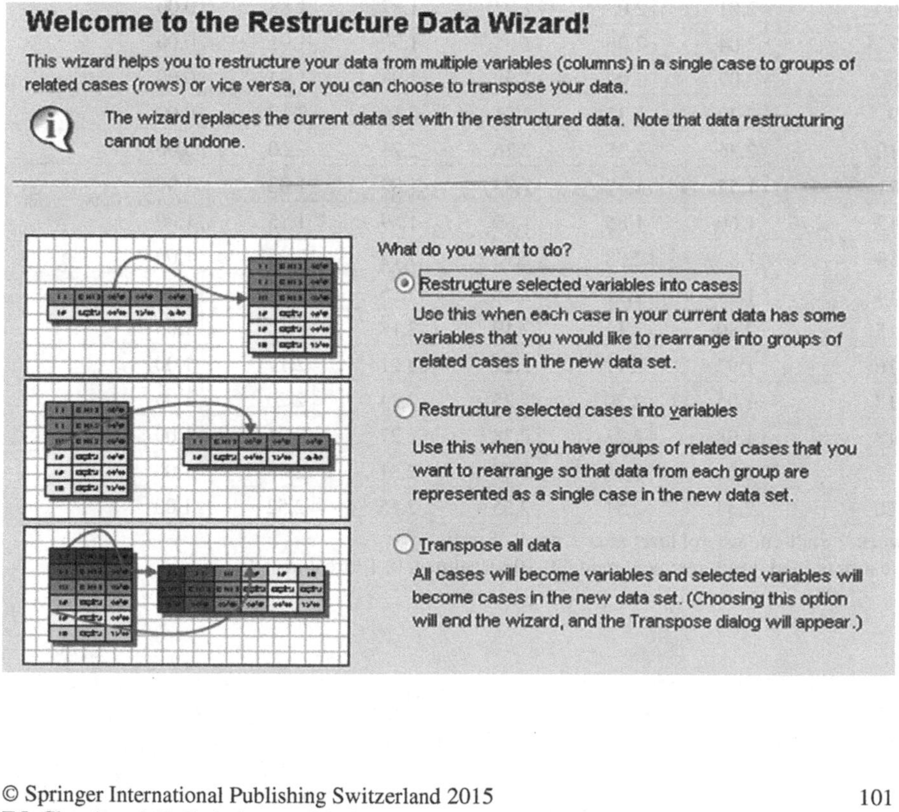

Welcome to the Restructure Data Wizard!
This wizard helps you to restructure your data from multiple variables (columns) in a single case to groups of related cases (rows) or vice versa, or you can choose to transpose your data.
The wizard replaces the current data set with the restructured data. Note that data restructuring cannot be undone.
What do you want to do?
Restructure selected variables into cases
Use this when each case in your current data has some variables that you would like to rearrange into groups of related cases in the new data set.
Restructure selected cases into variables
Use this when you have groups of related cases that you want to rearrange so that data from each group are represented as a single case in the new data set.
Transpose all data
All cases will become variables and selected variables will become cases in the new data set. (Choosing this option will end the wizard, and the Transpose dialog will appear.)

T.J. Cleophas, A.H. Zwinderman, *Machine Learning in Medicine - a Complete Overview*, DOI 10.1007/978-3-319-15195-3_17

Suppose in a study the treatment outcome has been measured several times instead of once. In current clinical research repeated measures in a single subject are common. The problem with repeated measures is, that they are more close to one another than unrepeated measures. If this is not taken into account, then data analysis will lose power. The underneath table gives an example of a 2 group parallel-group study comparing two treatments for cholesterol reduction of 5 weeks. The example is taken from Chap. 6, Mixed linear models, pp 65–77, in: Machine learning in medicine part one, Springer Heidelberg Germany, 2013, from the same authors.

It shows that 5 different variables present the 5 subsequent outcome measurements in each patient. In order to analyze these data in appropriately the table has to be restructured with each week given a separate row. This is a pretty laborious exercise, and it will get really annoying if you have 100 or more patients instead of 20. The restructure data wizard, however, should do the job within seconds.

patient no	week 1	week 2	week 3	week 4	week 5	treatment modality
1	1,66	1,62	1,57	1,52	1,50	0,00
2	1,69	1,71	1,60	1,55	1,56	0,00
3	1,92	1,94	1,83	1,78	1,79	0,00
4	1,95	1,97	1,86	1,81	1,82	0,00
5	1,98	2,00	1,89	1,84	1,85	0,00
6	2,01	2,03	1,92	1,87	1,88	0,00
7	2,04	2,06	1,95	1,90	1,91	0,00
8	2,07	2,09	1,98	1,93	1,94	0,00
9	2,30	2,32	2,21	2,16	2,17	0,00
10	2,36	2,35	2,26	2,23	2,20	0,00
11	1,57	1,82	1,83	1,83	1,82	1,00
12	1,60	1,85	1,89	1,89	1,85	1,00
13	1,83	2,08	2,12	2,12	2,08	1,00
14	1,86	2,11	2,16	2,15	2,11	1,00
15	2,80	2,14	2,19	2,18	2,14	1,00
16	1,92	2,17	2,22	2,21	2,17	1,00
17	1,95	2,20	2,25	2,24	2,20	1,00
18	1,98	2,23	2,28	2,27	2,24	1,00
19	2,21	2,46	2,57	2,51	2,48	1,00
20	2,34	2,51	2,55	2,55	2,52	1,00

week 1 = hdl-cholesterol level after 1 week of trial
treatment modality = treatment modality (0 = treatment 0, 1 = treatment 1)

Primary Scientific Question

Can the restructure data wizard provide a table suitable for testing treatment efficacies adjusted for the repeated nature of the outcome data.

Example

The above data file is entitled "restructure.sav", and is in extras.springer.com. Start by opening the data file in SPSS statistical software.

Command:

click Data....click Restructure....mark Restructure selected variables into cases.... click Next....mark One (for example, w1, w2, and w3)....click Next....Name: id (the patient id variable is already provided)....Target Variable: enter "firstweek, secondweek...... fifthweek"....Fixed Variable(s): enter treatment....click Next.... How many index variables do you want to create?....mark One....click Next....click Next again....click Next again....click Finish....Sets from the original data will still be in use…click OK.

Return to the main screen and observe that there are now 100 rows instead of 20 in the data file. The first 10 rows are given underneath.

id	treatment	Index1	Trans1
1	0,00	1	1,66
1	0,00	2	1,62
1	0,00	3	1,57
1	0,00	4	1,52
1	0,00	5	1,50
2	0,00	1	1,69
2	0,00	2	1,71
2	0,00	3	1,60
2	0,00	4	1,55
2	0,00	5	1,56

id = patient id
treatment = treatment modality
Index1 = week of treatment (1–5)
Trans1 = outcome values

We will now perform a mixed linear analysis of the data.

Command:

Analyze....mixed models....linear....specify subjects and repeated....subject: enter id ....continue....linear mixed model....dependent: Trans1....factors: Index1, treatment....fixed....build nested term....treatment ....add....Index1....add.... Index1 build term by* treatment....Index1 *treatment....add....continue....OK (* = sign of multiplication).

The underneath table shows the main results from the above analysis. After adjustment for the repeated nature of the outcome data the treatment modality 0 performs much better than the treatment modality 1. The results from alternative analyses for these data were not only less appropriate but also less sensitive. The discussion of this is beyond the scope of the current chapter, but it can found in the Chap. 6, Mixed linear models, pp 65–77, in: Machine learning in medicine part one, Springer Heidelberg Germany, 2013, from the same authors.

Type III tests of fixed effects[a]

Source	Numerator df	Denominator df	F	Sig.
Intercept	1	76,570	6988,626	,000
Week	4	31,149	,384	,818
Treatment	1	76,570	20,030	,000
Week*treatment	4	31,149	1,337	,278

[a]Dependent variable: outcome

Conclusion

The restructure data wizard provides a table suitable for testing treatment efficacies adjusted for the repeated nature of the outcome data. It is particularly pleasant if your data file is big, and has many (repeated) observations.

Note

More background, theoretical and mathematical information of restructuring data files is in the Chap. 6, Mixed linear models, pp 65–77, in: Machine learning in medicine part one, Springer Heidelberg Germany, 2013, from the same authors.

Chapter 18
Control Charts for Quality Control of Medicines (164 Tablet Desintegration Times)

General Purpose

A consistent quality of a process or product, like the manufacturing of tablets is, traditionally, tested by 1 sample chi-square tests of their weights, diameters, desintegration times. E.g., tablets may only be approved, if the standard deviation of their diameters is less than 0.7 mm. E.g., a 50 tablet sample with a standard deviation of 0.9 mm is significantly different from 0.7 (^ = symbol of power term).

$$\text{Chi}-\text{square} = (50-1)0.9\wedge 2/0.7\wedge 2 = 81$$
$$50-1\,\text{degrees of freedom}$$
$$p < 0.01(\text{one sided})$$

The example is from the Chap. 44, entitled "Clinical data where variability is more important than averages", pp 487–497, (in: Statistics applied to clinical studies 5th edition, Springer Heidelberg Germany, 2012, from the same authors). Nowadays, we live in an era of machine learning, and ongoing quality control, instead of testing now and then, has become more easy, and, in addition, provides information of process variations over time and process performance. Control charts available in SPSS and other data mining software is helpful to that aim.

Primary Scientific Question

Control charts are currently routinely applied for the process control of larger factories, but they are, virtually, unused in the medical field. We will assess, whether they can be helpful to process control of pharmaceuticals.

T.J. Cleophas, A.H. Zwinderman, *Machine Learning in Medicine - a Complete Overview*, DOI 10.1007/978-3-319-15195-3_18

Example

A important quality criterion of tablets is the desintegration time in water of 37 °C within 30 min or so. If it is considerably longer, the tablet will be too hard for consumption, if shorter it will be too soft for storage. 164 Tablets were tested over a period of 40 days.

day	desintegration (min)
1	33,2
1	31,0
1	32,7
1	30,8
1	32,2
1	31,3
2	30,1
2	31,5
2	33,6
2	32,2
4	32,9
4	32,2

The desintegration times of the first 11 tablets are above. The entire data file is in "qolcontrol.sav", and is in extras.springer.com. We will start the analysis by opening the data file in SPSS statistical software.

Command:

Analyze....Quality Control....Control Charts....mark Cases are units....click Define.... Process Measurement: enter "desintegration"....Subgroups Defined by: enter "days"....click Control Rules....mark: Above +3 sigma,

Below − 3 sigma,

2 out of last 3 above + 2 sigma,

2 out of last 3 below − 2 sigma,

4 out of 5 last above + 1 sigma,

4 out of last 5 below − 1 sigma

....click Continue....click Statistics....Specification Limits: Upper: type 36,0.... Lower: type 30,0....Target: type 33,0....mark Actual % outside specification limits.... Process Capability Indices....in Capacity Indices mark

CP

CpL

CpU

k

CpM....

....in Performance Indices mark

PP
PpL
PpU
PpM....

....click continue....click OK.

In the output sheets are two pivot figures and two pivot tables. Many details of the analyses can be called up after double-clicking them, then clicking the term pivot in the menu bar, and closing the upcoming pivoting tray. Drop boxes appear everywhere, and are convenient to visualize statistical details and textual explanations about what is going on (see the Chap. 15 for additional information on the use of pivoting figures and tables).

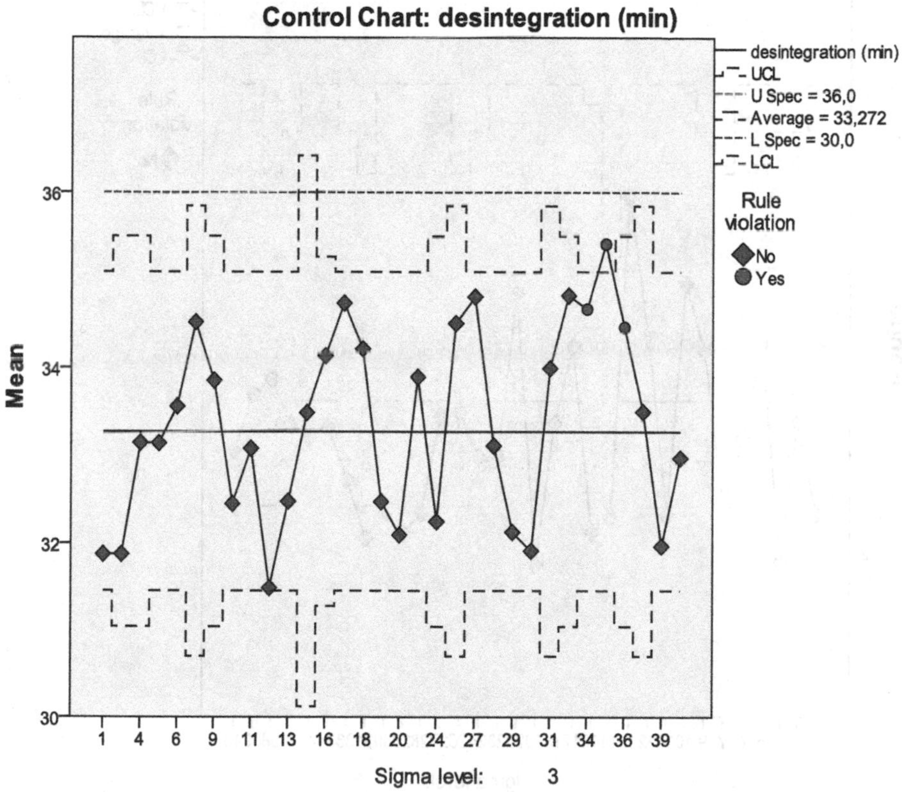

The above pivot figure shows a pattern of the mean desintegration times of the daily subsamples. The pattern is mostly within the 3 standard deviation limits. The straight interrupted lines give upper and lower specification limits (= overall mean

± 3 standard deviations, the lower one coincides with the x-axis, and is therefore not visible). The UCL (upper control limit) and LCL (lower control limit) curves describe sample ranges used to monitor spread in the daily subsamples. There are just three violations of the above set control rules of ±3 sigmas (= standard deviations) etc. The underneath table gives the details of the violations.

Rule violations for X-bar	
Day	Violations for points
34	2 points out of the last 3 above +2 sigma
35	Greater than +3 sigma
35	2 points out of the last 3 above +2 sigma
36	4 points out of the last 5 above +1 sigma

3 points violate control rules

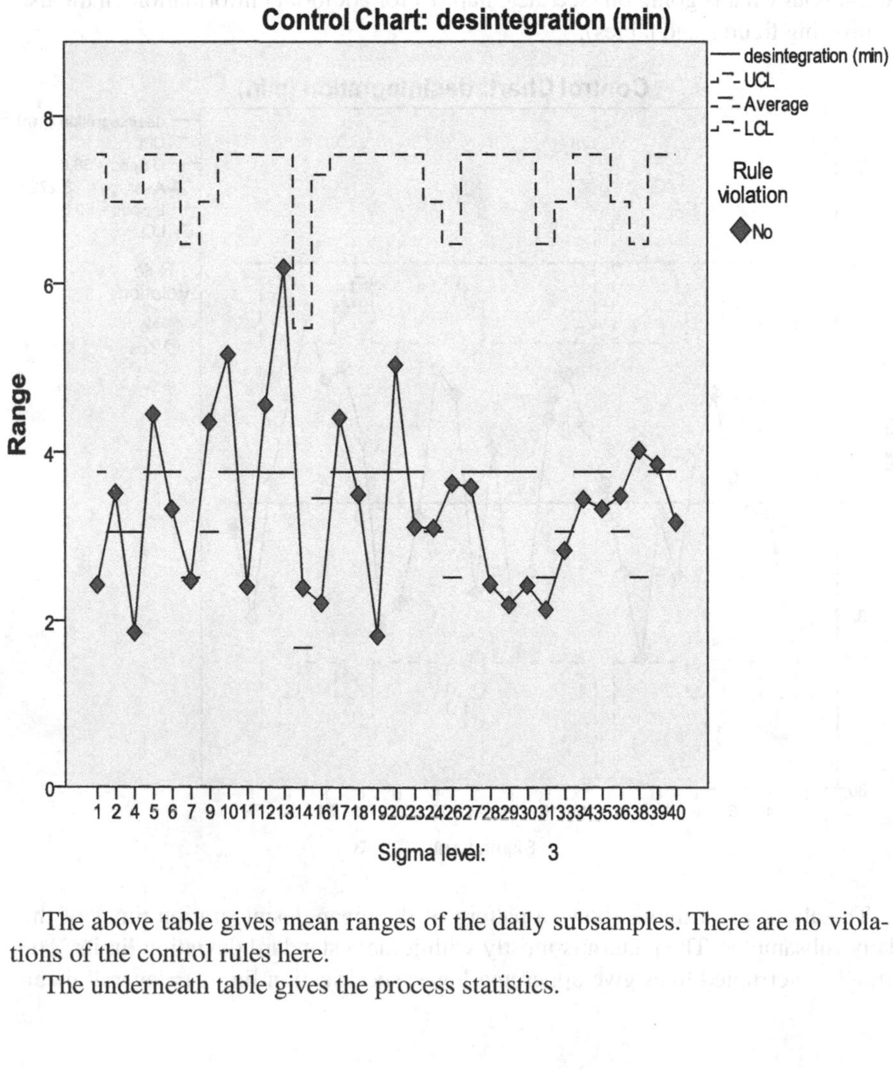

The above table gives mean ranges of the daily subsamples. There are no violations of the control rules here.

The underneath table gives the process statistics.

Process statistics		
Act. % outside SL		8,5 %
Capability indices	CP[a]	,674
	CpL[a]	,735
	CpU[a]	,613
	K	,091
	CpM[a,b]	,663
Performance indices	PP	,602
	PpL	,657
	PpU	,548
	PpM[b]	,594

The normal distribution is assumed. LSL = 30,0 and USL = 36,0
[a]The estimated capability sigma is based on the mean of the sample group ranges
[b]The target value is 33,0

Regarding the process capability indices:

CP ratio of differences between the specification limits and the observed process variation, it should be >1, <1 indicates too much variation.

CpL and CpU answer whether the process variations are symmetric, they should be close to CP.

K measure of capability of the data, which should have their centers close to the specified target, a small K value is good (particularly if CP is >1).

CpM same meaning as K, it should be close to CP.

Regarding the process performance indices:

The values are similar to those of the process capability indices, but a bit smaller, because they overall instead of sample variability is taken into account. If a lot smaller, they indicate selection bias in the data.

PP similar meaning as CP.

PpL and PpU similar meaning as CpL and CpU.

The above table shows that the process stability is pretty bad with CP and PP values a lot < 1. K is small, which is good, because it indicates that the center of the data is close to the specified target.

Conclusion

The above analysis shows that control charts methodology may be helpful to process control of pharmaceuticals. The example data were largely in control, and the process mean was close to the specified target value of 33,0 min. Nonetheless, statistics of process stability were pretty weak, and precision of the data was pretty bad.

Note

More background, theoretical and mathematical information of the SPSS module Quality Control is in the Chap. 62. More information of process quality control is also in the Chap. 44, entitled "Clinical data where variability is more important than averages", pp 487–497, in: Statistics applied to clinical studies 5th edition, Springer Heidelberg Germany 2012, from the same authors.

Part II
(Log) Linear Models

Chapter 19
Linear, Logistic, and Cox Regression for Outcome Prediction with Unpaired Data (20, 55, and 60 Patients)

General Purpose

To assess whether linear, logistic and Cox modeling can be used to train clinical data samples to make predictions about groups and individual patients.

Specific Scientific Question

How many hours will patients sleep, how large is the risk for patients to fall out of bed, how large is the hazard for patients to die.

This chapter was previously published in "Machine learning in medicine-cookbook 1" as Chap. 4, 2013.

T.J. Cleophas, A.H. Zwinderman, *Machine Learning in Medicine - a Complete Overview*, DOI 10.1007/978-3-319-15195-3_19

Linear Regression, the Computer Teaches Itself to Make Predictions

Var 1	Var 2	Var 3	Var 4	Var 5
0,00	6,00	65,00	0,00	1,00
0,00	7,10	75,00	0,00	1,00
0,00	8,10	86,00	0,00	0,00
0,00	7,50	74,00	0,00	0,00
0,00	6,40	64,00	0,00	1,00
0,00	7,90	75,00	1,00	1,00
0,00	6,80	65,00	1,00	1,00
0,00	6,60	64,00	1,00	0,00
0,00	7,30	75,00	1,00	0,00
0,00	5,60	56,00	0,00	0,00
1,00	5,10	55,00	1,00	0,00
1,00	8,00	85,00	0,00	1,00
1,00	3,80	36,00	1,00	0,00
1,00	4,40	47,00	0,00	1,00
1,00	5,20	58,00	1,00	0,00
1,00	5,40	56,00	0,00	1,00
1,00	4,30	46,00	1,00	1,00
1,00	6,00	64,00	1,00	0,00
1,00	3,70	33,00	1,00	0,00
1,00	6,20	65,00	0,00	1,00

Var 1 = treatment 0 is placebo, treatment 1 is sleeping pill
Var 2 = hours of sleep
Var 3 = age
Var 4 = gender
Var 5 = comorbidity

SPSS 19.0 is used for analysis, with the help of an XML (eXtended Markup Language) file. The data file is entitled "linoutcomeprediction" and is in extras.springer.com. Start by opening the data file.

Command:

Click Transform....click Random Number Generators....click Set Starting Point ....click Fixed Value (2000000)....click OK....click Analyze....Regression.... Linear....Dependent: enter hoursofsleep....Independent: enter treatment and age.... click Save....Predicted Values: click Unstandardized....in XML Files click Export final model....click Browse....File name: enter "exportlin"....click Save....click Continue....click OK.

Coefficients[a]

Model		Unstandardized coefficients		Standardized coefficients		
		B	Std. Error	Beta	t	Sig.
1	(Constant)	,989	,366		2,702	,015
	Treatment	–,411	,143	–,154	–2,878	,010
	Age	,085	,005	,890	16,684	,000

[a]Dependent variable: hoursofsleep

The output sheets show in the coefficients table that both treatment and age are significant predictors at $p<0.10$. Returning to the data file we will observe that SPSS has computed predicted values and gives them in a novel variable entitled PRE_1. The saved XML file will now be used to compute the predicted hours of sleep in 4 novel patients with the following characteristics. For convenience the XML file is given in extras.springer.com.

Var 1	Var 2	Var 3	Var 4	Var 5
,00	6,00	66,00	,00	1,00
,00	7,10	74,00	,00	1,00
,00	8,10	86,00	,00	,00
,00	7,50	74,00	,00	,00

Var 1 = treatment 0 is placebo, treatment 1 is sleeping pill
Var 2 = hours of sleep
Var 3 = age
Var 4 = gender
Var 5 = comorbidity

Enter the above data in a new SPSS data file.

Command:

Utilities….click Scoring Wizard….click Browse….click Select….Folder: enter the exportlin.xml file….click Select….in Scoring Wizard click Next….click Use value substitution….click Next….click Finish.

The above data file now gives individually predicted hours of sleep as computed by the linear model with the help of the XML file.

Var 1	Var 2	Var 3	Var 4	Var 5	Var 6
,00	6,00	66,00	,00	1,00	6,51
,00	7,10	74,00	,00	1,00	7,28
,00	8,10	86,00	,00	,00	8,30
,00	7,50	74,00	,00	,00	7,28

Var 1 = treatment 0 is placebo, treatment 1 is sleeping pill
Var 2 = hours of sleep
Var 3 = age
Var 4 = gender
Var 5 = comorbidity
Var 6 = predicted hours of sleep

Conclusion

The module linear regression can be readily trained to predict hours of sleep both in groups and, with the help of an XML file, in individual future patients.

Note

More background, theoretical and mathematical information of linear regression is available in Statistics applied to clinical studies, 5th edition, Chaps. 14 and 15, entitled "Linear regression basic approach" and "Linear regression for assessing precision, confounding, interaction", pp 161–176 and 177–185, Springer Heidelberg Germany 2012, from the same authors.

Logistic Regression, the Computer Teaches Itself to Make Predictions

Var 1	Var 2	Var 3	Var 4	Var 5
,00	1,00	50,00	,00	1,00
,00	1,00	76,00	,00	1,00
,00	1,00	57,00	1,00	1,00
,00	1,00	65,00	,00	1,00
,00	1,00	46,00	1,00	1,00
,00	1,00	36,00	1,00	1,00
,00	1,00	98,00	,00	,00
,00	1,00	56,00	1,00	,00
,00	1,00	44,00	,00	,00
,00	1,00	76,00	1,00	1,00
,00	1,00	75,00	1,00	1,00
,00	1,00	74,00	1,00	1,00
,00	1,00	87,00	,00	,00

Var 1 department type
Var 2 falling out of bed (1 = yes)
Var 3 age
Var 4 gender
Var 5 letter of complaint (1 = yes)

Only the first 13 patients are given, the entire data file is entitled "logoutcomeprediction" and is in extras.springer.com.

SPSS 19.0 is used for analysis, with the help of an XML (eXtended Markup Language) file. Start by opening the data file.

Command:

Click Transform....click Random Number Generators....click Set Starting Point ....click Fixed Value (2000000)....click OK....click Analyze....Regression .... Binary Logistic....Dependent: enter fallingoutofbed ....Covariates: enter departmenttype and letterofcomplaint....click Save....in Predicted Values click Probabilities....in Export model information to XML file click Browse.... File name: enter "exportlog"....click Save....click Continue....click OK.

Variables in the equation

		B	S.E.	Wald	df	Sig.	Exp(B)
Step 1[a]	Departmenttype	1,349	,681	3,930	1	,047	3,854
	Letterofcomplaint	2,039	,687	8,816	1	,003	7,681
	Constant	−1,007	,448	5,047	1	,025	,365

[a]Variable(s) entered on step 1: departmenttype, letterofcomplaint

In the above output table it is shown that both department type and letter of complaint are significant predictors of the risk of falling out of bed. Returning to the data file we will observe that SPSS has computed predicted values and gives them in a novel variable entitled PRE_1. The saved XML file will now be used to compute the predicted hours of sleep in 5 novel patients with the following characteristics. For convenience the XML file is given in extras.springer.com.

Var 1	Var 2	Var 3	Var 4	Var 5
,00	,00	67,00	,00	,00
1,00	1,00	54,00	1,00	,00
1,00	1,00	65,00	1,00	,00
1,00	1,00	74,00	1,00	1,00
1,00	1,00	73,00	,00	1,00

Var 1 department type
Var 2 falling out of bed (1 = yes)
Var 3 age
Var 4 gender
Var 5 letter of complaint (1 = yes)

Enter the above data in a new SPSS data file.

Command:

Utilities....click Scoring Wizard....click Browse....click Select....Folder: enter the exportlog.xml file....click Select....in Scoring Wizard click Next....mark Probability of Predicted Category....click Next....click Finish.

The above data file now gives individually predicted probabilities of falling out of bed as computed by the logistic model with the help of the XML file.

Var 1	Var 2	Var 3	Var 4	Var 5	Var 6
,00	,00	67,00	,00	,00	,73
1,00	1,00	54,00	1,00	,00	,58
1,00	1,00	65,00	1,00	,00	,58
1,00	1,00	74,00	1,00	1,00	,92
1,00	1,00	73,00	,00	1,00	,92

Var 1 department type
Var 2 falling out of bed (1 = yes)
Var 3 age
Var 4 gender
Var 5 letter of complaint (1 = yes)
Var 6 Predicted Probability

Conclusion

The module binary logistic regression can be readily trained to predict probability of falling out of bed both in groups and, with the help of an XML file, in individual future patients.

Note

More background, theoretical and mathematical information of binary logistic regression is available in Statistics applied to clinical studies 5th edition, Chaps. 17, 19, and 65, entitled "Logistic and Cox regression, Markov models, Laplace transformations", "Post-hoc analyses in clinical trials", and "Odds ratios and multiple regression", pp 199–218, 227–231, and 695–711, Springer Heidelberg Germany 2012, from the same authors.

Cox Regression, the Computer Teaches Itself to Make Predictions

Var 1	Var 2	Var 3	Var 4
1,00	1,00	,00	65,00
1,00	1,00	,00	66,00
2,00	1,00	,00	73,00
2,00	1,00	,00	91,00

Var 1	Var 2	Var 3	Var 4
2,00	1,00	,00	86,00
2,00	1,00	,00	87,00
2,00	1,00	,00	54,00
2,00	1,00	,00	66,00
2,00	1,00	,00	64,00
3,00	,00	,00	62,00
4,00	1,00	,00	57,00
5,00	1,00	,00	85,00
6,00	1,00	,00	85,00

Var 1 follow up in months
Var 2 event (1 = yes)
Var 3 treatment modality
Var 4 age

Only the first 13 patients are given, the entire data file is entitled "Coxoutcomeprediction" and is in extras.springer.com.

SPSS 19.0 is used for analysis, with the help of an XML (eXtended Markup Language) file. Start by opening the data file.

Command:

Click Transform….click Random Number Generators….click Set Starting Point ….click Fixed Value (2000000)….click OK….click Analyze….Survival….Cox Regression….Time: followupmonth….Status: event….Define event: enter 1…. Covariates: enter treatment and age….click Save….mark: Survival function…. In Export Model information to XML file click Browse…. File name: enter "export-Cox"….click Save….click Continue….click OK.

Variables in the equation

	B	SE	Wald	df	Sig.	Exp(B)
Treatment	–,791	,332	5,686	1	,017	,454
Age	,028	,012	5,449	1	,020	1,028

In the above output table it is shown that both treatment modality and age are significant predictors of survival. Returning to the data file we will now observe that SPSS has computed individual probabilities of survival and gave them in a novel variable entitled SUR_1. The probabilities vary from 0.00 to 1.00. E.g., for the first patient, based on follow up of 1 month, treatment modality 0, and age 65, the computer has computed a mean survival chance at the time of observation of 0.95741 (= over 95 %). Other patients had much less probability of survival. If you would have limited sources for further treatment in this population, it would make sense not to burden with continued treatment those with, e.g., less than 20 % survival probability. We should emphasize that the probability is based on the information of the variables 1, 3, 4, and is assumed to be measured just prior to the event, and the event is not taken into account here.

Var 1	Var 2	Var 3	Var 4	SUR_1
1,00	1,00	,00	65,00	,95741

The saved XML file will now be used to compute the predicted probabilities of survival in 5 novel patients with the following characteristics. For convenience the XML file is given in extras.springer.com. We will skip the variable 2 for the above reason.

Var 1	Var 2	Var 3	Var 4
30,00		1,00	88,00
29,00		1,00	67,00
29,00		1,00	56,00
29,00		1,00	54,00
28,00		1,00	57,00

Var 1 follow up in months
Var 2 event (1 = yes)
Var 3 treatment modality
Var 4 age

Enter the above data in a new SPSS data file.

Command:

Utilities....click Scoring Wizard....click Browse....click Select....Folder: enter the exportCox.xml file....click Select....in Scoring Wizard click Next....mark Predicted Value....click Next....click Finish.

The above data file now gives individually predicted probabilities of survival as computed by the Cox regression model with the help of the XML file.

Var 1	Var 2	Var 3	Var 4	Var 5 PredictedValue
30,00		1,00	88,00	,18
29,00		1,00	67,00	,39
29,00		1,00	56,00	,50
29,00		1,00	54,00	,51
28,00		1,00	57,00	,54

Var 1 follow up in months
Var 2 event (1 = yes)
Var 3 treatment modality
Var 4 age
Var 5 predicted probability of survival (0.0–1.0)

Conclusion

The module Cox regression can be readily trained to predict probability of survival both in groups and, with the help of an XML file, in individual future patients. Like outcome prediction with linear and logistic regression models, Cox regression is an important method to determine with limited health care sources, who of the patients will be recommended expensive medications and other treatments.

Note

More background, theoretical and mathematical information of binary logistic regression is available in Statistics applied to clinical studies 5th edition, Chaps. 17 and 31, entitled "Logistic and Cox regression, Markov models, Laplace transformations", and "Time-dependent factor analysis", pp 199–218, and pp 353–364, Springer Heidelberg Germany 2012, from thc same authors.

Chapter 20
Generalized Linear Models for Outcome Prediction with Paired Data (100 Patients and 139 Physicians)

General Purpose

With linear and logistic regression *unpaired* data can be used for outcome prediction. With generalized linear models *paired* data can be used for the purpose.

Specific Scientific Question

Can crossover studies (1) of sleeping pills and (2) of lifestyle treatments be used as training samples to predict hours of sleep and lifestyle treatment in groups and individuals.

Generalized Linear Modeling, the Computer Teaches Itself to Make Predictions

Var 1	Var 2	Var 3	Var 4
6,10	79,00	1,00	1,00
5,20	79,00	1,00	2,00
7,00	55,00	2,00	1,00
7,90	55,00	2,00	2,00
8,20	78,00	3,00	1,00

(continued)

This chapter was previously published in "Machine learning in medicine-cookbook 1" as Chap. 5, 2013.

T.J. Cleophas, A.H. Zwinderman, *Machine Learning in Medicine - a Complete Overview*, DOI 10.1007/978-3-319-15195-3_20

Var 1	Var 2	Var 3	Var 4
3,90	78,00	3,00	2,00
7,60	53,00	4,00	1,00
4,70	53,00	4,00	2,00
6,50	85,00	5,00	1,00
5,30	85,00	5,00	2,00
8,40	85,00	6,00	1,00
5,40	85,00	6,00	2,00

Var 1 = outcome (hours of sleep after sleeping pill or placebo)
Var 2 = age
Var 3 = patientnumber (patientid)
Var 4 = treatment modality (1 sleeping pill, 2 placebo)

Only the data from first 6 patients are given, the entire data file is entitled "generalizedlm-pairedcontinuous" and is in extras.springer.com. SPSS 19.0 is used for analysis, with the help of an XML (eXtended Markup Language) file. Start by opening the data file.

Command:

Click Transform....click Random Number Generators....click Set Starting Point ....click Fixed Value (2000000)....click OK....click Analyze....Generalized Linear Models....again click Generalized Linear models....click Type of Model....click Linear....click Response....Dependent Variable: enter Outcome....Scale Weight Variable: enter patientid....click Predictors....Factors: enter treatment.... Covariates: enter age....click Model: Model: enter treatment and age....click Save: mark Predicted value of linear predictor....click Export....click Browse....File name: enter "exportpairedcontinuous"....click Save....click Continue....click OK.

Parameter estimates

			95 % Wald confidence interval		Hypothesis test		
Parameter	B	Std. Error	Lower	Upper	Wald Chi- Square	df	Sig.
(Intercept)	6,178	,5171	5,165	7,191	142,763	1	,000
[treatment = 1,00]	2,003	,2089	1,593	2,412	91,895	1	,000
[treatment = 2,00]	0[a]						
age	−,014	,0075	−,029	,001	3,418	1	,064
(Scale)	27,825[b]	3,9351	21,089	36,713			

Dependent variable: outcome
Model: (Intercept), treatment, age
[a]Set to zero because this parameter is redundant
[b]Maximum likelihood estimate

The output sheets show that both treatment and age are significant predictors at $p < 0.10$. Returning to the data file we will observe that SPSS has computed predicted values of hours of sleep, and has given them in a novel variable entitled XBPredicted

(predicted values of linear predictor). The saved XML file (entitled "exportpairedcontinuous") will now be used to compute the predicted hours of sleep in five novel patients with the following characteristics. For convenience the XML file is given in extras.springer.com.

Var 2	Var 3	Var 4
79,00	1,00	1,00
55,00	2,00	1,00
78,00	3,00	1,00
53,00	4,00	2,00
85,00	5,00	1,00

Var 2 = age
Var 3 = patientnumber (patientid)
Var 4 = treatment modality (1 sleeping pill, 2 placebo)

Enter the above data in a new SPSS data file.

Command:

Utilities….click Scoring Wizard….click Browse….click Select….Folder: enter the exportpairedcontinuous.xml file….click Select….in Scoring Wizard click Next…. click Use value substitution….click Next….click Finish.

The above data file now gives individually predicted hours of sleep as computed by the linear model with the help of the XML file.

Var 2	Var 3	Var 4	Var 5
79,00	1,00	1,00	7,09
55,00	2,00	1,00	7,42
78,00	3,00	1,00	7,10
53,00	4,00	2,00	5,44
85,00	5,00	1,00	7,00

Var 2 = age
Var 3 = patientnumber (patientid)
Var 4 = treatment modality (1 sleeping pill, 2 placebo)
Var 5 = predicted values of hours of sleep in individual patient

Conclusion

The module generalized linear models can be readily trained to predict hours of sleep in groups, and, with the help of an XML file, in individual future patients.

Generalized Estimation Equations, the Computer Teaches Itself to Make Predictions

Var 1	Var 2	Var 3	Var 4
,00	89,00	1,00	1,00
,00	89,00	1,00	2,00
,00	78,00	2,00	1,00
,00	78,00	2,00	2,00
,00	79,00	3,00	1,00
,00	79,00	3,00	2,00
,00	76,00	4,00	1,00
,00	76,00	4,00	2,00
,00	87,00	5,00	1,00
,00	87,00	5,00	2,00
,00	84,00	6,00	1,00
,00	84,00	6,00	2,00
,00	84,00	7,00	1,00
,00	84,00	7,00	2,00
,00	69,00	8,00	1,00
,00	69,00	8,00	2,00
,00	77,00	9,00	1,00
,00	77,00	9,00	2,00
,00	79,00	10,00	1,00
,00	79,00	10,00	2,00

Var 1 outcome (lifestyle advise given 0 = no, 1 = yes)
Var 2 physicians' age
Var 3 physicians' id
Var 4 prior postgraduate education regarding lifestyle advise (1 = no, 2 = yes)

Only the first 10 physicians are given, the entire data file is entitled "generalized-pairedbinary" and is in extras.springer.com. All physicians are assessed twice, once before lifestyle education and once after. The effect of lifestyle education on the willingness to provide lifestyle advise was the main objective of the study.

SPSS 19.0 is used for analysis, with the help of an XML (eXtended Markup Language) file. Start by opening the data file.

Command:

Click Transform….click Random Number Generators….click Set Starting Point ….click Fixed Value (2000000)….click OK….click Analyze….Generalized Linear Models….Generalized Estimating Equations….click Repeated….in Subjects variables enter physicianid....in Within-subject variables enter lifestyle advise....in Structure enter Unstructured....click Type of Model....mark Binary logistic....click Response....in Dependent Variable enter outcome....click Reference Category.... mark First....click Continue....click Predictors....in Factors enter lifestyleadvise.... in Covariates enter age....click Model....in Model enter lifestyle and age....click Save....mark Predicted value of mean of response....click Export ....mark Export model in XML....click Browse.... In File name: enter "exportpairedbinary"....in Look in: enter the appropriate map in your computer for storage....click Save.... click Continue....click OK.

Parameter estimates

Parameter	B	Std. Error	95 % Wald confidence interval		Hypothesis test		
			Lower	Upper	Wald Chi- Square	df	Sig.
(Intercept)	2,469	,7936	,913	4,024	9,677	1	,002
[lifestyleadvise=1,00]	–,522	,2026	–,919	–,124	6,624	1	,010
[lifestyleadvise=2,00]	0[a]						
age	–,042	,0130	–.068	–,017	10,563	1	,001
(Scale)	1						

Dependent variable: outcome
Model: (Intercept), lifestyleadvise, age
[a]Set to zero because this parameter is redundant

The output sheets show that both prior lifestyle education and physicians' age are very significant predictors at $p<0.01$. Returning to the data file we will observe that SPSS has computed predicted probabilities of lifestyle advise given or not by each physician in the data file, and a novel variable is added to the data file for the purpose. It is given the name MeanPredicted. The saved XML file entitled "exportpairedbinary" will now be used to compute the predicted probability of receiving lifestyle advise based on physicians' age and the physicians' prior lifestyle education in twelve novel physicians. For convenience the XML file is given in extras.springer.com.

Var 2	Var 3	Var 4
64,00	1,00	2,00
64,00	2,00	1,00
65,00	3,00	1,00
65,00	3,00	2,00
52,00	4,00	1,00
66,00	5,00	1,00
79,00	6,00	1,00
79,00	6,00	2,00

53,00	7,00	1,00
53,00	7,00	2,00
55,00	8,00	1,00
46,00	9,00	1,00

Var 2 age
Var 3 physicianid
Var 4 lifestyleadvise (prior postgraduate education regarding lifestyle advise (1 = no, 2 = yes))

Enter the above data in a new SPSS data file.

Command:

Utilities….click Scoring Wizard….click Browse….click Select….Folder: enter the exportpairedbinary.xml file….click Select….in Scoring Wizard click Next….mark Probability of Predicted Category….click Next….click Finish.

The above data file now gives individually predicted probabilities of receiving lifestyle advise as computed by the logistic model with the help of the XML file.

Var 2	Var 3	Var 4	Var 5
64,00	1,00	2,00	,56
64,00	2,00	1,00	,68
65,00	3,00	1,00	,69
65,00	3,00	2,00	,57
52,00	4,00	1,00	,56
66,00	5,00	1,00	,70
79,00	6,00	1,00	,80
79,00	6,00	2,00	,70
53,00	7,00	1,00	,57
53,00	7,00	2,00	,56
55,00	8,00	1,00	,59
46,00	9,00	1,00	,50

Var 2 age
Var 3 physicianid
Var 4 lifestyleadvise
Var 5 probability of predicted category (between 0.0 and 1.0)

Conclusion

The module generalized estimating equations can be readily trained to predict with paired data the probability of physicians giving lifestyle advise as groups and, with the help of an XML file, as individual physicians.

Note

More background, theoretical and mathematical information of paired analysis of binary data is given in SPSS for starters part one, Chap. 13, entitled "Paired binary (McNemar test)", pp 47–49, Springer Heidelberg Germany, 2010, from the same authors.

Chapter 21
Generalized Linear Models Event-Rates (50 Patients)

General Purpose

To assess whether in a longitudinal study event rates, defined as numbers of events per person per period, can be analyzed with the generalized linear model module.

Specific Scientific Question

Can generalized linear modeling be trained to predict rates of episodes of paroxysmal atrial fibrillation both in groups and in individual future patients.

Example

Fifty patients were followed for numbers of episodes of paroxysmal atrial fibrillation (PAF), while on treated with two parallel treatment modalities. The data file is below.

This chapter was previously published in "Machine learning in medicine-cookbook 1" as Chap. 6, 2013.

T.J. Cleophas, A.H. Zwinderman, *Machine Learning in Medicine - a Complete Overview*, DOI 10.1007/978-3-319-15195-3_21

Var 1	Var 2	Var 3	Var 4	Var 5
1	56,99	42,45	73	4
1	37,09	46,82	73	4
0	32,28	43,57	76	2
0	29,06	43,57	74	3
0	6,75	27,25	73	3
0	61,65	48,41	62	13
0	56,99	40,74	66	11
1	10,39	15,36	72	7
1	50,53	52,12	63	10
1	49,47	42,45	68	9
0	39,56	36,45	72	4
1	33,74	13,13	74	5

Var 1 = treatment modality
Var 2 = psychological score
Var 3 = social score
Var 4 = days of observation
Var 5 = number of episodes of paroxysmal atrial fibrillation (PAF)

The first 12 patients are shown only, the entire data file is entitled "generalizedlmeventrates" and is in extras.springer.com.

The Computer Teaches Itself to Make Predictions

SPSS 19.0 is used for training and outcome prediction. It uses XML (eXtended Markup Language) files to store data. We will perform the analysis with a linear regression analysis of variable 5 as outcome variable and the other 4 variables as predictors. Start by opening the data file.

Command:

Analyze….Regression….Linear….Dependent Variable: episodes of paroxysmal atrial fibrillation….Independent: treatment modality, psychological score, social score, days of observation….OK.

Coefficients[a]

Model		Unstandardized coefficients		Standardized coefficients		
		B	Std. Error	Beta	t	Sig.
1	(Constant)	49,059	5,447		9,006	,000
	Treat	−2,914	1,385	−,204	−2,105	,041
	Psych	,014	,052	,036	,273	,786

(continued)

Coefficients[a]						
		Unstandardized coefficients		Standardized coefficients		
Model		B	Std. Error	Beta	t	Sig.
	Soc	–,073	,058	–,169	–1,266	,212
	Days	–,557	,074	–,715	–7,535	,000

[a]Dependent variable: paf

The above table shows that treatment modality is weakly significant, and psychological and social scores are not. Furthermore, days of observation is very significant. However, it is not entirely appropriate to include this variable if your outcome is the numbers of events per person per time unit. Therefore, we will perform a linear regression, and adjust the outcome variable for the differences in days of observation using weighted least square regression.

Coefficients[a,b]						
		Unstandardized coefficients		Standardized coefficients		
Model		B	Std. Error	Beta	t	Sig.
1	(Constant)	10,033	2,862		3,506	,001
	Treat	–3,502	1,867	–.269	–1,876	,067
	Psych	,033	,069	,093	,472	,639
	Soc	–,093	,078	–,237	–1,194	,238

[a]Dependent variable: paf
[b]Weighted least squares regression -Weighted by days

Command:

Analyze....Regression....Linear....Dependent: episodes of paroxysmal atrial fibrillation....Independent: treatment modality, psychological score, social score .... WLS Weight: days of observation.... OK.

The above table shows the results. A largely similar pattern is observed, but treatment modality is no more statistically significant. We will use the generalized linear modeling module to perform a Poisson regression which is more appropriate for rate data. The model applied will also be stored and reapplied for making predictions about event rates in individual future patients.

Command:

Click Transform....click Random Number Generators....click Set Starting Point.... click Fixed Value (2000000)....click OK....click Generalized Linear Models .... click again Generalized Linear Models....mark: Custom....Distribution: Poisson..... Link function: Log....Response: Dependent variable: numbers of episodes of PAF....Scale Weight Variable: days of observation....Predictors: Main Effect: treatment modality....Covariates: psychological score, social score.... Model: main effects: treatment modality, psychological score, social score.... Estimation: mark Model-based Estimation ....click Save....mark Predicted value of mean of response....click Export....mark Export model in XML....click Browse.... in File name enter "exportrate"....in Look in: enter the appropriate map in your computer for storage....click Save....click OK.

Parameter estimates

Parameter	B	Std. Error	95 % Wald confidence interval Lower	Upper	Hypothesis test Wald Chi- Square	df	Sig.
(Intercept)	1,868	,0206	1,828	1,909	8256,274	1	,000
[treat=0]	,667	,0153	,637	,697	1897,429	1	,000
[treat=1]	0[a]						
psych	,006	,0006	,005	,008	120,966	1	,000
soc	–,019	,0006	–.020	–,017	830,264	1	,000
(Scale)	1[b]						

Dependent variable: paf
Model: (Intercept), treat, psych, soc
[a]Set to zero because this parameter is redundant
[b]Fixed at the displayed value

The outcome sheets give the results. All of a sudden, all of the predictors including treatment modality, psychological and social score are very significant predictors of the PAF rate. When minimizing the output sheets the data file returns and now shows a novel variable entitled "PredictedValues" with the mean rates of PAF episodes per patient (per day). The saved XML file will now be used to compute the predicted PAF rate in 5 novel patients with the following characteristics. For convenience the XML file is given in extras.springer.com.

Var 1	Var 2	Var 3	Var 4	Var 5
1,00	56,99	42,45	73,00	4,00
1,00	30,09	46,82	34,00	4,00
,00	32,28	32,00	76,00	2,00
,00	29,06	40,00	36,00	3,00
,00	6,75	27,25	73,00	3,00

Var 1 = treatment modality
Var 2 = psychological score
Var 3 = social score
Var 4 = days of observation
Var 5 = number of episodes of paroxysmal atrial fibrillation (PAF)

Enter the above data in a new SPSS data file.

Command:

Utilities….click Scoring Wizard….click Browse….click Select….Folder: enter the exportrate.xml file….click Select….in Scoring Wizard click Next….click Use value substitution….click Next….click Finish.

The above data file now gives individually predicted rates of PAF as computed by the linear model with the help of the XML file. Enter the above data in a new SPSS data file.

Var 1	Var 2	Var 3	Var 4	Var 5	Var 6
1,00	56,99	42,45	73,00	4,00	4,23
1,00	30,09	46,82	34,00	4,00	3,27
,00	32,28	32,00	76,00	2,00	8,54
,00	29,06	40,00	36,00	3,00	7,20
,00	6,75	27,25	73,00	3,00	7,92

Var 1 = treatment modality
Var 2 = psychological score
Var 3 = social score
Var 4 = days of observation
Var 5 = number of episodes of paroxysmal atrial fibrillation (PAF)
Var 6 = individually predicted mean rates of PAF (per day)

Conclusion

The module generalized linear models can be readily trained to predict event rate of PAF episodes both in groups, and, with the help of an XML file, in individual patients.

Note

More background, theoretical and mathematical information of generalized linear modeling is available in SPSS for Starters part two, Chap. 10, entitled "Poisson regression", pp 43–48, Springer Heidelberg Germany 2012, from the same authors.

Chapter 22
Factor Analysis and Partial Least Squares (PLS) for Complex-Data Reduction (250 Patients)

General Purpose

A few unmeasured factors, otherwise called latent factors, are identified to explain a much larger number of measured factors, e.g., highly expressed chromosome-clustered genes. Unlike factor analysis, partial least squares (PLS) identifies not only exposure (x-value), but also outcome (y-value) variables.

Specific Scientific Question

Twelve highly expressed genes are used to predict drug efficacy. Is factor analysis/ PLS better than traditional analysis for regression data with multiple exposure and outcome variables.

This chapter was previously published in "Machine learning in medicine-cookbook 1" as Chap. 7, 2013.

T.J. Cleophas, A.H. Zwinderman, *Machine Learning in Medicine - a Complete Overview*, DOI 10.1007/978-3-319-15195-3_22

G1	G2	G3	G4	G16	G17	G18	G19	G24	G25	G26	G27	O1	O2	O3	O4
8	8	9	5	7	10	5	6	9	9	6	6	6	7	6	7
9	9	10	9	8	8	7	8	8	9	8	8	8	7	8	7
9	8	8	8	8	9	7	8	9	8	9	9	9	8	8	8
8	9	8	9	6	7	6	4	6	6	5	5	7	7	7	6
10	10	8	10	9	10	10	8	8	9	9	9	8	8	8	7
7	8	8	8	8	7	6	5	7	8	8	7	7	6	6	7
5	5	5	5	5	6	4	5	5	6	6	5	6	5	6	4
9	9	9	9	8	8	8	8	9	8	3	8	8	8	8	8
9	8	9	8	9	8	7	7	7	7	5	8	8	7	6	6
10	10	10	10	10	10	10	10	10	8	8	10	10	10	9	10
2	2	8	5	7	8	8	8	9	3	9	8	7	7	7	6
7	8	8	7	8	6	6	7	8	8	8	7	8	7	8	8
8	9	9	8	10	8	8	7	8	8	9	9	7	7	8	8

Var G1-27 highly expressed genes estimated from their arrays' normalized ratios
Var O1-4 drug efficacy scores (the variables 20–23 from the initial data file)

The data from the first 13 patients are shown only (see extras.springer.com for the entire data file entitled "optscalingfactorplscanonical").

Factor Analysis

First the reliability of the model was assessed by assessing the test-retest reliability of the original predictor variables using the correlation coefficients after deletion of one variable: all of the data files should produce at least by 80 % the same result as that of the non-deleted data file (alphas > 80 %). SPSS 19.0 is used. Start by opening the data file.

Command:

Analyze....Scale....Reliability Analysis....transfer original variables to Variables box....click Statistics....mark Scale if item deleted....mark Correlations .... Continue....OK.

Item-total statistics

	Scale mean if item deleted	Scale variance if item deleted	Corrected item-total correlation	Squared multiple correlation	Cronbach's alpha if item deleted
Geneone	80,8680	276,195	,540	,485	,902
Genetwo	80,8680	263,882	,700	,695	,895
Genethree	80,7600	264,569	,720	,679	,895
Genefour	80,7960	282,002	,495	,404	,904

(continued)

Item-total statistics					
	Scale mean if item deleted	Scale variance if item deleted	Corrected item-total correlation	Squared multiple correlation	Cronbach's alpha if item deleted
Genesixteen	81,6200	258,004	,679	,611	,896
Geneseventeen	80,9800	266,196	,680	,585	,896
Geneeighteen	81,5560	263,260	,606	,487	,899
Genenineteen	82,2040	255,079	,696	,546	,895
Genetwentyfour	81,5280	243,126	,735	,632	,893
Genetwentyfive	81,2680	269,305	,538	,359	,902
Genetwentysix	81,8720	242,859	,719	,629	,894
Genetwentyseven	81,0720	264,501	,540	,419	,903

None of the original variables after deletion reduce the test-retest reliability. The data are reliable. We will now perform the principal components analysis with three components, otherwise called latent variables.

Command:

Analyze....Dimension Reduction....Factor....enter variables into Variables box.... click Extraction....Method: click Principle Components....mark Correlation Matrix, Unrotated factor solution....Fixed number of factors: enter 3....Maximal Iterations plot Convergence: enter 25....Continue....click Rotation....Method: click Varimax.... mark Rotated solution....mark Loading Plots....Maximal Iterations: enter 25.... Continue....click Scores.... mark Display factor score coefficient matrix ....OK.

Rotated component matrix[a]			
	Component		
	1	2	3
Geneone	,211	,810	,143
Genetwo	,548	,683	,072
Genethree	,624	,614	,064
Genefour	,033	,757	,367
Genesixteen	,857	,161	,090
Geneseventeen	,650	,216	,338
Geneeighteen	,526	,297	,318
Genenineteen	,750	,266	,170
Genetwentyfour	,657	,100	,539
Genetwentyfive	,219	,231	,696
Genetwentysix	,687	,077	,489
Genetwentyseven	,188	,159	,825

Extraction method: Principal component analysis
Rotation method: Varimax with Kaiser normalization
[a]Rotation converged in eight iterations

The best fit coefficients of the original variables constituting three new factors (unmeasured, otherwise called latent, factors) are given. The latent factor 1 has a very strong correlation with the genes 16–19, the latent factor 2 with the genes 1–4, and the latent factor 3 with the genes 24–27.

When returning to the data file, we now observe, that, for each patient, the software program has produced the individual values of these novel predictors.

In order to fit these novel predictors with the outcome variables, the drug efficacy scores (variables O1-4), multivariate analysis of variance (MANOVA) should be appropriate. However, the large number of columns in the design matrix caused integer overflow, and the command was not executed. Instead we will perform a univariate multiple linear regression with the add-up scores of the outcome variables (using the Transform and Compute Variable command) as novel outcome variable.

Command:

Transform….Compute Variable….transfer outcomeone to Numeric Expression box….click+….outcometwo idem….click+….outcomethree idem….click+…. outcomefour idem….Target Variable: enter "summaryoutcome"….click OK.

In the data file the summaryoutcome values are displayed as a novel variable.

Command:

Analyze….Regression….Dependent: enter summaryoutcome….Independent: enter Fac 1, Fac 2, and Fac 3….click OK.

Coefficients[a]

Model		Unstandardized coefficients B	Unstandardized coefficients Std. error	Standardized coefficients Beta	t	Sig.
1	(Constant)	27,332	,231		118,379	,000
	REGR factor score 1 for analysis 1	5,289	,231	,775	22,863	,000
	REGR factor score 2 for analysis 1	1,749	,231	,256	7,562	,000
	REGR factor score 3 for analysis 1	1,529	,231	,224	6,611	,000

[a]Dependent variable: summaryoutcome

All of the three latent predictors were, obviously, very significant predictors of the summary outcome variable.

Partial Least Squares Analysis (PLS)

Because PLS is not available in the basic and regression modules of SPSS, the software program R Partial Least Squares, a free statistics and forecasting software available on the internet as a free online software calculator was used (www.wessa.

net/rwasp). The data file is imported directly from the SPSS file entitled "optscalingfactorplscanonical" (cut/past commands).

Command:

List the selected clusters of variables: latent variable 2 (here G16-19), latent variable 1 (here G24-27), latent variable 4 (here G1-4), and latent outcome variable 3 (here O 1-4).

A square boolean matrix is constructed with "0 or 1" values if fitted correlation coefficients to be included in the model were "no or yes" according to the underneath table.

	Latent variable	1	2	3	4
Latent variable	1	0	0	0	0
	2	0	0	0	0
	3	1	1	0	0
	4	0	0	1	0

Click "compute". After 15 s of computing the program produces the results. First, the data were validated using the GoF (goodness of fit) criteria. GoF= √ [mean of r-square values of comparisons in model * r-square overall model], where * is the sign of multiplication. A GoF value varies from 0 to 1 and values larger than 0.8 indicate that the data are adequately reliable for modeling.

GoF value	
Overall	0.9459
Outer model (including manifest variables)	0.9986
Inner model (including latent variables)	0.9466.

The data are, thus, adequately reliable. The calculated best fit r-values (correlation coefficients) are estimated from the model, and their standard errors would be available from second derivatives. However, the problem with the second derivatives is that they require very large data files in order to be accurate. Instead, distribution free standard errors are calculated using bootstrap resampling.

Latent variables	Original r-value	Bootstrap r-value	Standard error	t-value
1 versus 3	0.57654	0.57729	0.08466	6.8189
2 versus 3	0.67322	0.67490	0.04152	16.2548
4 versus 3	0.18322	0.18896	0.05373	3.5168

All of the three correlation coefficients (r-values) are very significant predictors of the latent outcome variable.

Traditional Linear Regression

When using the summary scores of the main components of the three latent variables instead of the above modeled latent variables (using the above Transform and Compute Variable commands), the effects remained statistically significant, however, at lower levels of significance.

Command:

Analyze….Regression….Linear….Dependent: enter summaryoutcome…. Independent: enter the three summary factors 1-3….click OK.

Coefficients[a]

Model		Unstandardized coefficients		Standardized coefficients		
		B	Std. Error	Beta	t	Sig.
1	(Constant)	1,177	1,407		,837	,404
	Summaryfac1	,136	,059	,113	2,316	,021
	Summaryfac2	,620	,054	,618	11,413	,000
	Summaryfac3	,150	,044	,170	3,389	,001

[a]Dependent variable: summaryoutcome

The partial least squares method produces smaller t-values than did factor analysis (t=3.5–16.3 versus 6.6–22.9), but it is less biased, because it is a multivariate analysis adjusting relationships between the outcome variables. Both methods provided better t-values than did the above traditional regression analysis of summary variables (t=2.3–11.4).

Conclusion

Factor analysis and PLS can handle many more variables than the standard methods, and account the relative importance of the separate variables, their interactions and differences in units. Partial least squares method is parsimonious to principal components analysis, because it can separately include outcome variables in the model.

Note

More background, theoretical and mathematical information of the three methods is given in Machine learning in medicine part one, Chaps. 14 and 16, Factor analysis pp 167–181, and Partial least squares, pp 197–212, Springer Heidelberg Germany 2013, from the same authors.

Chapter 23
Optimal Scaling of High-Sensitivity Analysis of Health Predictors (250 Patients)

General Purpose

In linear models of health predictors (x-values) and health outcomes (y-values), better power of testing can sometimes be obtained, if continuous predictor variables are converted into the best fit discretized ones.

Specific Scientific Question

Highly expressed genes were used to predict drug efficacy. The example from chap. 22 was used once more. The gene expression levels were scored on a scale of 0–10, but some scores were rarely observed. Can the strength of prediction be improved by optimal scaling.

This chapter was previously published in "Machine learning in medicine-cookbook 1" as Chap. 8, 2013.

T.J. Cleophas, A.H. Zwinderman, *Machine Learning in Medicine - a Complete Overview*, DOI 10.1007/978-3-319-15195-3_23

G1	G2	G3	G4	G16	G17	G18	G19	G24	G25	G26	G27	O1	O2	O3	O4
8	8	9	5	7	10	5	6	9	9	6	6	6	7	6	7
9	9	10	9	8	8	7	8	8	9	8	8	8	7	8	7
9	8	8	8	8	9	7	8	9	8	9	9	9	8	8	8
8	9	8	9	6	7	6	4	6	6	5	5	7	7	7	6
10	10	8	10	9	10	10	8	8	9	9	9	8	8	8	7
7	8	8	8	8	7	6	5	7	8	8	7	7	6	6	7
5	5	5	5	5	6	4	5	5	6	6	5	6	5	6	4
9	9	9	9	8	8	8	8	9	8	3	8	8	8	8	8
9	8	9	8	9	8	7	7	7	7	5	8	8	7	6	6
10	10	10	10	10	10	10	10	10	8	8	10	10	10	9	10
2	2	8	5	7	8	8	8	9	3	9	8	7	7	7	6
7	8	8	7	8	6	6	7	8	8	8	7	8	7	8	8
8	9	9	8	10	8	8	7	8	8	9	9	7	7	8	8

Var G1-27 highly expressed genes estimated from their arrays' normalized ratios
Var O1-4 drug efficacy scores (sum of the scores is used as outcome)

Only the data from the first 13 patients are shown. The entire data file entitled "optscalingfactorplscanonical" can be downloaded from extra.springer.com.

Traditional Multiple Linear Regression

SPSS 19.0 is used for data analysis. Open the data file and command.

Command:

Analyze….Regression….Linear….Dependent: enter the 12 highly expressed genes….Independent: enter the summary scores of the 4 outcome variables (use Transform and Compute Variable command)….click OK.

Coefficients[a]

Model		Unstandardized coefficients		Standardized coefficients		
		B	Std. Error	Beta	t	Sig.
1	(Constant)	3,293	1,475		2,232	,027
	Geneone	–,122	,189	–,030	–.646	,519
	Genetwo	,287	,225	,078	1,276	,203
	Genethree	,370	,228	,097	1,625	,105
	Genefour	,063	,196	,014	,321	,748
	Genesixteen	,764	,172	,241	4,450	,000
	Geneseventeen	,835	,198	,221	4,220	,000

(continued)

Coefficients[a]						
		Unstandardized coefficients		Standardized coefficients		
Model		B	Std. Error	Beta	t	Sig.
	Geneeighteen	,088	,151	,027	,580	,563
	Genenineteen	,576	,154	,188	3,751	,000
	Genetwentyfour	,403	,146	,154	2,760	,006
	Genetwentyfive	,028	,141	,008	,198	,843
	Genetwentysix	,320	,142	,125	2,250	,025
	Genetwentyseven	–,275	,133	–,092	–2,067	,040

[a]Dependent variable: summaryoutcome

The number of statistically significant p-values (indicated here with Sig.), (<0.10) was 6 out of 12. In order to improve this result the Optimal Scaling program of SPSS is used. Continuous predictor variables are converted into best fit discretized ones.

Optimal Scaling Without Regularization

Command:

Analyze....Regression....Optimal Scaling....Dependent Variable: Var 28 (Define Scale: mark spline ordinal 2.2)....Independent Variables: Var 1, 2, 3, 4, 16, 17, 18, 19, 24, 25, 26, 27 (all of them Define Scale: mark spline ordinal 2.2)....Discretize: Method Grouping....OK.

Coefficients					
	Standardized coefficients				
	Beta	Bootstrap (1000) estimate of Std. Error	df	F	Sig.
Geneone	–,109	,110	2	,988	,374
Genetwo	,193	,107	3	3,250	,023
Genethree	–,092	,119	2	,591	,555
Genefour	,113	,074	3	2,318	,077
Genesixteen	,263	,087	4	9,065	,000
Geneseventeen	,301	,114	2	6,935	,001
Geneeighteen	,113	,136	1	,687	,408
Genenineteen	,145	,067	1	4,727	,031
Genetwentyfour	,220	,097	2	5,166	,007
Genetwentyfive	–,039	,094	1	,170	,681
Genetwentysix	,058	,107	2	,293	,746
Genetwentyseven	–.127	,104	2	1,490	,228

Dependent variable: summaryoutcome

There is no intercept anymore and the t-tests have been replaced with F-tests. The optimally scaled model without regularization shows similarly sized effects.

The number of p-values < 0.10 is 6 out of 12. In order to fully benefit from optimal scaling a regularization procedure for the purpose of correcting overdispersion (more spread in the data than compatible with Gaussian data) is desirable. Ridge regression minimizes the b-values such that $b_{ridge} = b\ /(1 + \text{shrinking factor})$. With shrinking factor = 0, $b_{ridge} = b$, with ∞, $b_{ridge} = 0$.

Optimal Scaling With Ridge Regression

Command:

Analyze….Regression….Optimal Scaling….Dependent Variable: Var 28 (Define Scale: mark spline ordinal 2.2)….Independent Variables: Var 1, 2, 3, 4, 16, 17, 18, 19, 24, 25, 26, 27 (all of them Define Scale: mark spline ordinal 2.2)….Discretize: Method Grouping, Number categories 7….click Regularization….mark Ridge…. OK.

Coefficients

	Standardized coefficients				
	Beta	Bootstrap (1000) estimate of Std. Error	df	F	Sig.
Geneone	,032	,033	2	,946	,390
Genetwo	,068	,021	3	10,842	,000
Genethree	,051	,030	1	2,963	,087
Genefour	,064	,020	3	10,098	,000
Genesixteen	,139	,024	4	34,114	,000
Geneseventeen	,142	,025	2	31,468	,000
Geneeighteen	,108	,040	2	7,236	,001
Genenineteen	,109	,020	2	30,181	,000
Genetwentyfour	,109	,021	2	27,855	,000
Genetwentyfive	,041	,038	3	1,178	,319
Genetwentysix	,098	,023	2	17,515	,000
Genetwentyseven	–,017	,047	1	,132	,716

Dependent variable: 20–23

The sensitivity of this model is better than the above two methods with 7 p-values < 0.0001, and 9 p-values < 0.10, while the traditional and unregularized Optimal Scaling only produced 6 and 6 p-values < 0.10. Also the lasso regularization model is possible (Var = variable). It shrinks the small b values to 0.

Optimal Scaling With Lasso Regression

Command:

Analyze....Regression....Optimal Scaling....Dependent Variable: Var 28 (Define Scale: mark spline ordinal 2.2)....Independent Variables: Var 1, 2, 3, 4, 16, 17, 18, 19, 24, 25, 26, 27 (all of them Define Scale: mark spline ordinal 2.2).... Discretize: Method Grouping, Number categories 7....click Regularization.... mark Lasso.... OK.

Coefficients

	Standardized coefficients				
	Beta	Bootstrap (1000) estimate of Std. Error	df	F	Sid.
Geneone	,000	,020	0	,000	
Genetwo	,054	,046	3	1,390	,247
Genethree	,000	,026	0	,000	
Genefour	,011	,036	3	,099	,960
Genesixteen	,182	,084	4	4,684	,001
Geneseventeen	,219	,095	3	5,334	,001
Geneeighteen	,086	,079	2	1,159	,316
Genenineteen	,105	,063	2	2,803	,063
Genetwentyfour	,124	,078	2	2,532	,082
Genetwentyfive	,000	,023	0	,000	
Genetwentysix	,048	,060	2	,647	,525
Genetwentyseven	,000	,022	0	,000	

Dependent variable: 20–23

The b-values of the genes 1, 3, 25 and 27 are now shrunk to zero, and eliminated from the analysis. Lasso is particularly suitable if you are looking for a limited number of predictors and improves prediction accuracy by leaving out weak predictors. Finally, the elastic net method is applied. Like lasso it shrinks the small b-values to 0, but it performs better with many predictor variables.

Optimal Scaling With Elastic Net Regression

Command:

Analyze....Regression....Optimal Scaling....Dependent Variable: Var 28 (Define Scale: mark spline ordinal 2.2)....Independent Variables: Var 1, 2, 3, 4, 16, 17, 18, 19, 24, 25, 26, 27 (all of them Define Scale: mark spline ordinal 2.2)....Discretize: Method Grouping, Number categories 7....click Regularization....mark Elastic Net....OK.

Coefficients

	Standardized coefficients				
	Beta	Bootstrap (1000) estimate of Std. Error	df	F	Sig.
Geneone	,000	,016	0	,000	
Genetwo	,029	,039	3	,553	,647
Genethree	,000	,032	3	,000	1,000
Genefour	,000	,015	0	,000	
Genesixteen	,167	,048	4	12,265	,000
Geneseventeen	,174	,051	3	11,429	,000
Geneeighteen	,105	,055	2	3,598	,029
Genenineteen	,089	,048	3	3,420	,018
Genetwentyfour	,113	,053	2	4,630	,011
Genetwentyfive	,000	,012	0	,000	
Genetwentysix	,062	,046	2	1,786	,170
Genetwentyseven	,000	,018	0	,000	

Dependent variable: 20–23

The results are pretty much the same, as it is with lasso. Elastic net does not provide additional benefit in this example but works better than lasso if the number of predictors is larger than the number of observations.

Conclusion

Optimal scaling of linear regression data provides little benefit due to overdispersion. Regularized optimal scaling using ridge regression provides excellent results. Lasso optimal scaling is suitable if you are looking for a limited number of strong predictors. Elastic net optimal scaling works better than lasso if the number of predictors is large.

Note

More background, theoretical and mathematical information of optimal scaling with or without regularization is available in Machine learning in medicine part one, Chaps. 3 and 4, entitled “Optimal scaling: discretization”, and “Optimal scaling: regularization including ridge, lasso, and elastic net regression”, pp 25–37, and pp 39–53, Springer Heidelberg Germany, 2013, from the same authors.

Chapter 24
Discriminant Analysis for Making a Diagnosis from Multiple Outcomes (45 Patients)

General Purpose

To assess whether discriminant analysis can be used to make a diagnosis from multiple outcomes both in groups and in individual patients.

Specific Scientific Question

Laboratory screenings were performed in patients with different types of sepsis (urosepsis, bile duct sepsis, and airway sepsis). Can discriminant analysis of laboratory screenings improve reliability of diagnostic processes.

Var 1	Var 2	Var 3	Var 4	Var 5	Var 6	Var 7	Var 8	Var 9	Var 10	Var 11
8,00	5,00	28,00	4,00	2,50	79,00	108,00	19,00	18,00	16,00	2,00
11,00	10,00	29,00	7,00	2,10	94,00	89,00	18,00	15,00	15,00	2,00
7,00	8,00	30,00	7,00	2,20	79,00	96,00	20,00	16,00	14,00	2,00
4,00	6,00	16,00	6,00	2,60	80,00	120,00	17,00	17,00	19,00	2,00
1,00	6,00	15,00	6,00	2,20	84,00	108,00	21,00	18,00	20,00	2,00
23,00	5,00	14,00	6,00	2,10	78,00	120,00	18,00	17,00	21,00	3,00
12,00	10,00	17,00	5,00	3,20	85,00	100,00	17,00	20,00	18,00	3,00
31,00	8,00	27,00	5,00	,20	68,00	113,00	19,00	15,00	18,00	3,00
22,00	7,00	26,00	5,00	1,20	74,00	98,00	16,00	16,00	17,00	3,00
30,00	6,00	25,00	4,00	2,40	69,00	90,00	20,00	18,00	16,00	3,00

(continued)

This chapter was previously published in "Machine learning in medicine-cookbook 1" as Chap. 9, 2013.

T.J. Cleophas, A.H. Zwinderman, *Machine Learning in Medicine - a Complete Overview*, DOI 10.1007/978-3-319-15195-3_24

Var 1	Var 2	Var 3	Var 4	Var 5	Var 6	Var 7	Var 8	Var 9	Var 10	Var 11
2,00	12,00	21,00	4,00	2,80	75,00	112,00	11,00	14,00	19,00	1,00
10,00	21,00	20,00	4,00	2,90	70,00	100,00	12,00	15,00	20,00	1,00

Var 1 gammagt
Var 2 asat
Var 3 alat
Var 4 bilirubine
Var 5 ureum
Var 6 creatinine
Var 7 creatinine clearance
Var 8 erythrocyte sedimentation rate
Var 9 c-reactive protein
Var 10 leucocyte count
Var 11 type of sepsis (1–3 as described above)

The first 12 patients are shown only, the entire data file is entitled "optscalingfactorplscanonical" and is in extras.springer.com.

The Computer Teaches Itself to Make Predictions

SPSS 19.0 is used for training and outcome prediction. It uses XML (eXtended Markup Language) files to store data. Start by opening the data file.

Command:

Click Transform….click Random Number Generators….click Set Starting Point…. click Fixed Value (2000000)….click OK….click Analyze….Classify…. Discriminant Analysis….Grouping Variable: enter diagnosisgroup….Define Range: Minimum enter 1…Maximum enter 3….click Continue….Independents: enter all of the 10 laboratory variables….click Statistics….mark Unstandardized ….mark Separate-groups covariance….click Continue….click Classify….mark All groups equal….mark Summary table….mark Within-groups….mark Combined groups…. click Continue….click Save….mark Predicted group memberships….in Export model information to XML file enter: exportdiscriminant….click Browse and save the XML file in your computer….click Continue….click OK.

The scientific question "is the diagnosis group a significant predictor of the outcome estimated with 10 lab values" is hard to assess with traditional multivariate methods due to interaction between the outcome variables. It is, therefore, assessed with the question "is the clinical outcome a significant predictor of the odds of having had a particular prior diagnosis. This reasoning may seem incorrect, using an outcome for making predictions, but, mathematically, it is no problem. It is just a matter of linear cause-effect relationships, but just the other way around, and it works very conveniently with "messy" outcome variables like in the example given. However, first, the numbers of outcome variables have to be reduced. SPSS accomplishes this by orthogonal modeling of the outcome variables, which produces novel composite outcome variables. They are the y-values of linear equations. The x-values of these linear equations are the original outcome variables, and their regression coefficients are given in the underneath table.

Structure matrix		
	Function	
	1	2
As at	,574*	,184
Gammagt	,460*	,203
C-reactive protein	–.034	,761*
Leucos	,193	,537*
Ureum	,461	,533*
Creatinine	,462	,520*
Alat	,411	,487*
Bili	,356	,487*
Esr	,360	,487*
Creatinine clearance	–,083	–.374*

Pooled within-groups correlations between discriminating variables and standardized canonical discriminant functions
Variables ordered by absolute size of correlation within function.
*Largest absolute correlation between each variable and any discriminant function

Wilks' Lambda				
Test of function(s)	Wilks' Lambda	Chi-square	df	Sig.
1 through 2	,420	32,500	20	,038
2	,859	5,681	9	,771

The two novel outcome variables significantly predict the odds of having had a prior diagnosis with p=0.038 as shown above. When minimizing the output sheets we will return to the data file and observe that the novel outcome variables have been added (the variables entitled Dis1_1 and Dis1_2), as well as the predicted diagnosis group predicted from the discriminant model (the variable entitled Dis_1). For convenience the XML file entitled "exportdiscriminant" is stored in extras.springer. com.

The saved XML file can now be used to predict the odds of having been in a particular diagnosis group in five novel patients whose lab values are known but whose diagnoses are not yet obvious.

Var 1	Var 2	Var 3	Var 4	Var 5	Var 6	Var 7	Var 8	Var 9	Var 10
1049,00	466,00	301,00	268,00	59,80	213,00	−2,00	109,00	121,00	42,00
383,00	230,00	154,00	120,00	31,80	261,00	13,00	80,00	58,00	30,00
9,00	9,00	31,00	204,00	34,80	222,00	10,00	60,00	57,00	34,00
438,00	391,00	479,00	127,00	31,80	372,00	9,00	69,00	56,00	33,00
481,00	348,00	478,00	139,00	21,80	329,00	15,00	49,00	47,00	32,00

Var 1 gammagt
Var 2 asat
Var 3 alat
Var 4 bilirubine
Var 5 ureum
Var 6 creatinine
Var 7 creatinine clearance
Var 8 erythrocyte sedimentation rate
Var 9 c-reactive protein
Var 10 leucocyte count

Enter the above data in a new SPSS data file.

Command:

Utilities….click Scoring Wizard….click Browse….click Select….Folder: enter the exportdiscriminant.xml file….click Select….in Scoring Wizard click Next….click Use value substitution….click Next….click Finish.

The above data file now gives predicted odds of having been in a particular diagnosis group computed by the discriminant analysis module with the help of the xml file.

Var 1	Var 2	Var 3	Var 4	Var 5	Var 6	Var 7	Var 8	Var 9	Var 10	Var 11
1049,00	466,00	301,00	268,00	59,80	213,00	−2,00	109,00	121,00	42,00	2,00
383,00	230,00	154,00	120,00	31,80	261,00	13,00	80,00	58,00	30,00	2,00
9,00	9,00	31,00	204,00	34,80	222,00	10,00	60,00	57,00	34,00	1,00
438,00	391,00	479,00	127,00	31,80	372,00	9,00	69,00	56,00	33,00	1,00
481,00	348,00	478,00	139,00	21,80	329,00	15,00	49,00	47,00	32,00	2,00

Var 1 gammagt
Var 2 asat
Var 3 alat
Var 4 bilirubine
Var 5 ureum
Var 6 creatinine
Var 7 creatinine clearance
Var 8 erythrocyte sedimentation rate
Var 9 c-reactive protein
Var 10 leucocyte count
Var 11 predicted odds of having been in a particular diagnosis group

Conclusion

The discriminant analysis module can be readily trained to provide from the laboratory values of individual patients the best fit odds of having been in a particular diagnosis group. In this way discriminant analysis can support the hard work of physicians trying to make a diagnosis.

Note

More background, theoretical and mathematical information of discriminant analysis is available in Machine learning part one, Chap. 17, entitled "Discriminant analysis for supervised data", pp 215–224, Springer Heidelberg Germany, 2013, from the same authors.

Chapter 25
Weighted Least Squares for Adjusting Efficacy Data with Inconsistent Spread (78 Patients)

General Purpose

Linear regression assumes that the spread of the outcome-values is homoscedastic: it is the same for each predictor value. This assumption is, however, not warranted in many real life situations. This chapter is to assess the advantages of *weighted* least squares (WLS) instead of *ordinary* least squares (OLS) linear regression analysis.

Specific Scientific Question

The effect of prednisone on peak expiratory flow was assumed to be more variable with increasing dosages. Can it, therefore, be measured with more precision if linear regression is replaced with weighted least squares procedure.

Var 1	Var 2	Var 3	Var 4
1	29	1,40	174
2	15	2,00	113
3	38	0,00	281
4	26	1,00	127
5	47	1,00	267
6	28	0,20	172
7	20	2,00	118
8	47	0,40	383
9	39	0,40	97
10	43	1,60	304

(continued)

This chapter was previously published in "Machine learning in medicine-cookbook 1" as Chap. 10, 2013.

T.J. Cleophas, A.H. Zwinderman, *Machine Learning in Medicine - a Complete Overview*, DOI 10.1007/978-3-319-15195-3_25

Var 1	Var 2	Var 3	Var 4
11	16	0,40	85
12	35	1,80	182
13	47	2,00	140
14	35	2,00	64
15	38	0,20	153
16	40	0,40	216

Var 1 Patient no
Var 2 prednisone (mg/24 h)
Var 3 peak flow (ml/min)
Var 4 beta agonist (mg/24 h)

Only the first 16 patients are given, the entire data file is entitled "weightedleastsquares" and is in extras.springer.com. SPSS 19.0 is used for data analysis. We will first make a graph of prednisone dosages and peak expiratory flows. Start with opening the data file.

Weighted Least Squares

Command:

click Graphs....Legacy Dialogs....Scatter/Dot....click Simple Scatter....click Define....Y Axis enter peakflow....X Axis enter prednisone....click OK.

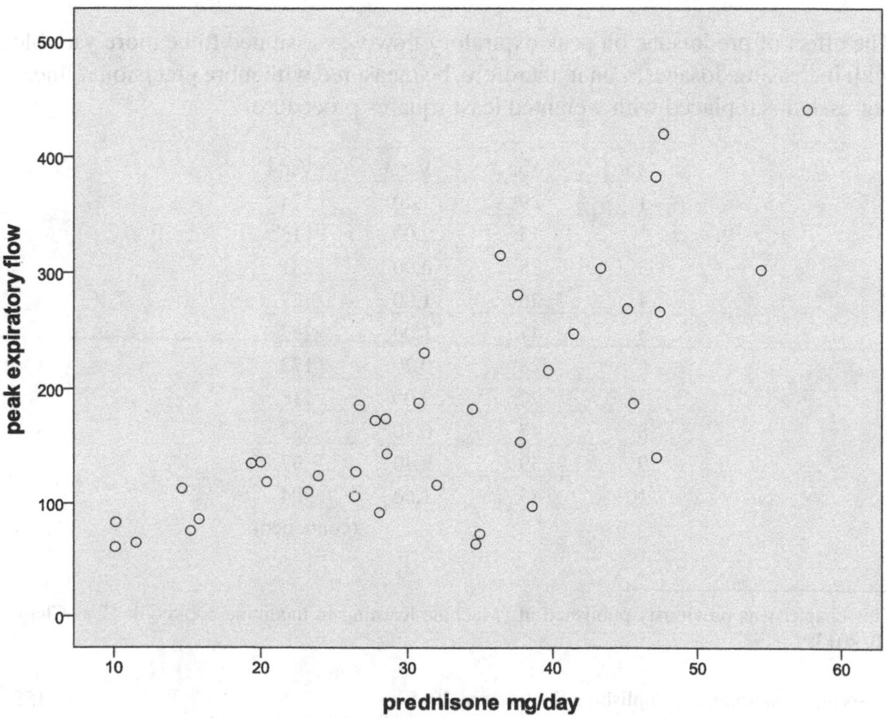

The output sheet shows that the spread of the y-values is small with low dosages and gradually increases. We will, therefore, perform both a traditional and a weighted least squares analysis of these data.

Command:

Analyze....Regression....Linear....Dependent: enter peakflow....
Independent: enter prednisone, betaagonist....OK.

Model Summary[a]				
Model	R	R square	Adjusted R square	Std. Error of the estimate
1	,763[b]	,582	,571	65,304

[a]Dependent variable: peak expiratory flow
[b]Predictors: (Constant), beta agonist mg/24 h, prednisone mg/day

Coefficients[a]						
		Unstandardized coefficients		Standardized coefficients		
Model		B	Std. Error	Beta	t	Sig.
1	(Constant)	–22,534	22,235		–1,013	,314
	Prednisone mg/day	6,174	,604	,763	10,217	,000
	Beta agonist mg/24 h	6,744	11,299	,045	,597	,552

[a]Dependent variable: peak expiratory flow

In the output sheets an R value of 0.763 is observed, and the linear effects of prednisone dosages are a statistically significant predictor of the peak expiratory flow, but, surprisingly, the beta agonists dosages are not.

We will, subsequently, perform a WLS analysis.

Command:

Analyze....Regression....Weight Estimation.... select: Dependent: enter peakflow .... Independent(s): enter prednisone, betaagonist....select prednisone also as Weight variable....Power range: enter 0 through 5 by 0.5....click Options....select Save best weights as new variable....click Continue....click OK.

In the output sheets it is observed that the software has calculated likelihoods for different powers, and the best likelihood value is chosen for further analysis. When returning to the data file again a novel variable is added, the WGT_1 variable (the weights for the WLS analysis). The next step is to perform again a linear regression, but now with the weight variable included.

Command:

Analyze....Regression....Linear.... select: Dependent: enter peakflow.... Independent(s) : enter prednisone, betaagonist....select the weights for the wls analysis (the GGT_1) variable as WLS Weight....click Save....select Unstandardized in Predicted Values....deselect Standardized in Residuals....click Continue....click OK.

Model Summary[a,b]				
Model	R	R Square	Adjusted R Square	Std. Error of the estimate
1	,846[c]	,716	,709	,125

[a]Dependent Variable: peak expiratory flow
[b]Weighted Least Squares Regression-Weighted by Weight for peakflow from WLS, MOD_6 PREDNISONE** -3,500
[c]Predictors: (Constant), beta agonist mg/24 h, prednisone mg/day

Coefficients[a,b]						
		Unstandardized coefficients		Standardized coefficients		
Model		B	Std. Error	Beta	t	Sig.
1	(Constant)	5,029	7,544		,667	,507
	Prednisone mg/day	5,064	,369	,880	13,740	,000
	Beta agonist mg/24 h	10,838	3,414	203	3,174	,002

[a]Dependent Variable: peak expiratoryflow
[b]Weighted Least Squares Regression – Weighted by Weight for peakflow from WLS, M0D_6 PREDNISONE"-3,500

The output table now shows an R value of 0.846. It has risen from 0.763, and provides thus more statistical power. The above lower table shows the effects of the two medicine dosages on the peak expiratory flows. The t-values of the medicine predictors have increased from approximately 10 and 0.5 to 14 and 3.2. The p-values correspondingly fell from 0.000 and 0.552 to respectively 0.000 and 0.002. Larger prednisone dosages and larger beta agonist dosages significantly and independently increased peak expiratory flows. After adjustment for heteroscedasticity, the beta agonist became a significant independent determinant of peak flow.

Conclusion

The current paper shows that, even with a sample of only 78 patients, WLS is able to demonstrate statistically significant linear effects that had been, previously, obscured by heteroscedasticity of the y-value.

Note

More background, theoretical and mathematical information of weighted least squares modeling is given in Machine learning in medicine part three, Chap. 10, Weighted least squares, pp 107–116, Springer Heidelberg Germany, 2013, from the same authors.

Chapter 26
Partial Correlations for Removing Interaction Effects from Efficacy Data (64 Patients)

General Purpose

The outcome of cardiovascular research is generally affected by many more factors than a single one, and multiple regression assumes that these factors act independently of one another, but why should they not affect one another. This chapter is to assess whether partial correlation can be used to remove interaction effects from linear data.

Specific Scientific Question

Both calorie intake and exercise are significant independent predictors of weight loss. However, exercise makes you hungry and patients on weight training are inclined to reduce (or increase) their calorie intake. Can partial correlations methods adjust the interaction between the two predictors.

Var 1	Var 2	Var 3	Var 4	Var 5
1,00	0,00	1000,00	0,00	45,00
29,00	0,00	1000,00	0,00	53,00
2,00	0,00	3000,00	0,00	64,00
1,00	0,00	3000,00	0,00	64,00
28,00	6,00	3000,00	18000,00	34,00
27,00	6,00	3000,00	18000,00	25,00
30,00	6,00	3000,00	18000,00	34,00

(continued)

This chapter was previously published in "Machine learning in medicine-cookbook 1" as Chap. 11, 2013.

T.J. Cleophas, A.H. Zwinderman, *Machine Learning in Medicine - a Complete Overview*, DOI 10.1007/978-3-319-15195-3_26

Var 1	Var 2	Var 3	Var 4	Var 5
27,00	6,00	1000,00	6000,00	45,00
29,00	0,00	2000,00	0,00	52,00
31,00	3,00	2000,00	6000,00	59,00
30,00	3,00	1000,00	3000,00	58,00
29,00	3,00	1000,00	3000,00	47,00
27,00	0,00	1000,00	0,00	45,00
28,00	0,00	1000,00	0,00	66,00
27,00	0,00	1000,00	0,00	67,00

Var 1 weight loss (kg)
Var 2 exercise (times per week)
Var 3 calorie intake (cal)
Var 4 interaction
Var 5 age (years)

Only the first fifteen patients are given, the entire file is entitled "partialcorrelations" and is in extras.springer.com.

Partial Correlations

We will first perform a linear regression of these data. SPSS 19.0 is used for the purpose. Start by opening the data file.

Command:

Analyze....Regression....Linear....Dependent variable: enter weightloss.... Independent variables: enter exercise and calorieintake....click OK.

Coefficients[a]

Model		Unstandardized coefficients		Standardized coefficients		
		B	Std. Error	Beta	t	Sig.
1	(Constant)	29,089	2,241		12,978	,000
	Exercise	2,548	,439	,617	5,802	,000
	Calorieintake	–,006	,001	–,544	–5,116	,000

[a]Dependent variable: weightloss

The output sheets show that both calorie intake and exercise are significant independent predictors of weight loss. However, interaction between exercise and calorie intake is not accounted. In order to check, an interaction variable (x_3=calorie intake * exercise, with * symbol of multiplication) is added to the model.

Command:

Transform data....Compute Variable....in Target Variable enter the term "interaction"....to Numeric Expression: transfer from Type & Label "exercise" ....click * ....transfer from Type & Label calorieintake....click OK.

The interaction variable is added by SPSS to the data file and is entitled "interaction". After the addition of the interaction variable to the regression model as third independent variable, the analysis is repeated.

Coefficients[a]

Model		Unstandardized coefficients		Standardized coefficients		
		B	Std. Error	Beta	t	Sig.
1	(Constant)	34,279	2,651		12,930	,000
	Interaction	,001	,000	,868	3,183	,002
	Exercise	–,238	,966	–,058	–,246	,807
	Calorieintake	–,009	,002	–,813	–6,240	,000

[a]Dependent variable: weightloss

The output sheet now shows that exercise is no longer significant and interaction on the outcome is significant at p=0.002. There is, obviously, interaction in the study, and the overall analysis of the data is, thus, no longer relevant. The best method to find the true effect of exercise would be to repeat the study with calorie intake held constant. Instead of this laborious exercise, a partial correlation analysis with calorie intake held artificially constant can be adequately performed, and would provide virtually the same result. Partial correlation analysis is performed using the SPSS module Correlations.

Command:

Analyze....Correlate....Partial....Variables: enter weight loss and calorie intake ....Controlling for: enter exercise....OK.

Correlations

Control variables			Weightloss	Calorieintake
Exercise	Weightloss	Correlation	1,000	–,548
		Significance (2-tailed)		,000
		df	0	61
	Calorieintake	Correlation	–,548	1,000
		Significance (2-tailed)	,000	
		df	61	0

Correlations

Control variables			Weightloss	Exercise
Calorieintake	Weightloss	Correlation	1,000	,596
		Significance (2-tailed)		,000
		df	0	61
	Exercise	Correlation	,596	1,000
		Significance (2-tailed)	,000	
		df	61	0

The upper table shows, that, with exercise held constant, calorie intake is a significant negative predictor of weight loss with a correlation coefficient of −0.548 and a p-value of 0.0001. Also partial correlation with exercise as independent and calorie intake as controlling factor can be performed.

Command:

Analyze….Correlate….Partial….Variables: enter weight loss and exercise…. Controlling for: enter calorie intake….OK.

The lower table shows that, with calorie intake held constant, exercise is a significant positive predictor of weight loss with a correlation coefficient of 0.596 and a p-value of 0.0001.

Why do we no longer have to account interaction with partial correlations. This is simply because, if you hold a predictor fixed, this fixed predictor can no longer change and interact in a multiple regression model.

Also higher order partial correlation analyses are possible. E.g., age may affect all of the three variables already in the model. The effect of exercise on weight loss with calorie intake and age fixed can be assessed.

Command:

Analyze….Correlate….Partial….Variables: enter weight loss and exercise…. Controlling for: enter calorie intake and age….OK.

Correlations

Control variables			Weightloss	Exercise
Age & calorieintake	Weightloss	Correlation	1,000	,541
		Significance (2-tailed)		,000
		df	0	60
	Exercise	Correlation	,541	1,000
		Significance (2-tailed)	,000	
		df	60	0

In the above output sheet it can be observed that the correlation coefficient is still very significant.

Conclusion

Without the partial correlation approach the conclusion from this study would have been: no definitive conclusion about the effects of exercise and calorie intake is possible, because of a significant interaction between exercise and calorie intake. The partial correlation analysis allows to conclude that both exercise and calorie intake have a very significant linear relationship with weight loss effect.

Note

More background, theoretical and mathematical information of partial correlations methods is given in Machine learning in medicine part one, Chap. 5, Partial correlations, pp 55–64, Springer Heidelberg Germany, 2013, from the same authors.

Chapter 27
Canonical Regression for Overall Statistics of Multivariate Data (250 Patients)

General Purpose

To assess in datasets with multiple predictor and outcome variables, whether canonical analysis, unlike traditional multivariate analysis of variance (MANOVA), can provide overall statistics of combined effects.

Specific Scientific Question

The example of the Chaps. 22 and 23 is used once again. Twelve highly expressed genes are used to predict four measures of drug efficacy. We are more interested in the combined effect of the predictor variables on the outcome variables than we are in the separate effects of the different variables.

G1	G2	G3	G4	G16	G17	G18	G19	G24	G25	G26	G27	O1	O2	O3	O4
8	8	9	5	7	10	5	6	9	9	6	6	6	7	6	7
9	9	10	9	8	8	7	8	8	9	8	8	8	7	8	7
9	8	8	8	8	9	7	8	9	8	9	9	9	8	8	8
8	9	8	9	6	7	6	4	6	6	5	5	7	7	7	6
10	10	8	10	9	10	10	8	8	9	9	9	8	8	8	7
7	8	8	8	8	7	6	5	7	8	8	7	7	6	6	7
5	5	5	5	5	6	4	5	5	6	6	5	6	5	6	4
9	9	9	9	8	8	8	8	9	8	3	8	8	8	8	8
9	8	9	8	9	8	7	7	7	7	5	8	8	7	6	6

(continued)

This chapter was previously published in "Machine learning in medicine-cookbook 1" as Chap. 12, 2013.

T.J. Cleophas, A.H. Zwinderman, *Machine Learning in Medicine - a Complete Overview*, DOI 10.1007/978-3-319-15195-3_27

(continued)

10	10	10	10	10	10	10	10	10	8	8	10	10	10	9	10
2	2	8	5	7	8	8	8	9	3	9	8	7	7	7	6
7	8	8	7	8	6	6	7	8	8	8	7	8	7	8	8
8	9	9	8	10	8	8	7	8	8	9	9	7	7	8	8

Var G1-27 highly expressed genes estimated from their arrays' normalized ratios
Var O1-4 drug efficacy scores (the variables 20–23 from the initial data file)

The data from the first 13 patients are shown only (see extra.springer.com for the entire data file entitled "optscalingfactorplscanonical"). First, MANOVA (multivariate analysis of variance) was performed with the four drug efficacy scores as outcome variables and the twelve gene expression levels as covariates. We can now use SPSS 19.0. Start by opening the data file.

Canonical Regression

Command:

click Analyze….click General Linear Model….click Multivariate….Dependent Variables: enter the four drug efficacy scores….Covariates: enter the 12 genes…. OK.

	Effect value	F	Hypothesis df	Error df	p-value
Intercept	0.043	2.657	4.0	234.0	0.034
Gene 1	0.006	0.362	4.0	234.0	0.835
Gene 2	0.27	1.595	4.0	234.0	0.176
Gene 3	0.042	2.584	4.0	234.0	0.038
Gene 4	0.013	0.744	4.0	234.0	0.563
Gene 16	0.109	7.192	4.0	234.0	0.0001
Gene 17	0.080	5.118	4.0	234.0	0.001
Gene 18	0.23	1.393	4.0	234.0	0.237
Gene 19	0.092	5.938	4.0	234.0	0.0001
Gene 24	0.045	2.745	4.0	234.0	0.029
Gene 25	0.017	1.037	4.0	234.0	0.389
Gene 26	0.027	1.602	4.0	234.0	0.174
Gene 27	0.045	2.751	4.0	234.0	0.029

The MANOVA table is given (F = F-value, df = degrees of freedom). It shows that MANOVA can be considered as another regression model with intercepts and regression coefficients. We can conclude that the genes 3, 16, 17, 19, 24, and 27 are significant predictors of all four drug efficacy outcome scores. Unlike ANOVA, MANOVA does not give overall p-values, but rather separate p-values for separate covariates. However, we are, particularly, interested in the combined effect of the set of predictors, otherwise called covariates, on the set of outcomes, rather than we are in modeling the separate variables. In order to asses the overall effect of the cluster of genes on the cluster of drug efficacy scores canonical regression is performed.

Command:

click File....click New....click Syntax....the Syntax Editor dialog box is displayed....enter the following text: "manova" and subsequently enter all of the outcome variables....enter the text "WITH"....then enter all of the gene-names.... then enter the following text: /discrim all alpha(1)/print=sig(eigen dim)....click Run.

Numbers variables (covariates v outcome variables)							
	Canon cor	Sq cor	Wilks L	F	Hypoth df	Error df	p
12 v 4	0.87252	0.7613	0.19968	9.7773	48.0	903.4	0.0001
7 v 4	0.87054	0.7578	0.21776	16.227	28.0	863.2	0.0001
7 v 3	0.87009	0.7571	0.22043	22.767	21.0	689.0	0.0001

The above table is given (cor = correlation coefficient, sq = squared, L = lambda, hypoth = hypothesis, df = degree of freedom, p = p-value, v = versus). The upper row, shows the result of the statistical analysis. The correlation coefficient between the 12 predictor and 4 outcome variables equals 0.87252. A squared correlation coefficient of 0.7613 means that 76 % of the variability in the outcome variables is explained by the 12 covariates. The cluster of predictors is a very significant predictor of the cluster of outcomes, and can be used for making predictions about individual patients with similar gene profiles. Repeated testing after the removal of separate variables gives an idea about relatively unimportant contributors as estimated by their coefficients, which are kind of canonical b-values (regression coefficients). The larger they are, the more important they are.

Canon Cor			
Raw Model	12 v 4	7 v 4	7 v 3
Outcome 1	−0.24620	−0.24603	0.25007
Outcome 2	−0.20355	−0.19683	0.20679
Outcome 3	−0.02113	−0.02532	
Outcome 4	−0.07993	−0.08448	0.09037
Gene 1	0.01177		
Gene 2	−0.01727		
Gene 3	−0.05964	−0.08344	0.08489
Gene 4	−0.02865		
Gene 16	−0.14094	−0.13883	0.13755
Gene 17	−0.12897	−0.14950	0.14845

(continued)

(continued)

Canon Cor			
Raw Model	12 v 4	7 v 4	7 v 3
Gene 18	−0.03276		
Gene 19	−0.10626	−0.11342	0.11296
Gene 24	−0.07148	−0.07024	0.07145
Gene 25	−0.00164		
Gene 26	−0.05443	−0.05326	0.05354
Gene 27	0.05589	0.04506	−0.04527
Standardized			
Outcome 1	−0.49754	−0.49720	0.50535
Outcome 2	−0.40093	−0.38771	0.40731
Outcome 3	−0.03970	−0.04758	
Outcome 4	−0.15649	−0.16539	0.17693
Gene 1	0.02003		
Gene 2	−0.03211		
Gene 3	−0.10663	−0.14919	0.15179
Gene 4	−0.04363		
Gene 16	−0.30371	−0.29918	0.29642
Gene 17	−0.23337	−0.27053	0.26862
Gene 18	−0.06872		
Gene 19	−0.23696	−0.25294	0.25189
Gene 24	−0.18627	−0.18302	0.18618
Gene 25	−0.00335		
Gene 26	−0.14503	−0.14191	0.14267
Gene 27	0.12711	0.10248	−0.10229

The above table left column gives an overview of raw and standardized (z transformed) canonical coefficients, otherwise called canonical weights (the multiple b-values of canonical regression), (Canon Cor = canonical correlation coefficient, v = versus, Model = analysis model after removal of one or more variables). The outcome 3, and the genes 2, 4, 18 and 25 contributed little to the overall result. When restricting the model by removing the variables with canonical coefficients smaller than 0.05 or larger than −0.05 (the middle and right columns of the table), the results were largely unchanged. And so were the results of the overall tests (the 2nd and 3rd rows). Seven versus three variables produced virtually the same correlation coefficient but with much more power (lambda increased from 0.1997 to 0.2204, the F value from 9.7773 to 22.767, in spite of a considerable fall in the degrees of freedom). It, therefore, does make sense to try and remove the weaker variables from the model ultimately to be used. The weakest contributing covariates of the MANOVA were virtually identical to the weakest canonical predictors, suggesting that the two methods are closely related and one method confirms the results of the other.

Conclusion

Canonical analysis is wonderful, because it can handle many more variables than MANOVA, accounts for the relative importance of the separate variables and their interactions, provides overall statistics. Unlike other methods for combining the effects of multiple variables like factor analysis/partial least squares (chap. 8), canonical analysis is scientifically entirely rigorous.

Note

More background, theoretical and mathematical information of canonical regression is given in Machine learning in medicine part one, Chap. 18, Canonical regression, pp 225–240, Springer Heidelberg Germany, 2013, from the same authors.

Chapter 28
Multinomial Regression for Outcome Categories (55 Patients)

General Purpose

To assess whether multinomial regression can be trained to make predictions about (1) patients being in a category and (2) the probability of it.

Specific Scientific Question

Patients from different hospital departments and ages are assessed for falling out of bed (0=no, 1=yes without injury, 2=yes with injury). The falloutofbed categories are the outcome, the department and ages are the predictors. Can a data file of such patients be trained to make predictions in future patients about their best fit category and probability of being in it.

department	falloutofbed	age(years)
,00	1	56,00
,00	1	58,00
,00	1	87,00
,00	1	64,00
,00	1	65,00
,00	1	53,00
,00	1	87,00
,00	1	77,00
,00	1	78,00
,00	1	89,00

This chapter was previously published in "Machine learning in medicine-cookbook 2" as Chap. 4, 2014.

T.J. Cleophas, A.H. Zwinderman, *Machine Learning in Medicine - a Complete Overview*, DOI 10.1007/978-3-319-15195-3_28

Only the first 10 patients are given, the entire data file is entitled "categoriesasoutcome" and is in extras.springer.com.

The Computer Teaches Itself to Make Predictions

SPSS versions 18 and later can be used. SPSS will produce an XML (eXtended Markup Language) file of the prediction model from the above data. We will start by opening the above data file.

Command:

click Transform....click Random Number Generators....click Set Starting Point.... click Fixed Value (2000000)....click OK....click Analyze.... Regression .... Multinomial Logistic Regression....Dependent: falloutofbed.... Factor: department....Covariate: age....click Save....mark: Estimated response probability, Predicted category, Predicted category probability, Actual category probability.... click Browse....various folders in your personal computer come up....in "File name" of the appropriate folder enter "exportcategoriesasoutcome"....click Save....click Continue....click OK.

Parameter estimates

								95 % Confidence interval for Exp (B)	
Fall with/out injury[a]		B	Std. error	Wald	df	Sig.	Exp(B)	Lower bound	Upper bound
0	Intercept	5,337	2,298	5,393	1	,020			
	Age	–,059	,029	4,013	1	,045	,943	,890	,999
	[department=,00]	–1,139	,949	1,440	1	,230	,320	,050	2,057
	[department=1,00]	0[b]			0				
1	Intercept	3,493	2,333	2,241	1	,134			
	Age	–,022	,029	,560	1	,454	,978	,924	1,036
	[department=,00]	–1,945	,894	4,735	1	,030	,143	,025	,824
	[department=1,00]	0[b]			0				

[a]The reference category is: 2
[b]This parameter is set to zero because it is redundant

The above table is in the output. The independent predictors of falloutofbed are given. Per year of age there are 0,943 less "no falloutofbeds" versus "falloutofbeds with injury". The department 0,00 has 0,143 less falloutofbeds with versus without injury. The respective p-values are 0,045 and 0,030. When returning to the main data view, we will observe that SPSS has provided 6 novel variables for each patient.

1. EST1_1 estimated response probability (probability of the category 0 for each patient)
2. EST2_1 idem for category 1

3. EST3_1 idem for category 2
4. PRE_1 predicted category (category with highest probability score)
5. PCP_1 predicted category probability (the highest probability score predicted by model)
6. ACP_1 actual category probability (the highest probability computed from data)

With the Scoring Wizard and the exported XML file entitled "exportcategoriesasoutcome" we can now try and predict from the department and age of future patients (1) the most probable category they are in, and (2) the very probability of it. The department and age of 12 novel patients are as follow.

department	age
,00	73,00
,00	38,00
1,00	89,00
,00	75,00
,00	84,00
,00	74,00
1,00	90,00
1,00	72,00
1,00	62,00
1,00	34,00
1,00	85,00
1,00	43,00

Enter the above data in a novel data file and command:

Utilities....click Scoring Wizard....click Browse....Open the appropriate folder with the XML file entitled "exportcategoriesasoutcome"....click on the latter and click Select....in Scoring Wizard double-click Next....mark Predicted category and Probability of it....click Finish.

department	age	probability of being in predicted category	predicted category
,00	73,00	,48	1,00
,00	38,00	,48	1,00
1,00	89,00	,36	2,00
,00	75,00	,47	1,00
,00	84,00	,48	2,00
,00	74,00	,48	1,00
1,00	90,00	,37	2,00
1,00	72,00	,55	,00
1,00	62,00	,65	,00
1,00	34,00	,84	,00

(continued)

department	age	probability of being in predicted category	predicted category
1,00	85,00	,39	,00
1,00	43,00	,79	,00

0 = no falloutofbed
1 = falloutofbed without injury
2 = falloutofbed with injury

In the data file SPSS has provided two novel variables as requested. The first patient from department 0,00 and 73 years of age has a 48 % chance of being in the "falloutofbed without injury". His/her chance of being in the other two categories is smaller than 48 %.

Conclusion

Multinomial, otherwise called polytomous, logistic regression can be readily trained to make predictions in future patients about their best fit category and the probability of being in it.

Note

More background theoretical and mathematical information of analyses using categories as outcome is available in Machine learning in medicine part two, Chap.10, Anomaly detection, pp 93–103, Springer Heidelberg Germany, 2013, from the same authors.

Chapter 29
Various Methods for Analyzing Predictor Categories (60 and 30 Patients)

General Purpose

Categories unlike continuous data need not have stepping functions. In order to apply regression analysis for their analysis we need to recode them into multiple binary (dummy) variables. Particularly, if Gaussian distributions in the outcome are uncertain, automatic non-parametric testing is an adequate and very convenient modern alternative.

Specific Scientific Questions

1. Does race have an effect on physical strength (the variable race has a categorical rather than linear pattern).
2. Are the hours of sleep / levels of side effects different in categories treated with different sleeping pills.

Example 1

The effects on physical strength (scores 0–100) assessed in 60 subjects of different races (hispanics (1), blacks (2), asians (3), and whites (4)), and ages (years), are in the left three columns of the data file entitled “categoriesaspredictor”.

This chapter was previously published in “Machine learning in medicine-cookbook 2” as Chap. 5, 2014.

T.J. Cleophas, A.H. Zwinderman, *Machine Learning in Medicine - a Complete Overview*, DOI 10.1007/978-3-319-15195-3_29

Patient number	physical strength	race	age
1	70,00	1,00	35,00
2	77,00	1,00	55,00
3	66,00	1,00	70,00
4	59,00	1,00	55,00
5	71,00	1,00	45,00
6	72,00	1,00	47,00
7	45,00	1,00	75,00
8	85,00	1,00	83,00
9	70,00	1,00	35,00
10	77,00	1,00	49,00

Only the first 10 patients are displayed above. The entire data file in www.springer.com. For the analysis we will use multiple linear regression.

Command:

Analyze....Regression....Linear....Dependent: physical strength score.... Independent: race, age, ...OK.

Coefficients[a]

		Unstandardized coefficients		Standardized coefficients		
Model		B	Std. Error	Beta	t	Sig.
1	(Constant)	92,920	7,640		12,162	,000
	Race	–,330	1,505	–,027	–,219	,827
	Age	–,356	,116	–,383	–3,071	,003

[a]Dependent variable: strengthscore

The above table shows that age is a significant predictor but race is not. However, the analysis is not adequate, because the variable race is analyzed as a stepwise function from 1 to 4, and the linear regression model assumes that the outcome variable will rise (or fall) linearly, but, in the data given, this needs not be necessarily so. It may, therefore, be more safe to recode the stepping variable into the form of a categorical variable. The underneath data overview shows in the right 4 columns how it is manually done.

patient number	physical strength	race	age	race 1	race 2	race 3	race 4
				hispanics	blacks	asians	whites
1	70,00	1,00	35,00	1,00	0,00	0,00	0,00
2	77,00	1,00	55,00	1,00	0,00	0,00	0,00
3	66,00	1,00	70,00	1,00	0,00	0,00	0,00
4	59,00	1,00	55,00	1,00	0,00	0,00	0,00
5	71,00	1,00	45,00	1,00	0,00	0,00	0,00
6	72,00	1,00	47,00	1,00	0,00	0,00	0,00
7	45,00	1,00	75,00	1,00	0,00	0,00	0,00
8	85,00	1,00	83,00	1,00	0,00	0,00	0,00
9	70,00	1,00	35,00	1,00	0,00	0,00	0,00
10	77,00	1,00	49,00	1,00	0,00	0,00	0,00

We, subsequently, use again linear regression, but now for categorical analysis of race.

Command:

click Transform….click Random Number Generators….click Set Starting Point…. click Fixed Value (2000000)….click OK….click Analyze….Regression ….Linear ….Dependent: physical strength score….Independent: race 1, race 3, race 4, age…. click Save….mark Unstandardized….in Export model information to XML (eXtended Markup Language) file: type "exportcategoriesaspredictor"….click Browse….File name: enter "exportcategoriesaspredictor"….click Continue….click OK.

Coefficients[a]

		Unstandardized coefficients		Standardized coefficients		
Model		B	Std. Error	Beta	t	Sig.
1	(Constant)	97,270	4,509		21,572	,000
	Age	–,200	,081	–,215	–2,457	,017
	Race1	–17,483	3,211	–,560	–5,445	,000
	Race3	–25,670	3,224	–,823	–7,962	,000
	Race4	–8,811	3,198	–,282	–2,755	,008

[a]Dependent variable: strengthscore

The above table is in the output. It shows that race 1, 3, 4 are significant predictors of physical strength compared to race 2. The results can be interpreted as follows.

The underneath regression equation is used:

$$y = a + b_1x_1 + b_2x_2 + b_3x_3 + b_4x_4$$

a = intercept
b_1 = regression coefficient for age
b_2 = hispanics
b_3 = asians
b_4 = white

If an individual is black (race 2), then x_2, x_3, and x_4 will turn into 0, and the regression equation becomes

$$y = a + b_1x_1$$

If hispanic, $$y = a + b_1x_1 + b_2x_2$$

If asian, $$y = a + b_1x_1 + b_3x_3$$

If white, $$y = a + b_1x_1 + b_4x_4.$$

So, e.g., the best predicted physical strength score of a white male of 25 years of age would equal

$$y = 97.270 + 0.20 * 25 - 8.811 * 1 = 93.459,$$
$$(* = \text{sign of multiplication}).$$

Obviously, all of the races are negative predictors of physical strength, but the blacks scored highest and the asians lowest. All of these results are adjusted for age.

If we return to the data file page, we will observe that SPSS has added a new variable entitled "PRE_1". It represents the individual strengthscores as predicted by the recoded linear model. They are pretty similar to the measured values.

We can now with the help of the Scoring Wizard and the exported XML (eXtended Markup Language) file entitled "exportcategoriesaspredictor" try and predict strength scores of future patients with known race and age.

race	age
1,00	40,00
2,00	70,00
3,00	54,00
4,00	45,00
1,00	36,00
2,00	46,00
3,00	50,00
4,00	36,00

First, recode the stepping variable race into 4 categorical variables.

race	age	race1	race3	race4
1,00	40,00	1,00	,00	,00
2,00	70,00	,00	,00	,00
3,00	54,00	,00	1,00	,00
4,00	45,00	,00	,00	1,00
1,00	36,00	1,00	,00	,00
2,00	46,00	,00	,00	,00
3,00	50,00	,00	1,00	,00
4,00	36,00	,00	,00	1,00

Then Command:

click Utilities….click Scoring Wizard….click Browse….click Select….Folder: enter the exportcategoriesaspredictor.xml file….click Select….in Scoring Wizard click Next….click Finish.

race	age	race1	race3	race4	predicted strength score
1,00	40,00	1,00	,00	,00	71,81
2,00	70,00	,00	,00	,00	83,30
3,00	54,00	,00	1,00	,00	60,83
4,00	45,00	,00	,00	1,00	79,48
1,00	36,00	1,00	,00	,00	72,60
2,00	46,00	,00	,00	,00	88,09
3,00	50,00	,00	1,00	,00	61,62
4,00	36,00	,00	,00	1,00	81,28

The above data file now gives predicted strength scores of the 8 future patients as computed with help of the XML file.

Also with a binary outcome variable categorical analysis of covariates is possible. Using logistic regression in SPSS is convenient for the purpose, we need not *manually* transform the quantitative estimator into a categorical one. For the analysis we have to apply the usual commands.

Command:

Analyze ....Regression....Binary logistic....Dependent variable.... Independent variables....then, open dialog box labeled Categorical Variables.... select the categorical variable and transfer it to the box Categorical Variables....then click Continue....OK.

Example 2

Particularly, if Gaussian distributions in the outcome are uncertain, automatic non-parametric testing is an adequate and very convenient modern alternative. Three parallel-groups were treated with different sleeping pills. Both hours of sleep and side effect score were assessed.

Group	efficacy	gender	comorbidity	side effect score
0	6,00	,00	1,00	45,00
0	7,10	,00	1,00	35,00
0	8,10	,00	,00	34,00
0	7,50	,00	,00	29,00
0	6,40	,00	1,00	48,00
0	7,90	1,00	1,00	23,00
0	6,80	1,00	1,00	56,00
0	6,60	1,00	,00	54,00
0	7,30	1,00	,00	33,00
0	5,60	,00	,00	75,00

Only the first ten patients are shown. The entire data file is in extras.springer.com and is entitled "categoriesaspredictor2". Automatic nonparametric tests is available in SPSS 18 and up. Start by opening the above data file.

Command:

Analyze....Nonparametric Tests....Independent Samples....click Objective....mark Automatically compare distributions across groups....click Fields....in Test fields: enter "hours of sleep" and "side effect score"....in Groups: enter "group"....click Settings....Choose Tests....mark "Automatically choose the tests based on the data"....click Run.

In the interactive output sheets the underneath table is given. Both the distribution of hours of sleep and side effect score are significantly different across the three categories of treatment. The traditional assessment of these data would have been a multivariate analysis of variance (MANOVA) with treatment-category as predictor and both hours of sleep and side effect score as outcome. However, normal distributions are uncertain in this example, and the correlation between the two outcome measures may not be zero, reducing the sensitivity of MANOVA. A nice thing about the automatic nonparametric tests is that, like discriminant analysis (Machine learning in medicine part one, Chap. 17, Discriminant analysis for supervised data, pp 215–224, Springer Heidelberg Germany, 2013, from the same authors), they assume orthogonality of the two outcomes, which means that the correlation level between the two does not have to be taken into account. By double-clicking the table you will obtain an interactive set of views of various details of the analysis, entitled the Model Viewer.

Hypothesis test summary

	Null hypothesis	Test	Sig.	Decision
1	The distribution of hours of sleep is the same across categories of group.	Independent-Samples Kruskal-Wallis Test	,001	Reject the null hypothesis.
2	The distribution of side effect score is the same across categories of group.	Independent-Samples Kruskal-Wallis Test	,036	Reject the null hypothesis.

Asymptotic significances are displayed. The significance level is,05

One view provides the box and whiskers graphs (medians, quartiles, and ranges) of hours of sleep of the three treatment groups. Group 0 seems to perform better than the other two, but we don't know where the significant differences are.

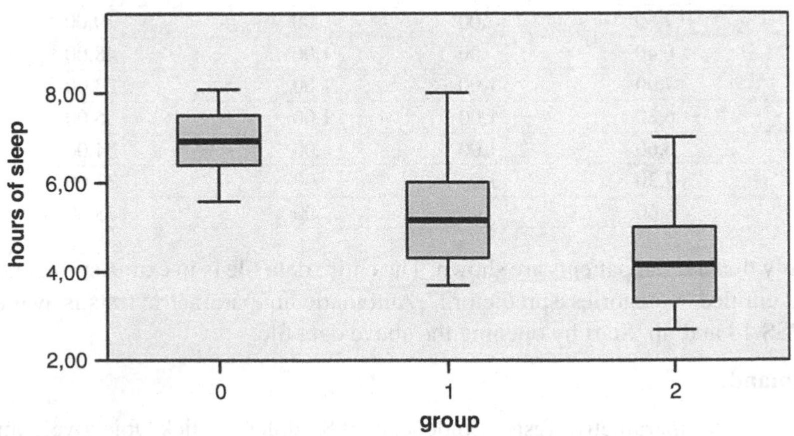

Also the box and whiskers graph of side effect scores is given. Some groups again seem to perform better than the other. However, we cannot see whether 0 vs 1, 1 vs 2, and/or 0 vs 2 are significantly different.

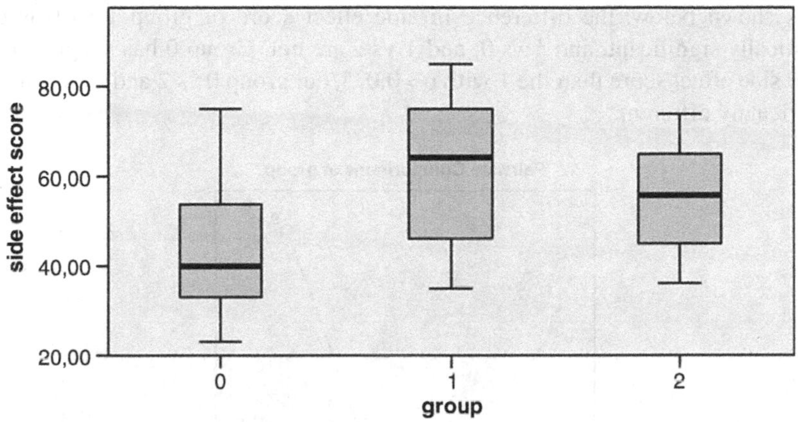

In the view space at the bottom of the auxiliary view (right half of the Model Viewer) several additional options are given. When clicking Pairwise Comparisons, a distance network is displayed with yellow lines corresponding to statistically significant differences, and black ones to insignificant ones. Obviously, the differences in hours of sleep of group 1 vs (versus) 0 and group 2 vs 0 are statistically significant, and 1 vs 2 is not. Group 0 had significantly more hours of sleep than the other two groups with p = 0.044 and 0.0001.

Pairwise Comparisons of group

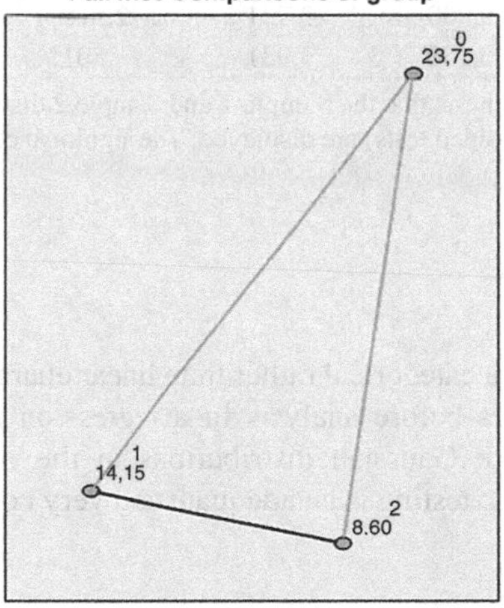

Each node shows the sample average rank of group

Sample1-	Sample2	Test statistic	Std. Error	Std. Test statistic	Sig.	Adj.Sig.
2-	1	5,550	3,936	1,410	,158	,475
2-	0	15,150	3,936	3,849	,000	,000
1-	0	9,600	3,936	2,439	,015	,044

Each row tests the null hypothesis that the Sample 1 and Sample 2 distributions are the same
Asymptotic significances (2-sided tests) are displayed. The significance level is ,05

As shown below, the difference in side effect score of group 1 vs 0 is also statistically significant, and 1 vs 0, and 1 vs 2 are not. Group 0 has a significantly better side effect score than the 1 with p=0.035, but group 0 vs 2 and 1 vs 2 are not significantly different.

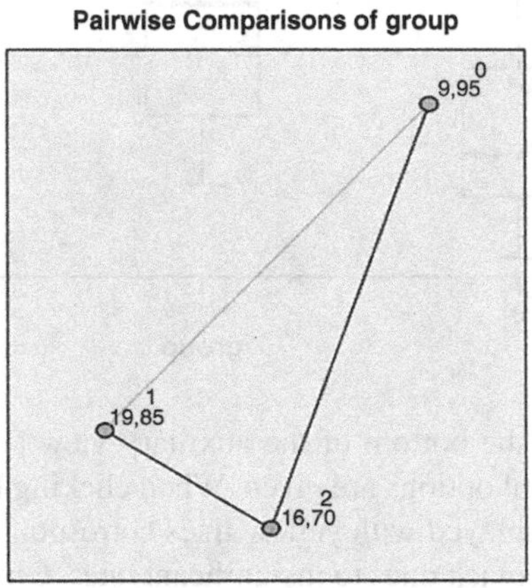

Each node shows the sample average rank of group

Sample1-	Sample2	Test statistic	Std. Error	Std. Test statistic	Sig.	Adj.Sig.
0-	2	−6,750	3,931	−1,717	,086	,258
0-	1	−9,900	3,931	−2,518	,012	,035
2-	1	3,150	3,931	,801	,423	1,000

Each row tests the null hypothesis that the Sample 1 and Sample 2 distributions are the same
Asymptotic significances (2-sided tests) are displayed. The significance level is ,05

Conclusion

Predictor variables with a categorical rather than linear character should be recoded into categorical variables before analysis in a regression model. An example is given. Particularly if the Gaussian distributions in the outcome are uncertain, automatic non-parametric testing is an adequate and very convenient alternative.

Note

More background theoretical and mathematical information of categories as predictor is given in SPSS for starters part two, Chap. 5, Categorical data, pp 21–24, and Statistics applied to clinical studies 5th edition, Chap. 21, Races as a categorical variable, pp 244–252, both from the same authors and edited by Springer Heidelberg Germany 2012.

Chapter 30
Random Intercept Models for Both Outcome and Predictor Categories (55 patients)

General Purpose

Categories are very common in medical research. Examples include age classes, income classes, education levels, drug dosages, diagnosis groups, disease severities, etc. Statistics has generally difficulty to assess categories, and traditional models require either binary or continuous variables. If in the outcome, categories can be assessed with multinomial regression (see the above Chap. 28), if as predictors, they can be assessed with automatic nonparametric tests (see the above Chap. 29). However, with multiple categories or with categories both in the outcome and as predictors, random intercept models may provide better sensitivity of testing. The latter models assume that for each predictor category or combination of categories x_1, x_2,…slightly different a-values can be computed with a better fit for the outcome category y than a single a-value.

$$y = a + b_1x_1 + b_2x_2 + \ldots.$$

We should add that, instead of the above linear equation, even better results were obtained with log-linear equations (log = natural logarithm).

$$\log y = a + b_1x_1 + b_2x_2 + \ldots.$$

This chapter was previously published in "Machine learning in medicine-cookbook 2" as Chap. 6, 2014.

T.J. Cleophas, A.H. Zwinderman, *Machine Learning in Medicine - a Complete Overview*, DOI 10.1007/978-3-319-15195-3_30

Specific Scientific Question

In a study three hospital departments (no surgery, little surgery, lot of surgery), and three patient age classes (young, middle, old) were the predictors of the risk class of falling out of bed (fall out of bed no, yes but no injury, yes and injury). Are the predictor categories significant determinants of the risk of falling out of bed with or without injury. Does a random intercept provide better statistics.

Example

department	falloutofbed	agecat	patient_id
0	1	1,00	1,00
0	1	1,00	2,00
0	1	2,00	3,00
0	1	1,00	4,00
0	1	1,00	5,00
0	1	,00	6,00
1	1	2,00	7,00
0	1	2,00	8,00
1	1	2,00	9,00
0	1	,00	10,00

Variable 1: department = department class (0 = no surgery, 1 = little surgery, 2 = lot of surgery)
Variable 2: falloutofbed = risk of falling out of bed (0 = fall out of bed no, 1 = yes but no injury, 2 = yes and injury)
Variable 3: agecat = patient age classes (young, middle, old)
Variable 4: patient_id = patient identification

Only the first 10 patients of the 55 patient file is shown above. The entire data file is in extras.springer.com and is entitled "randomintercept.sav". SPSS version 20 and up can be used for analysis. First, we will perform a fixed intercept log-linear analysis.

Command:

click Analyze….Mixed Models....Generalized Linear Mixed Models....click Data Structure….click "patient_id" and drag to Subjects on the Canvas….click Fields and Effects….click Target….Target: select "fall with/out injury"….click Fixed Effects….click "agecat"and "department" and drag to Effect Builder:….mark Include intercept….click Run.

The underneath results show that both the various regression coefficients as well as the overall correlation coefficients between the predictors and the outcome are, generally, statistically significant.

Source	F	df1	df2	Sig.
Corrected Model	9,398	4	10	,002
Agecat	6,853	2	10	,013
Department	9,839	2	10	,004

Probability distribution: Multinomial
Link function: Cumulative logit

Model Term		Coefficient	Sig.
	0	2,140	,028
Threshold for falloutofbed=	1	7,229	,000
Agecat=0		5,236	,005
Agecat=1		−0,002	,998
Agecat=2		0,000[a]	
Department=0		3,660	,008
Department=1		4,269	,002
Department=2		0,000[a]	

Probability distribution: Multinomial
Link function: Cumulative logit
[a]This coefficient is set to zero because it is redundant

Subsequently, a random intercept analysis is performed.

Command:

Analyze….Mixed Models....Generalized Linear Mixed Models....click Data Structure….click "patient_id" and drag to Subjects on the Canvas….click Fields and Effects….click Target….Target: select "fall with/out injury"….click Fixed Effects…. click "agecat"and "department" and drag to Effect Builder:….mark Include intercept….click Random Effects….click Add Block…mark Include intercept….Subject combination: select patient_id….click OK….click Model Options….click Save Fields…mark PredictedValue….mark PredictedProbability….click Save....click Run.

The underneath results show the test statistics of the random intercept model. The random intercept model shows better statistics:

$p = 0.007$ and 0.013 overall for age,
$p = 0.001$ and 0.004 overall for department,
$p = 0.003$ and 0.005 regression coefficients for age class 0 versus 2,
$p = 0.900$ and 0.998 for age class 1 versus 2,
$p = 0.004$ and 0.008 for department 0 versus 2, and
$p = 0.001$ and 0.0002 for department 1 versus 2.

Source	F	df1	df2	Sig.
Corrected Model	7,935	4	49	,000
Agecat	5,513	2	49	,007
Department	7,602	2	49	,001

Probability distribution: Multinomial
Link function: Cumulative logit

Model term		Coefficient	Sig.
Threshold for falloutofbed=	0	2,082	,015
	1	5,464	,000
Agecat=0		3,869	,003
Agecat=1		0,096	,900
Agecat=2		0,000[a]	
Department=0		3,228	,004
Department=1		3,566	,000
Department=2		0,000[a]	

Probability distribution: Multinomial
Link function: Cumulative logit
[a]This coefficient is set to zero because it is redundant

In the random intercept model we have also commanded predicted values (variable 7) and predicted probabilities of having the predicted values as computed by the software (variables 5 and 6).

1	2	3	4	5	6	7 (variables)
0	1	1,00	1,00	,224	,895	1
0	1	1,00	2,00	,224	,895	1
0	1	2,00	3,00	,241	,903	1
0	1	1,00	4,00	,224	,895	1
0	1	1,00	5,00	,224	,895	1
0	1	,00	6,00	,007	,163	2
1	1	2,00	7,00	,185	,870	1
0	1	2,00	8,00	,241	,903	1
1	1	2,00	9,00	,185	,870	1
0	1	,00	10,00	,007	,163	2

Variable 1: department
Variable 2: falloutofbed
Variable 3: agecat
Variable 4: patient_id
Variable 5: predicted probability of predicted value of target accounting the department score only
Variable 6: predicted probability of predicted value of target accounting both department and agecat scores
Variable 7: predicted value of target

Like automatic linear regression (see Chap. 31) and other generalized mixed linear models (see Chap. 33) random intercept models include the possibility to make XML files from the analysis, that can subsequently be used for making predictions about the chance of falling out of bed in future patients. However, SPSS uses here slightly different software called winRAR ZIP files that are "shareware". This means that you pay a small fee and be registered if you wish to use it. Note that winRAR ZIP files have an archive file format consistent of compressed data used by

Microsoft since 2006 for the purpose of filing XML (eXtended Markup Language) files. They are only employable for a limited period of time like e.g. 40 days.

Conclusion

Generalized linear mixed models are suitable for analyzing data with multiple categorical variables. Random intercept versions of these models provide better sensitivity of testing than fixed intercept models.

Note

More information on statistical methods for analyzing data with categories is in the Chaps. 28 and 29 of this book.

Chapter 31
Automatic Regression for Maximizing Linear Relationships (55 patients)

General Purpose

Automatic linear regression is in the Statistics Base add-on module SPSS version 19 and up. X-variables are automatically transformed in order to provide an improved data fit, and SPSS uses rescaling of time and other measurement values, outlier trimming, category merging and other methods for the purpose. This chapter is to assess whether automatic linear regression is helpful to obtain an improved precision of analysis of clinical trials.

Specific Scientific Question

In a clinical crossover trial an old laxative is tested against a new one. Numbers of stools per month is the outcome. The old laxative and the patients' age are the predictor variables. Does automatic linear regression provide better statistics of these data than traditional multiple linear regression does.

Data Example

Patno	newtreat	oldtreat	age categories
1,00	24,00	8,00	2,00
2,00	30,00	13,00	2,00

(continued)

This chapter was previously published in "Machine learning in medicine-cookbook 2" as Chap. 7, 2014.

T.J. Cleophas, A.H. Zwinderman, *Machine Learning in Medicine - a Complete Overview*, DOI 10.1007/978-3-319-15195-3_31

Patno	newtreat	oldtreat	age categories
3,00	25,00	15,00	2,00
4,00	35,00	10,00	3,00
5,00	39,00	9,00	3,00
6,00	30,00	10,00	3,00
7,00	27,00	8,00	1,00
8,00	14,00	5,00	1,00
9,00	39,00	13,00	1,00
10,00	42,00	15,00	1,00

patno = patient number
newtreat = frequency of stools on a novel laxative
oldtreat = frequency of stools on an old laxative
agecategories = patients' age categories (1 = young, 2 = middle-age, 3 = old)

Only the first 10 patients of the 55 patients are shown above. The entire file is in extras.springer.com and is entitled "automaticlinreg". We will first perform a standard multiple linear regression.

Command:

Analyze....Regression....Linear....Dependent: enter newtreat....Independent: enter oldtreat and agecategories....click OK.

Model summary

Model	R	R Square	Adjusted R Square	Std. error of the estimate
1	,429[a]	,184	,133	9,28255

[a]Predictors: (Constant), oldtreat, agecategories

ANOVA[a]

Model		Sum of squares	df	Mean square	F	Sig.
	Regression	622,869	2	311,435	3,614	,038[b]
1	Residual	2757,302	32	86,166		
	Total	3380,171	34			

[a]Dependent variable: newtreat
[b]Predictors: (Constant), oldtreat, agecategories

Coefficients[a]

	Unstandardized coefficients		Standardized coefficients		
Model	B	Std. Error	Beta	t	Sig.
(Constant)	20,513	5,137		3,993	,000
1 agecategories	3,908	2,329	,268	1,678	,103
oldtreat	,135	,065	,331	2,070	,047

[a]Dependent variable: newtreat

Automatic Data Preparation		
Target: newtreat		
Field	Role	Actions taken
(agecategories_transformed)	Predictor	Merge categories to maximize association with target
(oldtreat_transformed)	Predictor	Trim outliers

If the original field name is X, then the transformed field is displayed as (X_transformed) The original field is excluded from the analysis and the transformed field is included instead

An interactive graph shows the predictors as lines with thicknesses corresponding to their predictive power and the outcome in the form of a histogram with its best fit Gaussian pattern. Both of the predictors are now statistically very significant with a correlation coefficient at $p < 0.0001$, and regression coefficients at p-values of respectively 0.001 and 0.007.

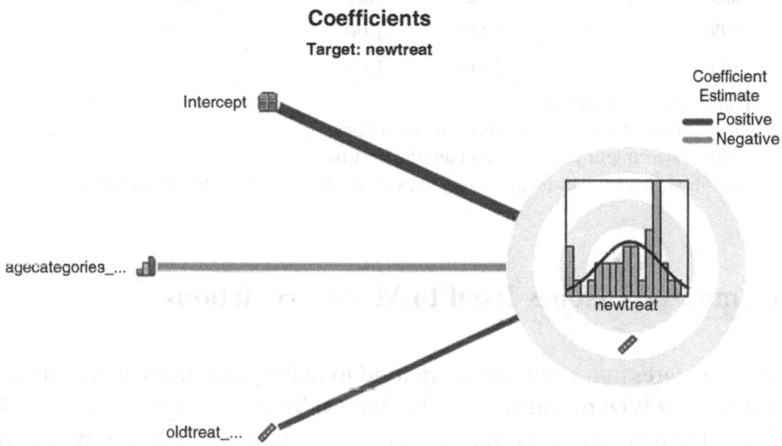

Coefficients			
Target: newtreat			
Model term	Coefficient ▶	Sig.	Importance
Intercept	35.926	.000	
Agecategories_transformed=0	−11.187	.001	0.609
Agecategories_transformed=1	0.000[a]		0.609
Oldtreat_transformed	0.209	.007	0.391

[a]This coefficient is set to zero because it is redundant

Effects					
Target: newtreat					
Source	Sum of squares	df	Mean square	F	Sig.
Corrected model ▶	1.289,960	2	644,980	9,874	,000
Residual	2.090,212	32	65,319		
Corrected total	3380,171	34			

Returning to the data view of the original data file, we now observe that SPSS has provided a novel variables with values for the new treatment as predicted from statistical model employed. They are pretty close to the real outcome values.

Patno	newtreat	oldtreat	age categories	Predicted Values
1,00	24,00	8,00	2,00	26,41
2,00	30,00	13,00	2,00	27,46
3,00	25,00	15,00	2,00	27,87
4,00	35,00	10,00	3,00	38,02
5,00	39,00	9,00	3,00	37,81
6,00	30,00	10,00	3,00	38,02
7,00	27,00	8,00	1,00	26,41
8,00	14,00	5,00	1,00	25,78
9,00	39,00	13,00	1,00	27,46
10,00	42,00	15,00	1,00	27,87

patno = patient number
newtreat = frequency of stools on a novel laxative
oldtreat = frequency of stools on an old laxative
agecategories = patients' age categories (1 = young, 2 = middle-age, 3 = old)

The Computer Teaches Itself to Make Predictions

The modeled regression coefficients are used to make predictions about future data using the Scoring Wizard and an XML (eXtended Markup Language) file (winRAR ZIP file) of the data file. Like random intercept models (see Chap. 6) and other generalized mixed linear models (see Chap. 9) automatic linear regression includes the possibility to make XML files from the analysis, that can subsequently be used for making outcome predictions in future patients. SPSS uses here software called winRAR ZIP files that are "shareware". This means that you pay a small fee and be registered if you wish to use it. Note that winRAR ZIP files have a archive file format consistent of compressed data used by Microsoft since 2006 for the purpose of filing XML files. They are only employable for a limited period of time like e.g. 40 days. Below the data of 9 future patients are given.

Newtreat	oldtreat	agecategory
	4,00	1,00
	13,00	1,00
	15,00	1,00
	15,00	1,00

(continued)

Newtreat	oldtreat	agecategory
	11,00	2,00
	80,00	2,00
	10,00	3,00
	18,00	2,00
	13,00	2,00

Enter the above data in a novel data file and command:

Utilities....click Scoring Wizard....click Browse....Open the appropriate folder with the XML file entitled "exportautomaticlinreg"....click on the latter and click Select....in Scoring Wizard double-click Next....mark Predicted Value....click Finish.

Newtreat	oldtreat	agecategory	predictednewtreat
	4,00	1,00	25,58
	13,00	1,00	27,46
	15,00	1,00	27,87
	15,00	1,00	27,87
	11,00	2,00	27,04
	80,00	2,00	41,46
	10,00	3,00	38,02
	18,00	2,00	28,50
	13,00	2,00	27,46

In the data file SPSS has provided the novel variable as requested. The first patient with only 4 stools per month on the old laxative and young of age will have over 25 stools on the new laxative.

Conclusion

SPSS' automatic linear regression can be helpful to obtain an improved precision of analysis of clinical trials and provided in the example given better statistics than traditional multiple linear regression did.

Note

More background theoretical and mathematical information of linear regression is available in Statistics applied to clinical studies 5th edition, Chap. 14, entitled Linear regression basic approach, and Chap. 15, Linear regression for assessing precision confounding interaction, Chap. 18, Regression modeling for improved precision, pp 161–176, 177–185, 219–225, Springer Heidelberg Germany, 2013, from the same authors.

Chapter 32
Simulation Models for Varying Predictors (9,000 Patients)

General Purpose

In medicine predictors are often varying, like, e.g., the numbers of complications and the days in hospital in patients with various conditions. This chapter is to assess, whether Monte Carlo simulation of the varying predictors can improve the outcome predictions.

Specific Scientific Question

The hospital costs for patients with heart infarction are supposed to be dependent on factors like patients' age, intensive care hours (ichours), numbers of complications. What percentage of patients will cost the hospital over 20,000 Euros, what percentage over 10,000. How will costs develop if the numbers of complications are reduced by 2 and the numbers of ichours by 20.

This chapter was previously published in "Machine learning in medicine-cookbook 2" as Chap. 8, 2014.

T.J. Cleophas, A.H. Zwinderman, *Machine Learning in Medicine - a Complete Overview*, DOI 10.1007/978-3-319-15195-3_32

Instead of Traditional Means and Standard Deviations, Monte Carlo Simulations of the Input and Outcome Variables are Used to Model the Data. This Enhances Precision, Particularly, With non-Normal Data

Age Years	complication number	ic hours	costs Euros
48	7	36	5488
66	7	57	8346
75	7	67	6976
72	6	45	5691
60	6	58	3637
84	9	54	16369
74	8	54	11349
42	9	26	10213
71	7	49	6474
73	10	35	30018
53	8	37	7632
79	6	46	6538
50	10	39	13797

Only the first 13 patients of this 9000 patient hypothesized data file is shown. The entire data file is in extras.springer.com and is entitled "simulation1.sav". SPSS 21 or 22 can be used. Start by opening the data file. We will first perform a traditional linear regression with the first three variables as input and the fourth variable as outcome.

Command:

click Transform….click Random Number Generators….click Set Starting Point ….click Fixed Value (2000000)….click OK….click Analyze ….Regression…. Linear….Dependent: costs…Independent: age, complication, ichours….click Save….click Browse….Select the desired folder in your computer….File name: enter "exportsimulation"….click Save….click Continue….click OK.

In the output sheets it is observed that all of the predictors are statistically very significant. Also a PMML (predictive model markup language) document, otherwise called XML (eXtended Markup Language) document has been produced and filed in your computer entitled "exportsimulation".

Coefficients[a]

	Unstandardized coefficients		Standardized coefficients		
Model	B	Std. Error	Beta	t	Sig.
(Constant)	−28570,977	254,044		−112,465	,000
age(years)	202,403	2,767	,318	73,136	,000
complications(n)	4022,405	21,661	,807	185,696	,000
ichours(hours)	−111,241	2,124	−,227	−52,374	,000

[a]Dependent variable: cost (Euros)

We will now perform the Monte Carlo simulation.

Command:

Analyze….Simulation….click Select SPSS Model File….click Continue….in Look in: select folder with "exportsimulation.xml" file….click Open….click Simulation Fields….click Fit All….click Save….mark Save the plan file for this simulation…. click Browse….in Look in: select the appropriate folder for storage of a simulation plan document and entitle it, e.g., "splan"….click Save….click Run.

In the output the underneath interactive probability density graph is exhibited. After double-clicking the vertical lines can be moved and corresponding areas under the curve percentages are shown.

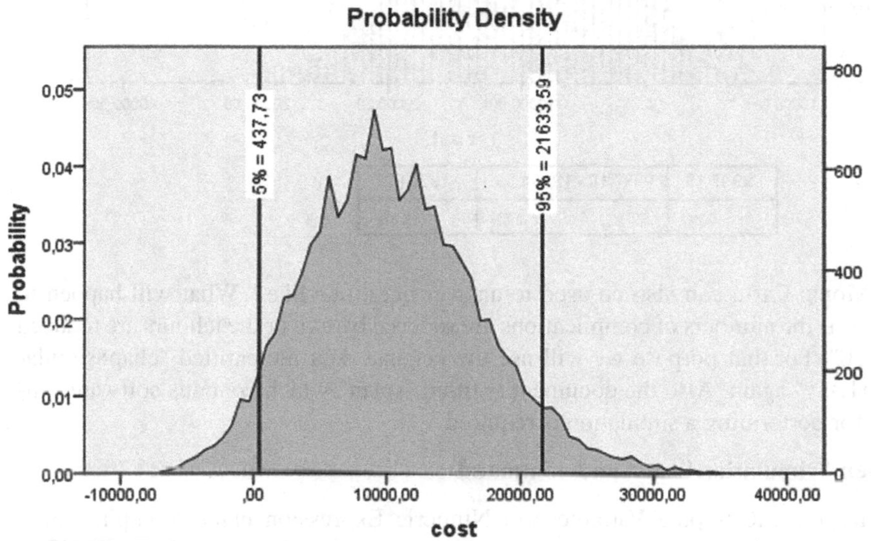

<437.73	437.73 - 21633.59	>21633.59
5%	90%	5%

Overall 90 % of the heart attacks patients will cost the hospital between 440 and 21.630 Euros. In the graph click Chart Options….in View click Histogram….click Continue.

The histogram below is displayed. Again the vertical lines can be moved as desired. It can, e.g., be observed that, around, 7.5 % of the heart attack patients will cost the hospital over 20.000 Euros, around 50 % of them will cost over 10.000 Euros.

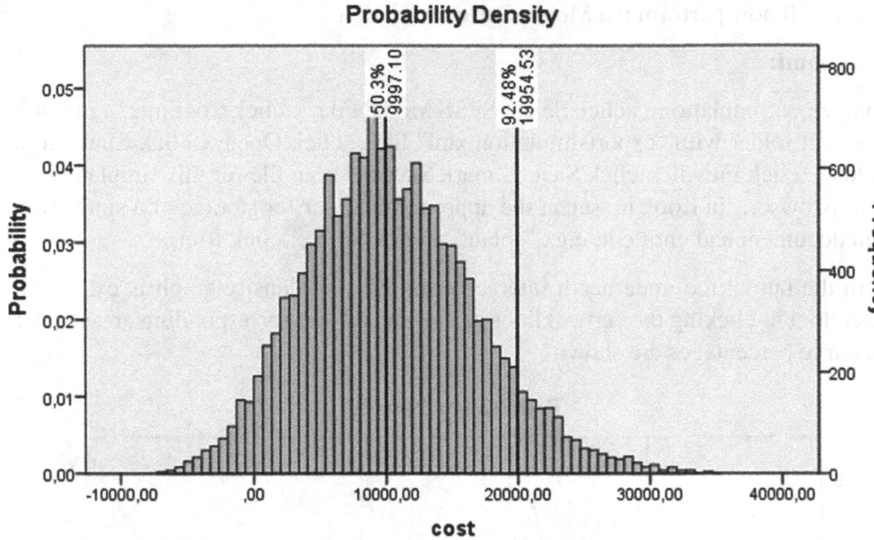

<9997.10	9997.10 - 19954.53	>19954.53
50%	42%	8%

Monte Carlo can also be used to answer questions like " What will happen to costs, if the numbers of complications are reduced by two or the ichours are reduced by 20". For that purpose we will use the original data file entitled "chap8simulation1.sav" again. Also the document entitled "splan" which contains software syntax for performing a simulation is required.

Open "simulation1.sav" and command:

Transform….Compute Variable….in Numeric Expression enter "complications" from the panel below Numeric Expressions enter "-" and "2"….in Target Variable type complications….click OK….in Change existing variable click OK.

In the data file all of the values of the variable "complications" have now been reduced by 2. This transformed data file is saved in the desired folder and entitled e.g. "simulation2.sav". We will now perform a Monte Carlo simulation of this transformed data file using the simulation plan "splan".

In "simulation2.sav" command: Analyze….Simulation….click Open an Existing Simulation Plan….click Continue….in Look in: find the appropriate folder in your computer….click "splan.splan"….click Open….click Simulation….click Fit All…. click Run.

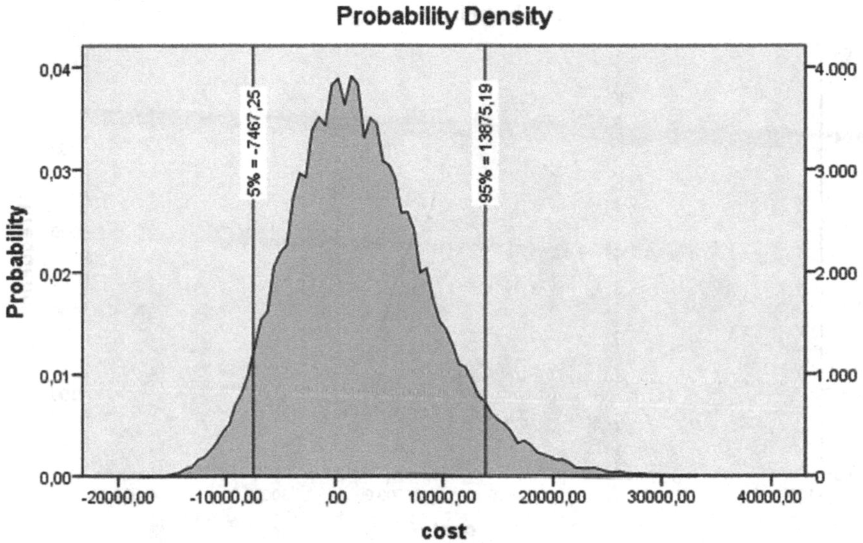

< -7467,25	-7467,25 - 13875,19	> 13875,19
5%	90%	5%

The above graph shows that fewer complications reduces the costs, e.g., 5 % of the patients cost over 13.875 Euros, while the same class costed over 21.633 Euros before.

What about the effect of the hours in the ic unit. For that purpose, in "simulation1.sav" perform the same commands as shown directly above, and transform the ichours variable by −20 hours. The transformed document can be named "simulation3.sav" and saved. The subsequent simulation procedure in this data file using again "splan.splan" produces the underneath output.

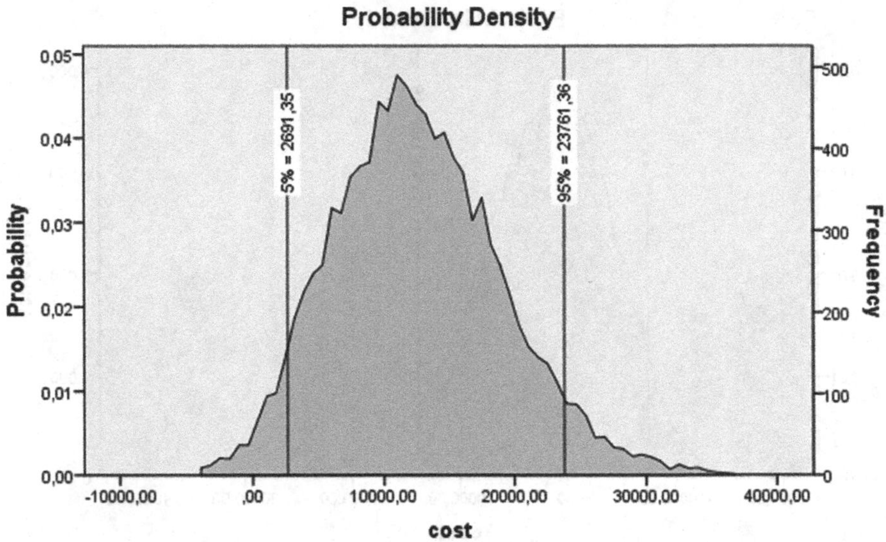

< 2691,35	2691,35 - 23761,36	> 23761,36
5%	90%	5%

It is observed that the costs are now not reduced, but rather somewhat increased with 5 % of the patients costing over 23.761 Euros instead of 21.633. This would make sense, nonetheless, because it is sometimes assumed by hospital managers that the reduction of stay-days in hospital is accompanied with more demanding type of care (Statistics Applied to Clinical Studies 5th edition, Chap. 44, Clinical data where variability is more important than averages, pp 487–498, Springer Heidelberg Germany, 2012).

Conclusion

Monte Carlo simulations of inputs where variability is more important than means can model outcome distributions with increased precision. This is, particularly, so with non-normal data. Also questions, like "how will hospital costs develop, if the numbers of complications are reduced by 2 or numbers of hours in the intensive care unit reduced by 20", can be answered.

Note

More background, theoretical and mathematical information of Monte Carlo simulation is provided in Statistics applied to clinical studies 5th edition, Chap. 44, Clinical data where variability is more important than averages, pp 487–498, Springer Heidelberg Germany, 2012, from the same authors as the current publication.

Chapter 33
Generalized Linear Mixed Models for Outcome Prediction from Mixed Data (20 Patients)

General Purpose

To assess whether generalized linear mixed models can be used to train clinical samples with both fixed and random effects about individual future patients

Specific Scientific Question

In a parallel-group study of two treatments, each patient was measured weekly for 5 weeks. As repeated measures in one patient are more similar than unrepeated ones, a random interaction effect between week and patient was assumed.

Example

In a parallel-group study of two cholesterol reducing compounds, patients were measured weekly for 5 weeks. As repeated measures in one patient are more similar than unrepeated ones, we assumed that a random interaction variable between week and patient would appropriately adjust this effect.

Patient_id	week	hdl-cholesterol (mmol/l)	treatment (0 or 1)
1	1	1,66	0
1	2	1,62	0
1	3	1,57	0
1	4	1,52	0
1	5	1,50	0
2	1	1,69	0

(continued)

This chapter was previously published in "Machine learning in medicine-cookbook 2" as Chap. 9, 2014.

T.J. Cleophas, A.H. Zwinderman, *Machine Learning in Medicine - a Complete Overview*, DOI 10.1007/978-3-319-15195-3_33

Patient_id	week	hdl-cholesterol (mmol/l)	treatment (0 or 1)
2	2	1,71	0
2	3	1,60	0
2	4	1,55	0
2	5	1,56	0

Only the first 2 patients of the data file is shown. The entire file entitled "fixedandrandomeffects" is in extras.springer.com. We will try and develop a mixed model (mixed means a model with both fixed and random predictors) for testing the data. Also, SPSS will be requested to produce a ZIP (compressed file that can be unzipped) file from the intervention study, which could then be used for making predictions about cholesterol values in future patients treated similarly. We will start by opening the intervention study's data file.

Command:

click Transform....click Random Number Generators....click Set Starting Point....click Fixed Value (2000000)....click OK....click Analyze....Mixed Linear....Generalized Mixed Linear Models....click Data Structure....click left mouse and drag patient_id to Subjects part of the canvas....click left mouse and drag week to Repeated Measures part of the canvas....click Fields and Effects....click Target....check that the variable outcome is already in the Target window....check that Linear model is marked....click Fixed Effects....drag treatment and week to Effect builder....click Random Effects.... click Add Block....click Add a custom term....move week*treatment (* is symbol multiplication and interaction) to the Custom term window....click Add term....click OK.... click Model Options....click Save Fields....mark Predicted Values....click Export model.... type exportfixedandrandom....click Browse....in the appropriate folder enter in File name: mixed....click Run.

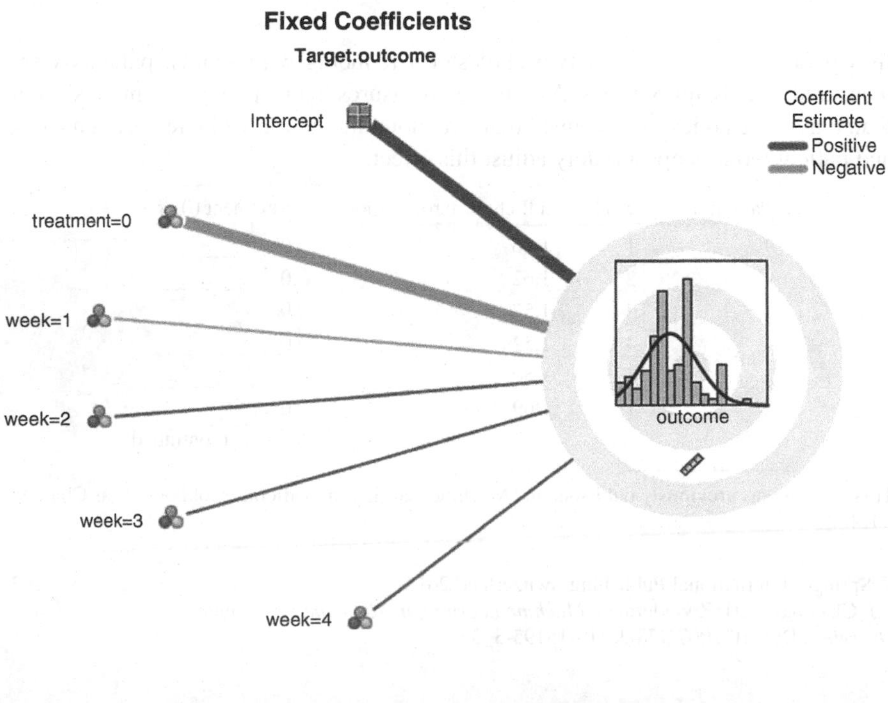

Source	F	df1	df2	Sig.
Corrected model	5,027	5	94	,000
Treatment	23,722	1	94	,000
Week	0,353	4	94	,041

Probability distribution:Normal
Link function:Identity

In the output sheet a graph is observed with the mean and standard errors of the outcome value displayed with the best fit Gaussian curve. The F-value of 23.722 indicates that one treatment is very significantly better than the other with p <0.0001. The thickness of the lines are a measure for level of significance, and so the significance of the 5 week is very thin and thus very weak. Week 5 is not shown. It is redundant, because it means absence of the other 4 weeks. If you click at the left bottom of the graph panel, a table comes up providing similar information in written form. The effect of the interaction variable is not shown, but implied in the analysis.

If we return to the data file page, we will observe that the software has produced a predicted value for each actually measured cholesterol value. The predicted and actual values are very much the same.

We will now use the ZIP file to make predictions about cholesterol values in future patients treated similarly.

week	treatment	patient_id
1	0	21
2	0	21
3	0	21
4	0	21
5	0	21
1	1	22
2	1	22
3	1	22
4	1	22
5	1	22

Command:

click Utilities....click Scoring Wizard....click Browse....click Select....Folder: enter the mixed ZIP file entitled "exportfixedandrandom"....click Select....in Scoring Wizard click Next....click Finish.

In the data file now the predicted cholesterol values are given.

week	treatment	patient_id	predicted cholesterol
1	0	21	1,88
2	0	21	1,96
3	0	21	1,94

(continued)

week	treatment	patient_id	predicted cholesterol
4	0	21	1,91
5	0	21	1,89
1	1	22	2,12
2	1	22	2,20
3	1	22	2,18
4	1	22	2,15
5	1	22	2,13

Conclusion

The module Generalized mixed linear models provides the possibility to handle both fixed and random effects, and is, therefore appropriate to adjust data with repeated measures and presumably a strong correlation between the repeated measures. Also individual future patients treated similarly can be assessed for predicted cholesterol values using a ZIP file.

Note

More background theoretical and mathematical information of models with both fixed and random variables is given in:

1. Machine learning in medicine part one, Chap. 6, Mixed linear models, pp 65–76, 2013,
2. Statistics applied to clinical studies 5th edition, Chap. 56, Advanced analysis of variance, random effects and mixed effects models, pp 607–618, 2012,
3. SPSS for starters part one, Chap. 7, Mixed models, pp 25–29, 2010, and,
4. Machine learning in medicine part three, Chap. 9, Random effects, pp 81–94, 2013.

All of these references are from the same authors and have been edited by Springer Heidelberg Germany.

Chapter 34
Two-Stage Least Squares (35 Patients)

General Purpose

The two stage least squares method assumes that the independent variable (x-variable) is problematic, meaning that it is somewhat uncertain. An additional variable can be argued to provide relevant information about the problematic variable, and is, therefore, called instrumental variable, and included in the analysis.

Primary Scientific Question

Non-compliance is a predictor of drug efficacy. Counseling causes improvement of patients' compliance and, therefore, indirectly improves the outcome drug efficacy.

$$y = \text{outcome variable}\left(\text{drug efficacy}\right)$$
$$x = \text{problematic variable}\left(\text{non}-\text{compliance}\right)$$
$$z = \text{instrumental variable}\left(\text{counseling}\right)$$

With two stage least squares the underneath stages are assessed.

$$1^{st}\ \text{stage}$$
$$x = \text{intercept} + \text{regression coefficient times}\ z$$

This chapter was previously published in "Machine learning in medicine-cookbook 2" as Chap. 10, 2014.

T.J. Cleophas, A.H. Zwinderman, *Machine Learning in Medicine - a Complete Overview*, DOI 10.1007/978-3-319-15195-3_34

With the help of the calculated intercept and regression coefficient from the above simple linear regression analysis improved x-values are calculated, e.g., for patient 1:

$$1^{st}\text{ stage}$$
$$x_{improved} = \text{intercept} + \text{regression coefficient times } 8 = 27.68$$
$$2^{nd}\text{ stage}$$
$$y = \text{intercept} + \text{regression coefficient times } x_{improved}$$

Example

Patients' non-compliance is a factor notoriously affecting the estimation of drug efficacy. An example is given of a simple evaluation study that assesses the effect of non-compliance (pills not used) on the outcome, the efficacy of a novel laxative with numbers of stools per month as efficacy estimator (the y-variable). The data of the first 10 of the 35 patients are in the table below. The entire data file is in extras.springer.com, and is entitled "twostageleastsquares".

Patient no	Instrumental variable (z)	Problematic predictor (x)	Outcome (y)
	Frequency counseling	Pills not used (non-compliance)	Efficacy estimator of new laxative (stools/month)
1.	8	25	24
2.	13	30	30
3.	15	25	25
4.	14	31	35
5.	9	36	39
6.	10	33	30
7.	8	22	27
8.	5	18	14
9.	13	14	39
10.	15	30	42

SPSS version 19 and up can be used for analysis. It uses the term explanatory variable for the problematic variable. Start by opening the data file.

Command:

Analyze….Regression….2 Stage Least Squares….Dependent: therapeutic efficacy….Explanatory: non-compliance…. Instrumental: counseling ….OK.

Model description		
		Type of variable
Equation 1	y	Dependent
	x	Ppredictor
	z	Instrumental

ANOVA						
		Sum of squares	df	Mean square	F	Sig.
Equation 1	Regression	1408,040	1	1408,040	4,429	,043
	Residual	10490,322	33	317,889		
	Total	11898,362	34			

Coefficients						
		Unstandardized coefficients				
		B	Std. Error	Beta	t	Sig.
Equation 1	(Constant)	–49,778	37,634		–1,323	,195
	x	2,675	1,271	1,753	2,105	,043

The result is shown above. The non-compliance adjusted for counseling is a statistically significant predictor of laxative efficacy with p = 0.043. This p-value has been automatically been adjusted for multiple testing. When we test the model without the help of the instrumental variable counseling the p-value is larger and the effect is no more statistically significant as shown underneath.

Command:

Analyze….Regression….Linear….Dependent: therapeutic efficacy ….Independent: non-compliance….OK.

ANOVA[a]						
Model		Sum of squares	df	Mean square	F	Sig.
1	Regression	334,482	1	334,482	3,479	,071[b]
	Residual	3172,489	33	96,136		
	Total	3506,971	34			

[a]Dependent variable: drug efficacy
[b]Predictors: (Constant), non-compliance

Coefficients[a]						
		Unstandardized coefficients		Standardized coefficients		
Model		B	Std. Error	Beta	t	Sig.
1	(Constant)	15,266	7,637		1,999	,054
	Non-compliance	,471	,253	,309	1,865	,071

[a]Dependent variable: drug efficacy

Conclusion

Two stage least squares with counseling as instrumental variable was more sensitive than simple linear regression with laxative efficacy as outcome and non-compliance as predictor. We should add that two stage least squares is at risk of overestimating the precision of the outcome, if the analysis is not adequately adjusted for multiple testing. However, in SPSS automatic adjustment for the purpose has been performed. The example is the simplest version of the procedure. And, multiple explanatory and instrumental variables can be included in the models.

Note

More background theoretical and mathematical information of two stage least squares analyses is given in Machine learning in medicine part two, Two-stage least squares, pp 9–15, Springer Heidelberg Germany, 2013, from the same authors.

Chapter 35
Autoregressive Models for Longitudinal Data (120 Mean Monthly Population Records)

General Purpose

Time series are encountered in every field of medicine. Traditional tests are unable to assess trends, seasonality, change points and the effects of multiple predictors like treatment modalities simultaneously. To assess whether autoregressive integrated moving average (ARIMA) methods are able to do all of that.

Specific Scientific Question

Monthly HbA1c levels in patients with diabetes type II are a good estimator for adequate diabetes control, and have been demonstrated to be seasonal with higher levels in the winter. A large patient population was followed for 10 year. The mean values are in the data. This chapter is to assess whether longitudinal summary statistics of a population can be used for the effects of seasons and treatment changes on populations with chronic diseases.

This chapter was previously published in "Machine learning in medicine-cookbook 2" as Chap. 11, 2014.

T.J. Cleophas, A.H. Zwinderman, *Machine Learning in Medicine - a Complete Overview*, DOI 10.1007/978-3-319-15195-3_35

Note:

No conclusion can here be drawn about individual patients. Autoregressive models can also be applied with data sets of individual patients, and with multiple outcome variables like various health outcomes.

Example

The underneath data are from the first year's observation data of the above diabetic patient data. The entire data file is in extras.springer.com, and is entitled "arimafile".

Date	HbA1	nurse	doctor	phone	self	meeting
01/01/1989	11,00	8,00	7,00	3	22	2
02/01/1989	10,00	8,00	9,00	3	27	2
03/01/1989	17,00	8,00	7,00	2	30	3
04/01/1989	7,00	8,00	9,00	2	29	2
05/01/1989	7,00	9,00	7,00	2	23	2
06/01/1989	10,00	8,00	9,00	3	27	2
07/01/1989	9,00	8,00	8,00	3	27	2
08/01/1989	10,00	8,00	7,00	3	30	2
09/01/1989	12,00	8,00	8,00	4	27	2
10/01/1989	13,00	9,00	11,00	3	32	2
11/01/1989	14,00	9,00	7,00	3	29	2
12/01/1989	23,00	10,00	11,00	5	39	3
01/01/1990	12,00	8,00	7,00	4	23	2
02/01/1990	8,00	8,00	6,00	2	25	3

Date = date of observation,
HbA1 = mean HbA1c of diabetes population,
nurse = mean number of diabetes nurse visits,
doctor = mean number of doctor visits,
phone = mean number of phone visits,
self = mean number of self-controls,
meeting = mean number of patient educational meetings

We will first assess the observed values along the time line. The analysis is performed using SPSS statistical software.

Command:

analyze….Forecast….Sequence Charts….Variables: enter HbA1c….Time Axis Labels: enter Date….OK.

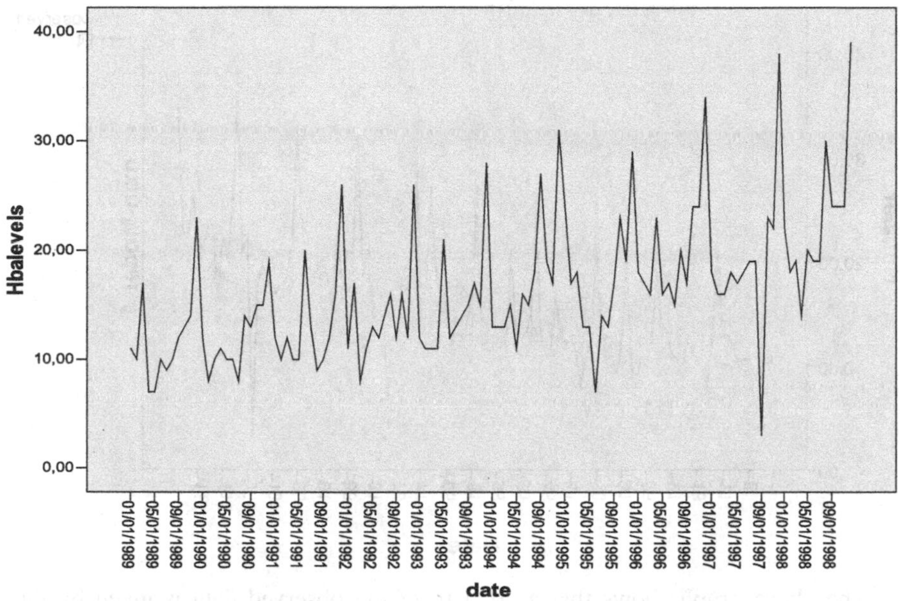

The above output sheets show the observed data. There are (1) numerous peaks, which are (2) approximately equally sized, and (3) there is an upward trend: (2) suggests periodicity which was expected from the seasonal pattern of HbA1c values, (3) is also expected, it suggests increasing HbA1c after several years due to beta-cell failure. Finally (4), there are several peaks that are not part of the seasonal pattern, and could be due to outliers.

ARIMA (autoregressive integrated moving average methodology) is used for modeling this complex data pattern. It uses the Export Modeler for outlier detection, and produces for the purpose XML (eXtended Markup Language) files for prediction modeling of future data.

Command:

Analyze….Forecast….Time Series Modeler….Dependent Variables: enter HbA1c….Independent Variables: enter nurse, doctor, phone, self control, and patient meeting….click Methods: Expert Modeler….click Criteria….Click Outlier Table….Select automatically ….Click Statistics Table….Select Parameter Estimates….mark Display forecasts….click Plots table….click Series, Observed values, Fit values….click Save….Predicted Values: mark Save….Export XML File: click Browse….various folders in your PC come up….in "File Name"of the appropriate folder enter "exportarima"….click Save….click Continue….click OK.

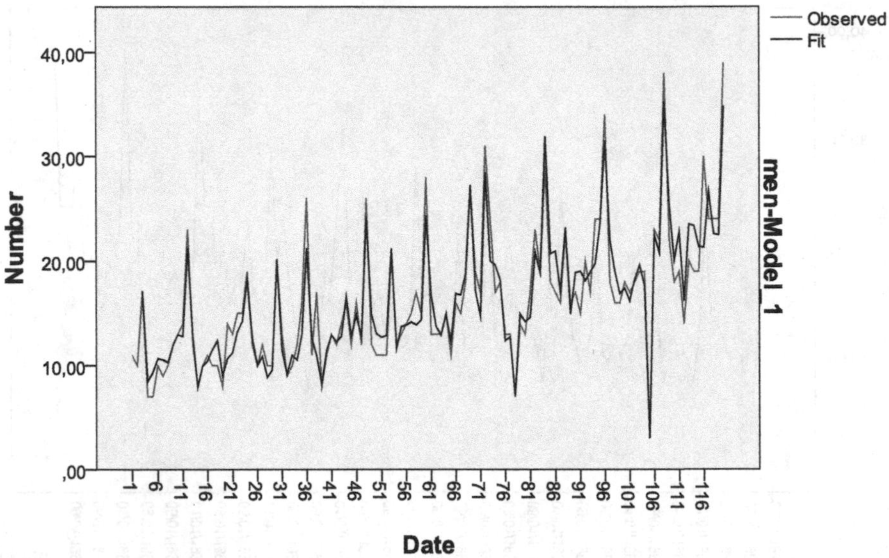

The above graph shows that a good fit of the observed data is given by the ARIMA model, and that an adequate predictive model is provided. The upward trend is in agreement with beta-cell failure after several years.

The underneath table shows that 3 significant predictors have been identified. Also the goodness of fit of the ARIMA (p, d, q) model is given, where p=number of lags, d=the trend (one upward trend means d=1), and q=number of moving averages (=0 here). Both Stationary R square, and Ljung-Box tests are insignificant. A significant test would have meant poor fit. In our example, there is an adequate fit, but the model has identified no less than 7 outliers. Phone visits, nurse visits, and doctor visits were significant predictors at $p<0.0001$, while self control and educational patient meetings were not so. All of the outliers are significantly more distant from the ARIMA model than could happen by chance. All of the p-values were very significant with $p<0.001$ and <0.0001.

Model statistics

Model	Number of predictors	Model Fit statistics	Ljung-BoxQ(18)			Number of outliers
		Stationary R-squared	Statistics	DF	Sig.	
men-Model_1	3	,898	17,761	18	,471	7

ARIMA model parameters

					Estimate	SE	t	Sig.
men-Model_1	men	Natural log	Constant		−2,828	,456	−6,207	,000
	phone	Natural log	Numerator	Lag 0	,569	,064	8,909	,000
	nurse	Natural log	Numerator	Lag 0	1,244	,118	10,585	,000
	doctor	Natural log	Numerator	Lag 0	,310	,077	4,046	,000
				Lag 1	−,257	,116	−2,210	,029
				Lag 2	−,196	,121	−1,616	,109
			Denominator	Lag 1	,190	,304	,623	,535

Outliers						
			Estimate	SE	t	Sig.
men-Model_1	3	Additive	,769	,137	5,620	,000
	30	Additive	,578	,138	4,198	,000
	53	Additive	,439	,135	3,266	,001
	69	Additive	,463	,135	3,439	,001
	78	Additive	–,799	,138	–5,782	,000
	88	Additive	,591	,134	4,409	,000
	105	Additive	–1,771	,134	–13,190	,000

When returning to the data view screen, we will observe that SPSS has added HbA1 values (except for the first two dates due to lack of information) as a novel variable. The predicted values are pretty similar to the measured values, supporting the adequacy of the model.

We will now apply the XML file and the Apply Models modus for making predictions about HbA1 values in the next 6 months, assuming that the significant variables nurse, doctor, phone are kept constant at their overall means.

First add the underneath data to the original data file and rename the file, e.g., "arimafile2", and store it at an appropriate folder in your computer.

Date	HbA1	nurse	doctor	phone	self	meeting
01/01/1999	10,00	8,00	4,00			
01/02/1999	10,00	8,00	4,00			
01/03/1999	10,00	8,00	4,00			
01/04/1999	10,00	8,00	4,00			
01/05/1999	10,00	8,00	4,00			
01/06/1999	10,00	8,00	4,00			

Then open "arimafile2.sav" and command:

Analyze….click Apply Models….click Reestimate from data….click First case after end of estimation period through a specified date….Observation: enter 01/06/1999….click Statistics: click Display Forecasts….click Save: Predicted Values mark Save….click OK.

The underneath table shows the predicted HbA1 values for the next 6 months and their upper and lower confidence limits (UCL and LCL).

Forecast							
Model		121	122	123	124	125	126
HbA1-Model_1	Forecast	17,69	17,30	16,49	16,34	16,31	16,30
	UCL	22,79	22,28	21,24	21,05	21,01	21,00
	LCL	13,49	13,19	12,58	12,46	12,44	12,44

For each model, forecasts start after the last non-missing in the range of the requested estimation period, and end at the last period for which non-missing values of all the predictors are available or at the end date of the requested forecast period, whichever is earlier

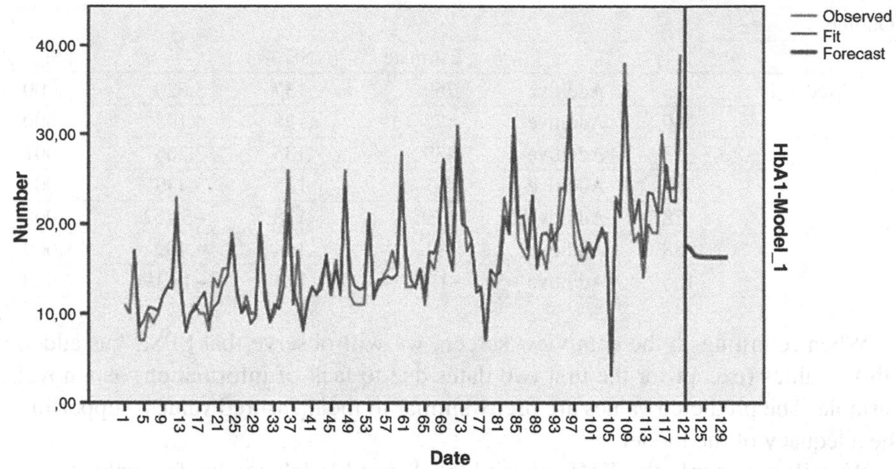

Also a graph of the HbA1 pattern after the estimation period is given as shown in the above graph. When returning to the data view of the arimafile2, we will observe that SPSS has added the predicted values as a novel variable.

Date	HbA1	nurse	doctor	phone	self	meeting	modeled HbA1	predicted HbA1
07/01/1998	19,00	11,00	8,00	5,00	28,00	4,00	21,35	21,35
08/01/1998	30,00	12,00	9,00	4,00	27,00	5,00	21,31	21,31
09/01/1998	24,00	13,00	8,00	5,00	30,00	5,00	26,65	26,65
10/01/1998	24,00	12,00	10,00	4,00	28,00	6,00	22,59	22,59
11/01/1998	24,00	11,00	8,00	5,00	26,00	5,00	22,49	22,49
12/01/1998	39,00	15,00	10,00	5,00	37,00	7,00	34,81	34,81
01/01/1999		10,00	8,00	4,00				17,69
01/02/1999		10,00	8,00	4,00				17,30
01/03/1999		10,00	8,00	4,00				16,49
01/04/1999		10,00	8,00	4,00				16,34
01/05/1999		10,00	8,00	4,00				16,31
01/06/1999		10,00	8,00	4,00				16,30

modeled HbA1 = calculated HbA1 values from the above arima model
Predicted HbA1 = the predicted HbA1 values using the XML file for future dates.

Conclusion

Autoregressive integrated moving average methods are appropriate for assessing trends, seasonality, and change points in a time series. In the example given no conclusion can be drawn about individual patients. Autoregressive models can, however, also be applied for data sets of individual patients. Also as a multivariate methodology it is appropriate for multiple instead of a single outcome variable like various health outcomes.

Note

More background theoretical and mathematical information of autoregressive models for longitudinal data is in Machine learning in medicine part two, Multivariate analysis of time series, pp 139–154, Springer Heidelberg Germany, 2013, from the same authors.

Chapter 36
Variance Components for Assessing the Magnitude of Random Effects (40 Patients)

General Purpose

If we have reasons to believe that in a study certain patients due to co-mobidity, co-medication and other factors will respond differently from others, then the spread in the data is caused not only by residual effect, but also by some subgroup property, otherwise called some random effect. Variance components analysis is able to assess the magnitudes of random effects as compared to that of the residual error of a study.

Primary Scientific Question

Can a variance components analysis by including the random effect in the analysis reduce the unexplained variance in a study, and, thus, increase the accuracy of the analysis model as used.

This chapter was previously published in "Machine learning in medicine-cookbook 3" as Chap. 3, 2014.

T.J. Cleophas, A.H. Zwinderman, *Machine Learning in Medicine - a Complete Overview*, DOI 10.1007/978-3-319-15195-3_36

Example

Variables

PAT	treat	gender	cad
52,00	,00	,00	2,00
48,00	,00	,00	2,00
43,00	,00	,00	1,00
50,00	,00	,00	2,00
43,00	,00	,00	2,00
44,00	,00	,00	1,00
46,00	,00	,00	2,00
46,00	,00	,00	2,00
43,00	,00	,00	1,00
49,00	,00	,00	2,00
28,00	1,00	,00	1,00
35,00	1,00	,00	2,00

PAT = episodes of paroxysmal atrial tachycardias
treat = treatment modality (0 = placebo treatment, 1 = active treatment)
gender = gender (0 = female)
cad = presence of coronary artery disease (1 no, 2 = yes)

The first 12 of a 40 patient parallel-group study of the treatment of paroxysmal tachycardia with numbers of episodes of PAT as outcome is given above. The entire data file is in "variancecomponents", and is available at extras.springer.com. We had reason to believe that the presence of coronary artery disease would affect the outcome, and, therefore, used this variable as a random rather than fixed variable. SPSS statistical software was used for data analysis. Start by opening the data file in SPSS.

Command:

Analyze....General Linear Model....Variance Components....Dependent Variable: enter "paroxtachyc"....Fixed Factor(s): enter "treat, gender"....Random Factor(s): enter "corartdisease"....Model: mark Custom....Model: enter "treat, gender, cad".... click Continue....click Options....mark ANOVA....mark Type III....mark Sums of squares....mark Expected mean squares....click Continue....click OK.

The output sheets are given underneath. The Variance Estimate table gives the magnitude of the Variance due to cad, and that due to residual error (unexplained variance, otherwise called Error). The ratio of the Var (cad)/[Var (Error) + Var (cad)] gives the proportion of variance in the data due to the random cad effect (5.844/(28 .426 + 5.844) = 0.206 = 20.6 %). This means that 79.4 % instead of 100 % of the error is now unexplained.

Variance estimates	
Component	Estimate
Var(cad)	5,844
Var(Error)	28,426

Dependent variable: paroxtach
Method: ANOVA (Type III sum of squares)

The underneath ANOVA table gives the sums of squares and mean squares of different effects. E.g. the mean square of cad = 139.469, and that of residual effect = 28.426.

ANOVA			
Source	Type III sum of squares	df	Mean square
Corrected model	727,069	3	242,356
Intercept	57153,600	1	57153,600
treat	515,403	1	515,403
gender	,524	1	,524
cad	139,469	1	139,469
Error	1023,331	36	28,426
Total	58904,000	40	
Corrected total	1750,400	39	

Dependent variable: paroxtach

The underneath Expected Mean Squares table gives the results of a special procedure, whereby variances of best fit quadratic functions of the variables are minimized to obtain the best unbiased estimate of the variance components. A little mental arithmetic is now required.

Expected mean squares			
	Variance component		
Source	Var(cad)	Var(Error)	Quadratic term
Intercept	20,000	1,000	Intercept, treat, gender
treat	,000	1,000	treat
gender	,000	1,000	gender
cad	19,000	1,000	
Error	,000	1,000	

Dependent variable: paroxtach
Expected mean squares are based on Type III sums of squares
For each source, the expected mean square equals the sum of the coefficients in the cells times the variance components, plus a quadratic term involving effects in the Quadratic Term cell

$$\begin{aligned}
&\text{EMS}(\text{expected mean square})\text{ of cad}(\text{the random effect})\\
&\qquad = 19 \times \text{Variance}(\text{cad}) + \text{Variance}(\text{Error})\\
&\qquad = 139.469\\
&\text{EMS of Error}(\text{the residual effect})\\
&\qquad = 0 + \text{Variance}(\text{Error})\\
&\qquad = 28.426\\
&\text{EMS of cad} \quad \text{Variance}(\text{Error})\\
&\qquad = 19 \times \text{Variance}(\text{cad})\\
&\qquad = 139.469 - 28.426\\
&\qquad = 110.043\\
&\text{Variance}(\text{cad})\\
&\qquad = 110.043/19\\
&\qquad = 5.844(\text{compare with the results of the above Variance Estimates table})
\end{aligned}$$

It can, thus, be concluded that around 20 % of the uncertainty is in the data is caused by the random effect.

Conclusion

If we have reasons to believe that in a study certain patients due to co-mobidity, co-medication and other factors will respond differently from others, then the spread in the data will be caused, not only by the residual effect, but also by the subgroup property, otherwise called the random effect. Variance components analysis, by including the random effect in the analysis, reduces the unexplained variance in a study, and, thus, increases the accuracy of the analysis model used.

Note

More background, theoretical and mathematical information of random effects models are given in Machine learning in medicine part three, Chap. 9, Random effects, pp 81–94, 2013, Springer Heidelberg Germany, from the same authors.

Chapter 37
Ordinal Scaling for Clinical Scores with Inconsistent Intervals (900 Patients)

General Purpose

Clinical studies often have categories as outcome, like various levels of health or disease. Multinomial regression is suitable for analysis (see Chap. 28). However, if one or two outcome categories in a study are severely underpresented, multinomial regression is flawed, and ordinal regression including specific link functions may provide a better fit for the data.

Primary Scientific Questions

This chapter is to assess how ordinal regression performs in studies where clinical scores have inconsistent intervals.

Example

In 900 patients the independent predictors for different degrees of feeling healthy were assessed. The predictors included were:

Variable	2	fruit consumption (times per week)
	3	unhealthy snacks (times per week)
	4	fastfood consumption (times per week)
	5	physical activities (times per week)
	6	age (number of years).

This chapter was previously published in "Machine learning in medicine-cookbook 3"as Chap. 4, 2014.

T.J. Cleophas, A.H. Zwinderman, *Machine Learning in Medicine - a Complete Overview*, DOI 10.1007/978-3-319-15195-3_37

Feeling healthy (Variable 1) was assessed as mutually elusive categories:

1 very much so
2 much so
3 not entirely so
4 not so
5 not so at all.

Underneath are the first 10 patients of the data file. The entire data file is in extras.springer.com, and is entitled "ordinalscaling".

Variables					
1	2	3	4	5	6
4	6	9	12	6	34
4	7	24	3	6	35
4	3	5	9	6	30
4	5	14	6	3	36
4	9	9	12	12	62
2	2	3	3	6	31
3	3	26	6	3	57
5	9	38	6	6	36
4	5	8	9	6	28
5	9	25	12	12	28

First, we will perform a multinomial regression analysis using SPSS statistical software. Open the data file in SPSS.

Command:

Analyze....Regression....Multinomial Logistic Regression....Dependent: enter feeling healthy....Covariates: enter fruitt/week, snacks.week, fastfood/week, physicalactivities/week, age in years....click OK.

Parameter estimates

								95 % Confidence interval for Exp (B)	
feeling healthy[a]		B	Std. Error	Wald	df	Sig.	Exp(B)	Lower bound	Upper bound
very much so	Intercept	−1,252	,906	1,912	1	,167			
	fruit	,149	,069	4,592	1	,032	1,161	1,013	1,330
	snacks	,020	,017	1,415	1	,234	1,020	,987	1,055
	fastfood	−,079	,057	1,904	1	,168	,924	,827	1,034
	physical	−,013	,056	,059	1	,809	,987	,885	1,100
	age	−,027	,017	2,489	1	,115	,974	,942	1,007

(continued)

Parameter estimates

								95 % Confidence interval for Exp (B)	
feeling healthy[a]		B	Std. Error	Wald	df	Sig.	Exp(B)	Lower bound	Upper bound
much so	Intercept	−2,087	,863	5,853	1	,016			
	fruit	,108	,071	2,302	1	,129	1,114	,969	1,280
	snacks	−.001	,019	,004	1	,950	,999	,962	1,037
	fastfood	,026	,057	,212	1	,645	1,026	,919	1,147
	physical	−,005	,051	,009	1	,925	,995	,900	1,101
	age	−.010	,014	,522	1	,470	,990	,962	1,018
not entirely so	Intercept	2,161	,418	26,735	1	,000			
	fruit	,045	,039	1,345	1	,246	1,046	,969	1,130
	snacks	−,012	,011	1,310	1	,252	,988	,968	1,009
	fastfood	−,037	,027	1,863	1	,172	,964	,914	1,016
	physical	−,040	,025	2,518	1	,113	,961	,914	1,010
	age	−.028	,007	14,738	1	,000	,972	,959	,986
no so	Intercept	,781	,529	2,181	1	,140			
	fruit	,100	,046	4,600	1	,032	1,105	1,009	1,210
	snacks	−,001	,012	,006	1	,939	,999	,975	1,024
	fastfood	−,038	,034	1,225	1	,268	,963	,901	1,029
	physical	−,037	,032	1,359	1	,244	,963	,905	1,026
	age	−,028	,010	8,651	1	,003	,972	,954	,991

[a]The reference category is: not so at all

The above table gives the analysis results. Twenty-four p-values are produced, and a few of them are statistically significant at $p<0.05$. For example, per fruit unit you may have 1.161 times more chance of feeling very healthy versus not healthy at all at $p=0.032$. And per year of age you may have 0.972 times less chance of feeling not entirely healthy versus not healthy at all at $p=0.0001$. We should add that the few significant p-values among the many insignificant ones could easily be due to type I errors (due to multiple testing). Also a flawed analysis due to inconsistent intervals has not yet been excluded. To assess this point a graph will be drawn.

Command:

Graphs....Legacy Dialogs....Bar....click Simple....mark Summary for groups of cases....click Define....Category Axis: enter "feeling healthy"....click OK.

The underneath graph is in the output sheet. It shows that, particularly the categories 1 and 2 are severily underpresented. Ordinal regression analysis with a complimentary log-log function gives little weight to small counts, and more weight to large counts, and may, therefore, better fit these data.

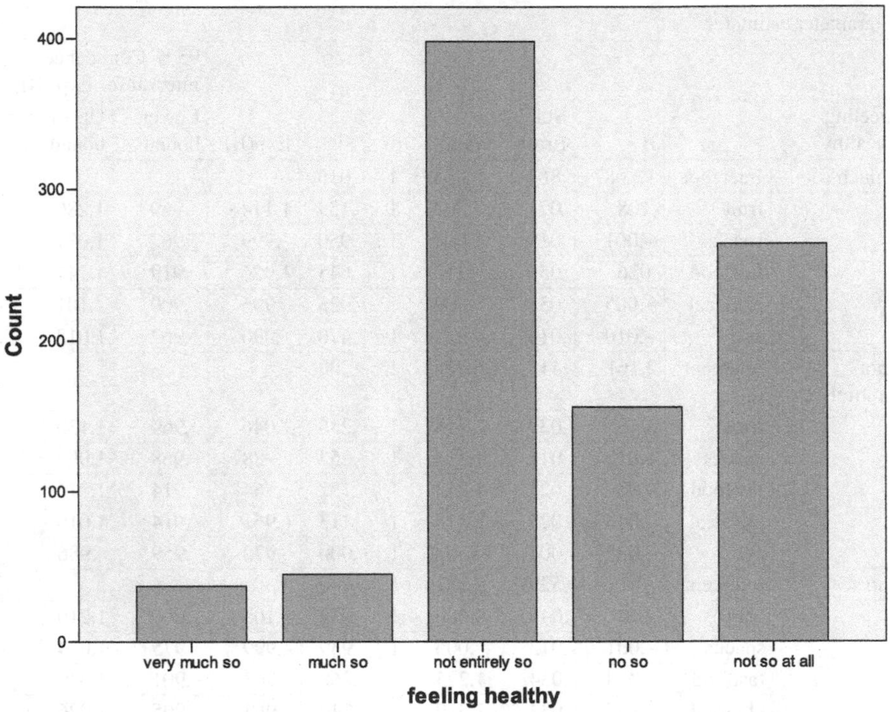

Command:

Analyze....Regression....Ordinal Regression....Dependent: enter feeling healthy.... Covariates: enter fruit/week, snacks.week, fastfood/week, physicalactivities/week, age in years....click Options....Link: click Complementary Log-log....click Continue....click OK.

Model fitting information

Model	–2 Log Likelihood	Chi-Square	df	Sig.
Intercept only	2349,631			
Final	2321,863	27,768	5	,000

Link function: Complementary Log-log

In the output sheets the model fitting table shows that the ordinal model provides an excellent fit for the data.

Parameter estimates								
		Estimate	Std. Error	Wald	df	Sig.	95 % Confidence interval Lower bound	Upper bound
Threshold	[feelinghealthy=1]	−2,427	,259	87,865	1	,000	−2,935	−1,920
	[feelinghealthy=2]	−1,605	,229	49,229	1	,000	−2,053	−1,156
	[feelinghealthy=3]	,483	,208	5,414	1	,020	,076	,890
	[feelinghealthy=4]	,971	,208	21,821	1	,000	,564	1,379
Location	fruit	−,036	,018	3,907	1	,048	−,072	,000
	snacks	,004	,005	,494	1	,482	−,006	,013
	fastfood	,017	,013	1,576	1	,209	−,009	,042
	physical	,017	,012	1,772	1	,183	−,008	,041
	age	,015	,004	15,393	1	,000	,008	,023

Link function: Complementary Log-log

The above table is also shown, and indicates that fruit and age are significant predictors of levels of feeling healthy. The less fruit/week, the more chance of feeling healthy versus not health at all (p=0.048), the higher the age the more chance of feeling healthy versus not healthy at all (p=0.0001).

Conclusion

Clinical studies often have categories as outcome, like various levels of health or disease. Multinomial regression is suitable for analysis, but, if one or two outcome categories in a study are severely underpresented, ordinal regression including specific link functions may better fit the data. The current chapter also shows that, unlike multinomial regression, ordinal regression tests the outcome categories as an overall function.

Note

More background, theoretical and mathematical information of multinomial regression is given in the Chap. 28.

Chapter 38
Loglinear Models for Assessing Incident Rates with Varying Incident Risks (12 Populations)

General Purpose

Data files that assess the effect of various predictors on frequency counts of morbidities/mortalities can be classified into multiple cells with varying incident risks (like, e.g., the incident risk of infarction). The underneath table gives an example:

In patients at risk of infarction with little soft drink consumption, and consumption of wine and other alcoholic beverages the incident risk of infarction equals 240/930 = 24.2 %, in those with lots of soft drinks, no wine, and no alcohol otherwise it is 285/1043 = 27.3 %.

soft drink (1 = little)	wine (0 = no)	alc beverages (0 = no)	infarcts number	Population number
1,00	1,00	1,00	240	993
1,00	1,00	,00	237	998
2,00	1,00	1,00	236	1016
2,00	1,00	,00	236	1011
3,00	1,00	1,00	221	1004
3,00	1,00	,00	221	1003
1,00	,00	1,00	270	939
1,00	,00	,00	269	940
2,00	,00	1,00	274	979
2,00	,00	,00	273	966
3,00	,00	1,00	284	1041
3,00	,00	,00	285	1043

This chapter was previously published in "Machine learning in medicine-cookbook 3" as Chap. 5, 2014.

T.J. Cleophas, A.H. Zwinderman, *Machine Learning in Medicine - a Complete Overview*, DOI 10.1007/978-3-319-15195-3_38

The general loglinear model using Poisson distributions (see Statistics applied to clinical studies 5th edition, Chap. 23, Poisson regression, pp 267–275, Springer Heidelberg Germany, 2012, from the same authors) is an appropriate method for statistical testing. This chapter is to assess this method, frequently used by banks and insurance companies but little by clinicians so far.

Primary Scientific Question

Can general loglinear modeling identify subgroups with significantly larger incident risks than other subgroups.

Example

The example in the above table will be applied. We wish to investigate the effect of soft drink, wine, and other alcoholic beverages on the risk of infarction. The data file is in extras.springer.com, and is entitled "loglinear". Start by opening the file in SPSS statistical software.

Command:

Analyze....Loglinear ....General Loglinear Analysis....Factor(s): enter softdrink, wine, other alc beverages....click "Data" in the upper textrow of your screen....click Weigh Cases....mark Weight cases by....Frequency Variable: enter "infarcts"....click OK....return to General Loglinear Analysis....Cell structure: enter "population".... Options ....mark Estimates....click Continue....Distribution of Cell Counts: mark Poisson....click OK.

Parameter estimates[a,b]

					95 % Confidence interval	
Parameter	Estimate	Std. Error	Z	Sig.	Lower bound	Upper bound
Constant	–1,513	,067	–22,496	,000	–1,645	–1,381
[softdrink=1,00]	,095	,093	1,021	,307	–,088	,278
[softdrink=2,00]	,053	,094	,569	,569	–,130	,237
[softdrink=3,00]	0[c]					
[wine=,00]	,215	,090	2,403	,016	,040	,391
[wine=1,00]	0[c]					
[alcbeverages=,00]	,003	,095	,029	,977	–,184	,189
[alcbeverages=1,00]	0[c]					
[softdrink=1,00] * [wine=,00]	–,043	,126	–,345	,730	–,291	,204
[softdrink=1,00] * [wine=1,00]	0[c]					
[softdrink=2,00] * [wine=,00]	–,026	,126	–,209	,834	–,274	,221
[softdrink=2,00] * [wine=1,00]	0[c]					

(continued)

Parameter estimates[a,b]

Parameter	Estimate	Std. Error	Z	Sig.	95 % Confidence interval Lower bound	Upper bound
[softdrink=3,00] * [wine=,00]	0[c]					
[softdrink=3,00] * [wine=1,00]	0[c]					
[softdrink=1,00] * [alcbeverages=,00]	–,021	,132	–,161	,872	–,280	,237
[softdrink=1,00] * [alcbeverages=1,00]	0[c]					
[softdrink=2,00] * [alcbeverages=,00]	,003	,132	,024	,981	–,256	,262
[softdrink=2,00] * [alcbeverages=1,00]	0[c]					
[softdrink=3,00] * [alcbeverages=,00]	0[c]					
[softdrink=3,00] * [alcbeverages=1,00]	0[c]					
[wine=,00] * [alcbeverages=,00]	–,002	,127	–,018	,986	–,251	,246
[wine=,00] * [alcbeverages=1,00]	0[c]					
[wine=1,00] * [alcbeverages=,00]	0[c]					
[wine=1,00] * [alcbeverages=1,00]	0[c]					
[softdrink=1,00] * [wine=,00] * [alcbeverages=,00]	,016	,178	,089	,929	–,334	,366
[softdrink=1,00] * [wine=,00] * [alcbeverages=1,00]	0[c]					
[softdrink=1,00] * [wine=1,00] * [alcbeverages=,00]	0[c]					
[softdrink=1,00] * [wine=1,0] * [alcbeverages=1,00]	0[c]					
[softdrink=2,00] * [winc=,00] * [alcbeverages=,00]	,006	,178	,036	,971	–,343	,356
[softdrink=2,00] * [wine=,00] * [alcbeverages=1,00]	0[c]					
[softdrink=2,00] * [wine=1,00] * [alcbeverages=,00]	0[c]					
[softdrink=2,00] * [wine=1,0]* [alcbeverages=1,00]	0[c]					
[softdrink=3,00] * [wine=,00] * [alcbeverages=,00]	0[c]					
[softdrink=3,00] * [wine=,00] * [alcbeverages=1,00]	0[c]					
[softdrink=3,00] * [wine=1,00] * [alcbeverages=,00]	0[c]					
[softdrink=3,00] * [wine=1,0] * [alcbeverages=1,00]	0[c]					

[a]Model: Poisson

[b]Design: Constant + softdrink + wine + alcbeverages + softdrink * wine + softdrink * alcbeverages + wine * alcbeverages + softdrink * wine * alcbeverages

[c]This parameter is set to zero because it is redundant

The above pretty dull table gives some wonderful information. The soft drink classes 1 and 2 are not significantly different from zero. These classes have, thus, no greater risk of infarction than class 3. However, the regression coefficient of no wine is greater than zero at $p = 0.016$. No wine drinkers have a significantly greater risk of infarction than the wine drinkers have. No "other alcoholic beverages" did not protect from infarction better than the consumption of it. The three predictors did not display any interaction effects. This result would be in agreement with the famous French paradox.

Conclusion

Data files that assess the effect of various predictors on frequency counts of morbidities/mortalities can be classified into multiple cells with varying incident risks (like, e.g., the incident risk of infarction). The general loglinear model using Poisson distributions is an appropriate method for statistical testing. It can identify subgroups with significantly larger incident risks than other subgroups.

Note

More background, theoretical and mathematical information Poisson regression is given in Statistics applied to clinical studies 5th edition, Chap. 23, Poisson regression, pp 267–275, Springer Heidelberg Germany, 2012, from the same authors.

Chapter 39
Loglinear Modeling for Outcome Categories (445 Patients)

General Purpose

Multinomial regression is adequate for identifying the main predictors of certain outcome categories, like different levels of injury or quality of life (QOL) (see also Chap. 28). An alternative approach is logit loglinear modeling. The latter method does not use continuous predictors on a case by case basis, but rather the weighted means of these predictors. This approach may allow for relevant additional conclusions from your data.

Primary Scientific Question

Does logit loglinear modeling allow for relevant additional conclusions from your categorical data as compared to polytomous / multinomial regression?

This chapter was previously published in "Machine learning in medicine-cookbook 3" as Chap. 6, 2014.

T.J. Cleophas, A.H. Zwinderman, *Machine Learning in Medicine - a Complete Overview*, DOI 10.1007/978-3-319-15195-3_39

Example

age	gender	married	lifestyle	qol
55	1	0	0	2
32	1	1	1	2
27	1	1	0	1
77	0	1	0	3
34	1	1	0	1
35	1	0	1	1
57	1	1	1	2
57	1	1	1	2
35	0	0	0	1
42	1	1	0	2
30	0	1	0	3
34	0	1	1	1

Variable
1 age (years)
2 gender (0=female)
3 married (0=no)
4 lifestyle (0=poor)
5 qol (quality of life levels 0=low, 2=high)

The above table show the data of the first 12 patiens of a 445 patient data file of qol (quality of life) levels and patient characteristics. The characteristics are the predictor variables of the qol levels (the outcome variable). The entire data file is in extras.springer.com, and is entitled "logitloglinear". We will first perform a traditional polynomial regression and then the logit loglinear model. SPSS statistical is used for analysis. Start by opening SPSS, and entering the data file.

Command:

Analyze....Regression....Multinomial Logistic Regression....Dependent: enter "qol"....Factor(s): enter "gender, married, lifestyle"....Covariate(s): enter "age"....OK.

The underneath table shows the main results. The following conclusions are appropriate.

Parameter estimates

qol[a]		B	Std. Error	Wald	df	Sig.	Exp(B)	95 % Confidence interval for Exp (B) Lower bound	Upper bound
Low	Intercept	28,027	2,539	121,826	1	,000			
	age	–,559	,047	143,158	1	,000	,572	,522	,626
	[gender=0]	,080	,508	,025	1	,875	1,083	,400	2,930
	[gender=1]	0[b]			0				
	[married=0]	2,081	,541	14,784	1	,000	8,011	2,774	23,140
	[married=1]	0[b]			0				
	[lifestyle=0]	–,801	,513	2,432	1	,119	,449	,164	1,228
	[lifestyle=1]	0[b]			0				
Medium	Intercept	20,133	2,329	74,743	1	,000			
	age	–,355	,040	79,904	1	,000	,701	,649	,758
	[gender=0]	,306	,372	,674	1	,412	1,358	,654	2,817
	[gender=1]	0[b]			0				
	[married=0]	,612	,394	2,406	1	,121	1,843	,851	3,992
	[married=1]	0[b]			0				
	[lifestyle=0]	–,014	,382	,001	1	,972	,987	,466	2,088
	[lifestyle=1]	0[b]			0				

[a]The reference category is: high
[b]This parameter is set to zero because it is redundant

1. The unmarried subjects have a greater chance of QOL level 0 than the married ones (the b-value is positive here).
2. The higher the age, the less chance of QOL levels 0 and 1 (the b-values are negative here). If you wish, you may also report the odds ratios (Exp (B).

   We will now perform a logit loglinear analysis.

Command:

Analyze.... Loglinear....Logit....Dependent: enter "qol"....Factor(s): enter "gender, married, lifestyle"....Cell Covariate(s): enter: "age"....Model: Terms in Model: enter: "gender, married, lifestyle, age"....click Continue....click Options....mark Estimates....mark Adjusted residuals....mark normal probabilities for adjusted residuals....click Continue....click OK.

The underneath table shows the observed frequencies per cell, and the frequencies to be expected, if the predictors had no effect on the outcome.

Cell counts and residuals[a,b]

Gender	Married	Lifestyle	qol	Observed		Expected		Residual	Standardized residual	Adjusted residual	Deviance
				Count	%	Count	%				
Male	Unmarried	Inactive	Low	7	23,3 %	9,111	30,4 %	−2,111	−,838	−1,125	−1,921
			Medium	16	53,3 %	14,124	47,1 %	1,876	,686	,888	1,998
			High	7	23,3 %	6,765	22,6 %	,235	,103	,127	,691
		Active	Low	29	61,7 %	25,840	55,0 %	3,160	,927	2,018	2,587
			Medium	5	10,6 %	10,087	21,5 %	−5,087	−1,807	−2,933	−2,649
			High	13	27,7 %	11,074	23,6 %	1,926	,662	2,019	2,042
	Married	Inactive	Low	9	11,0 %	10,636	13,0 %	−1,636	−,538	−,826	−1,734
			Medium	41	50,0 %	43,454	53,0 %	−2,454	−,543	−1,062	−2,183
			High	32	39,0 %	27,910	34,0 %	4,090	,953	2,006	2,958
		Active	Low	15	23,8 %	14,413	22,9 %	,587	,176	,754	1,094
			Medium	27	42,9 %	21,336	33,9 %	5,664	1,508	2,761	3,566
			High	21	33,3 %	27,251	43,3 %	−6,251	−1,590	−2,868	−3,308
Female	Unmarried	Inactive	Low	12	26,1 %	11,119	24,2 %	,881	,303	,627	1,353
			Medium	26	56,5 %	22,991	50,0 %	3,009	,887	1,601	2,529
			High	8	17,4 %	11,890	25,8 %	−3,690	−1,310	−1,994	−2,518
		Active	Low	18	54,5 %	19,930	60,4 %	−1,930	−,687	−,978	−1,915
			Medium	6	18,2 %	5,799	17,6 %	,201	,092	,138	,639
			High	9	27,3 %	7,271	22,0 %	1,729	,726	1,064	1,959
	Married	Inactive	Low	15	18,5 %	12,134	15,0 %	2,866	,892	1,670	2,522
			Medium	27	33,3 %	29,432	36,3 %	−2,432	−,562	−1,781	−2,158
			High	39	48,1 %	39,434	48,7 %	−,434	−,097	−,358	−,929
		Active	Low	16	25,4 %	17,817	28,3 %	−1,817	−,508	−1,123	−1,855
			Medium	24	38,1 %	24,779	39,3 %	−,779	−,201	−,882	−1,238
			High	23	36,5 %	20,404	32,4 %	2,596	,699	1,407	2,347

[a]Model: Multinomial logit

[b]Design: Constant + qol + qol * gender + qol * married + qol * lifestyle + qol * age

The two graphs below show the goodnesses of fit of the model, which are obviously pretty good, as both expected versus observed counts (first graph below) and q-q plot (second graph below) show excellent linear relationships (q-q plots are further explained in Chap. 42).

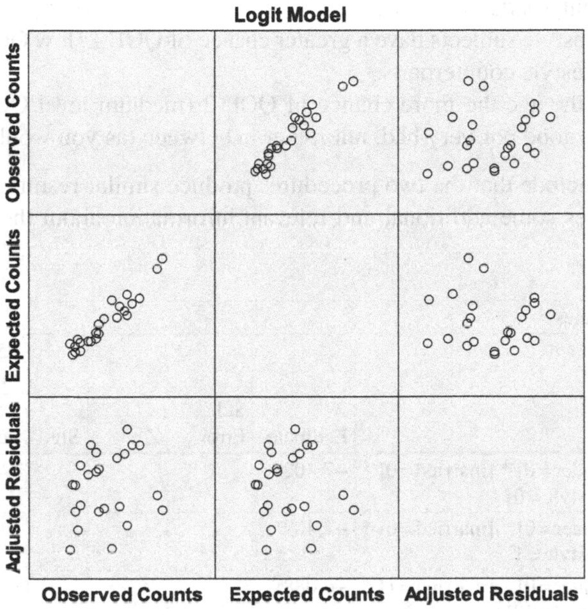

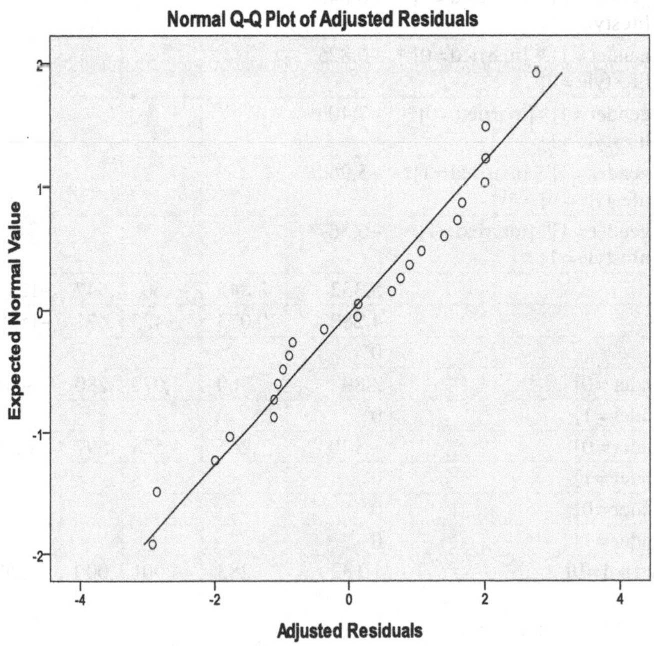

Note: the Q-Q plot (Q stands for quantile) shows here that the differences between observed and expected counts follow a normal distribution.

The next page table shows the results of the statistical tests of the data.

1. The unmarried subjects have a greater chance of QOL 1 (low QOL) than their married counterparts.
2. The poor lifestyle subjects have a greater chance of QOL 1 (low QOL) than their adequate-lifestyle counterparts.
3. The higher the age the more chance of QOL 2 (medium level QOL), which is neither very good nor very bad, nut rather in between (as you would expect).

We may conclude that the two procedures produce similar results, but the latter method provides some additional and relevant information about the lifestyle and age data.

Parameter estimates[c,d]

Parameter		Estimate	Std. Error	Z	Slg.	95 % Confidence interval Lower bound	Upper bound
Constant	[gender=0] * [married=0] * [lifestyle=0]	−7,402[a]					
	[gender=0] * [married=0] * [lifestyle=1]	−7,409[a]					
	[gender=0] * [married=1] * [lifestyle=0]	−6,088[a]					
	[gender=0] * [married=1]* [lifestyle=1]	−6,349[a]					
	[gender=1] * [married=0] * [lifestyle=0]	−6,825[a]					
	[gender=1]* [married=0]* [lifestyle=1]	−7,406[a]					
	[gender=1] * [married=1]* [lifestyle=0]	−5,960[a]					
	[gender=1]* [married=1]* [lifestyle=1]	−6,567[a]					
[qol=1]		5,332	8,845	,603	,547	−12,004	22,667
[qol=2]		4,280	10,073	,425	,671	−15,463	24,022
[qol=3]		0[b]					
[qol=1]* [gender=0]		,389	,360	1,079	,280	−,317	1,095
[qol=1]* [gender=1]		0[b]					
[qol=2]* [gender=0]		−,140	,265	−,528	,597	−,660	,380
[qol=2]* [gender=1]		0[b]					
[qol=3]* [gender=0]		0[b]					
[qol=3]* [gender=1]		0[b]					
[qol=1]* [married=0]		1,132	,283	4,001	,000	,578	1,687

(continued)

Parameter estimates[c,d]							
						95 % Confidence interval	
Parameter		Estimate	Std. Error	Z	Slg.	Lower bound	Upper bound
[qol=1]* [married=1]		0[b]					
[qol=2] * [married=0]		–,078	,294	–,267	,790	–,655	,498
[qol=2] * [married=1]		0[b]					
[qol=3] * [married=0]		0[b]					
[qol=3] * [married=1]		0[b]					
[qol=1]* [lifestyle=0]		–1,004	,311	–3,229	,001	–1,613	–,394
[qol=1] * [lifestyle=1]		0[b]					
[qol=2]* [lifestyle=0]		,016	,271	,059	,953	–,515	,547
[qol=2]* [lifestyle=1]		0[b]					
[qol=3]* [lifestyle=0]		0[b]					
[qol=3]* [lifestyle=1]		0[b]					
[qol=1] * age		,116	,074	1,561	,119	–,030	,261
[qol=2]* age		,114	,054	2,115	,034	,008	,219
[qol=3]* age		,149	,138	1,075	,282	–,122	,419

[a]Constants are not parameters under the multinomial assumption. Therefore, their standard errors are not calculated

[b]This parameter is set to zero because it is redundant

[c]Model: Multinomial logit

[d]Design: Constant + qol + qol * gender + qol * married + qol * lifestyle + qol * age

Conclusion

Multinomial regression is adequate for identifying the main predictors of certain outcome categories, like different levels of injury or quality of life An alternative approach is logit loglinear modeling. The latter method does not use continuous predictors on a case by case basis, but rather the weighted means. This approach allowed for relevant additional conclusions in the example given.

Note

More background, theoretical and mathematical information of polytomous/multinomial regression is given in the Chap. 28. More information of loglinear modeling is in the Chap. 38, entitled "Loglinear models for assessing incident rates with varying incident risks".

Chapter 40
Heterogeneity in Clinical Research: Mechanisms Responsible (20 Studies)

General Purpose

In clinical research similar studies often have different results. This may be due to differences in patient-characteristics and trial-quality-characteristics such as the use of blinding, randomization, and placebo-controls. This chapter is to assess whether 3-dimensional scatter plots and regression analyses with the treatment results as outcome and the predictors of heterogeneity as exposure are able to identify mechanisms responsible.

Primary Scientific Question

Are scatter plots and regression models able to identify the mechanisms responsible for heterogeneity in clinical research.

This chapter was previously published in "Machine learning in medicine-cookbook 3" as Chap. 7, 2014.

T.J. Cleophas, A.H. Zwinderman, *Machine Learning in Medicine - a Complete Overview*, DOI 10.1007/978-3-319-15195-3_40

Example

Variables			
1	2	3	4
% ADEs	study size	age	investigator type
21,00	106	1	1
14,40	578	1	1
30,40	240	1	1
6,10	671	0	0
12,00	681	0	0
3,40	28411	1	0
6,60	347	0	0
3,30	8601	0	0
4,90	915	0	0
9,60	156	0	0
6,50	4093	0	0
6,50	18820	0	0
4,10	6383	0	0
4,30	2933	0	0
3,50	480	0	0
4,30	19070	1	0
12,60	2169	1	0
33,20	2261	0	1
5,60	12793	0	0
5,10	355	0	0

ADEs = adverse drug effects
age 0 = young, 1 = elderly
investigator type, 0 = pharmacists, 1 = clinicians

In the above 20 studies the % of admissions to hospital due to adverse drug effects were assessed. The studies were very heterogeneous, because the percentages admissions due to adverse drug effects varied from 3.3 to 33.2. In order to identify possible mechanisms responsible, a scatter plot was first drawn. The data file is in extras.springer.com and is entitled "heterogeneity".

Start by opening the data file in SPSS statistical software.

Command:

click Graphs....click Legacy Dialogs....click Scatter/Dot....click 3-D Scatter....click Define....Y-Axis: enter percentage (ADEs)....X Axis: enter study-magnitude....Z Axis: enter clinicians =1....Set Markers by: enter elderly = 1....click OK.

The underneath figure is displayed, and it gives a 3-dimensional graph of the outcome (% adverse drug effects) versus study size versus investigator type (1 = clinician, 0 = pharmacist). A 4th dimension is obtained by coloring the circles (green = elderly, blue = young). Small studies tended to have larger results. Also clinician studies (clinicians = 1) tended to have larger results, while studies in elderly had both large and small effects.

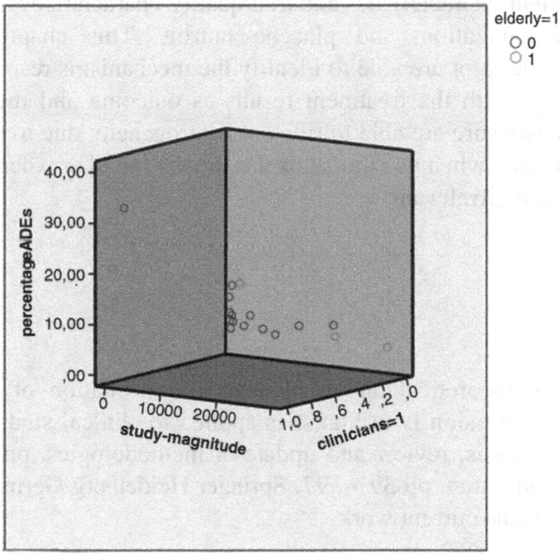

In order to test whether the observed trends were statistically significant, a linear regression is performed.

Command:

Analyze....Regression....Linear....Dependent: enter "percentage ADEs".... Independent(s): enter "study-magnitude, elderly = 1, clinicians = 1"....click OK.

Coefficients[a]

Model		Unstandardized coefficients		Standardized coefficients	t	Sig.
		B	Std. Error	Beta		
1	(Constant)	6,924	1,454		4,762	,000
	Study-magnitude	−7,674E-5	,000	−,071	−,500	,624
	Elderly = 1	−1,393	2,885	−,075	−,483	,636
	Clinicians = 1	18,932	3,359	,887	5,636	,000

[a]Dependent variable: percentage ADEs

The output sheets show the above table. The investigator type is the only statistically significant predictor of % of ADEs. Clinicians observed significantly more ADE admissions than did pharmacists at $p < 0.0001$. This is in agreement with the above graph

Conclusion

In clinical research similar studies often have different results. This may be due to differences in patient-characteristics and trial-quality-characteristics such as the use of blinding, randomization, and placebo-controls. This chapter shows that 3-dimensional scatter plot are able to identify the mechanisms responsible. Linear regression analyses with the treatment results as outcome and the predictors of heterogeneity as exposure are able to rule out heterogeneity due to chance. This is particularly important, when no clinical explanation is found or when heterogeneity seems to be clinically irrelevant.

Note

More background, theoretical and mathematical information of heterogeneous studies and meta-regression is in Statistics applied to clinical studies 5th edition, Chap. 33, Meta-analysis, review and update of methodologies, pp 379–390, and Chap. 34, Meta-regression, pp 391–397, Springer Heidelberg Germany, both from the same authors as the current work.

Chapter 41
Performance Evaluation of Novel Diagnostic Tests (650 and 588 Patients)

General Purpose

Both logistic regression and c-statistics can be used to evaluate the performance of novel diagnostic tests (see also Machine learning in medicine part two, Chap. 6, pp 45–52, Logistic regression for assessment of novel diagnostic tests against controls, Springer Heidelberg Germany, 2013, from the same authors). This chapter is to assess whether one method can outperform the other.

Primary Scientific Question

Is logistic regression with the odds of disease as outcome and test scores as covariate a better alternative for concordance (c)-statistics using the area under the curve of ROC (receiver operated characteristic) curves.

Example

In 650 patients with peripheral vascular disease a noninvasive vascular lab test was performed. The results of the first 10 patients are underneath.

test score	presence of peripheral vascular disease (0 = no, 1 = yes)
1,00	,00
1,00	,00

(continued)

This chapter was previously published in "Machine learning in medicine-cookbook 3" as Chap. 8, 2014.

T.J. Cleophas, A.H. Zwinderman, *Machine Learning in Medicine - a Complete Overview*, DOI 10.1007/978-3-319-15195-3_41

test score	presence of peripheral vascular disease (0 = no, 1 = yes)
2,00	,00
2,00	,00
3,00	,00
3,00	,00
3,00	,00
4,00	,00
4,00	,00
4,00	,00

The entire data file is in extras.springer.com, and is entitled “vascdisease1”. Start by opening the data file in SPSS.

Then Command:

Graphs....Legacy Dialogs....Histogram....Variable(s): enter "score"....Row(s): enter "disease"....click OK.

The underneath figure shows the output sheet. On the x-axis we have the vascular lab scores, on the y-axis “how often”. The scores in patients with (1) and without (0) the presence of disease according to the gold standard (angiography) are respectively in the lower and upper graph.

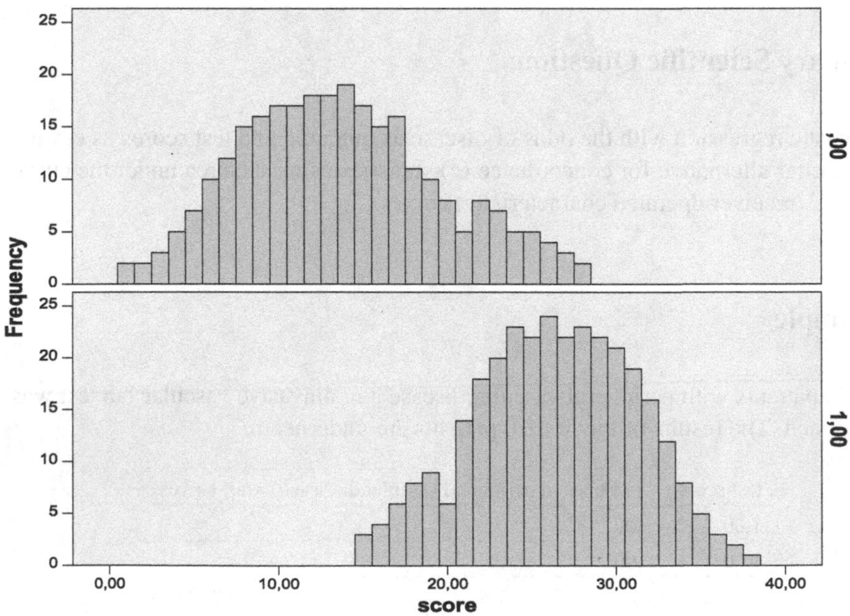

The second data file is obtained from a parallel-group population of 588 patients after the noninvasive vascular test has been improved. The first 10 patients are underneath.

test score	presence of peripheral vascular disease (0 = no, 1 = yes)
1,00	,00
2,00	,00
2,00	,00
3,00	,00
3,00	,00
3,00	,00
4,00	,00
4,00	,00
4,00	,00
4,00	,00

The entire data file is in extras.springer.com, and is entitled "vascdisease2". Start by opening the data file in SPSS.

Then Command:

Graphs....Legacy Dialogs....Histogram....Variable(s): enter "score"....Row(s): enter "disease"....click OK.

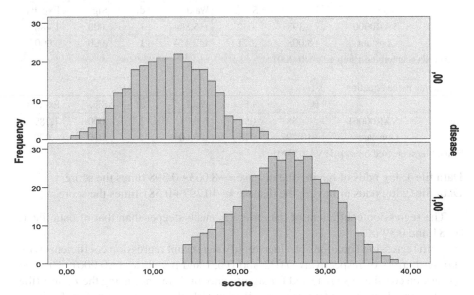

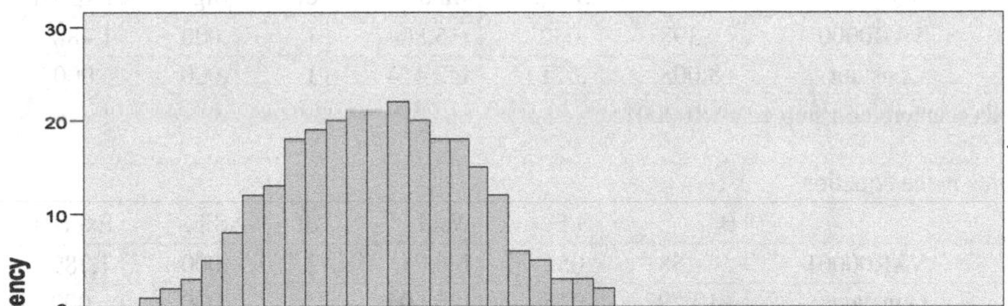

The above figure is in the output sheet.

The first test (upper figure) seems to perform less well than the second test (lower figure), because there may be more risk of false positives (the 0 disease curve is more skewed to the right in the upper than in the lower figure).

Binary Logistic Regression

Binary logistic regression is used for assessing this question. The following reasoning is used. If we move the threshold for a positive test to the right, then the proportion of false positive will decrease. The steeper the logistic regression line the faster this will happen. In contrast, if we move the threshold to the left, the proportion of false negatives will decrease. Again, the steeper the logistic regression line, the faster it will happen. And so, the steeper the logistic regression line, the fewer false negatives and false positives and thus the better the diagnostic test.

For both data files the above analysis is performed.

Command:

Analyze.... Regression....Binary logistic.... Dependent variable: disease.... Covariate: score....OK.

The output sheets show the best fit regression equations.

Variables in the equation

		B	S.E.	Wald	df	Sig.	Exp(B)
Step 1[a]	VAR00001	,398	,032	155,804	1	,000	1,488
	Constant	−8,003	,671	142,414	1	,000	,000

[a]Variable(s) entered on step 1: VAR00001

Variables in the equation

		B	S.E.	Wald	df	Sig.	Exp(B)
Step 1[a]	VAR00001	,581	,051	130,715	1	,000	1,789
	Constant	−10,297	,915	126,604	1	,000	,000

[a]Variable(s) entered on step 1: VAR00001

Data file 1: log odds of having the disease $= -8.003 + 0.398$ times the score
Data file 2: log odds of having the disease $= -10.297 + 0.581$ times the score.

The regression coefficient of data file 2 is much steeper than that of data file 1, 0.581 and 0.398.

Both regression equations produce highly significant regression coefficients with standard errors of respectively 0.032 and 0.051 and p-values of < 0.0001. The two regression coefficients are tested for significance of difference using the z – test (the z-test is in Chap. 2 of Statistics on a Pocket Calculator part 2, pp 3–5, Springer Heidelberg Germany, 2012, from the same authors):

$$z = (0.398 - 0.581) / \sqrt{(0.032^2 + 0.051^2)} = -0.183 / 0.060 = -3.05,$$

which corresponds with a p-value of < 0.01.

Obviously, test 2 produces a significantly steeper regression model, which means that it is a better predictor of the risk of disease than test 1. We can, additionally, calculate the odds ratios of successfully testing with test 2 versus test 1. The odds of disease with test 1 equals $e^{0.398} = 1.488$, and with test 2 it equals $e^{0.581} = 1.789$. The odds ratio = 1.789/1.488 = 1.202, meaning that the second test produces a 1.202 times better chance of rightly predicting the disease than test 1 does.

C-Statistics

C-statistics is used as a contrast test. Open data file 1 again.

Command:

Analyze....ROC Curve....Test Variable: enter "score"....State Variable: enter "disease"....Value of State Variable: type "1"....mark ROC Curve....mark Standard Error and Confidence Intervals....click OK.

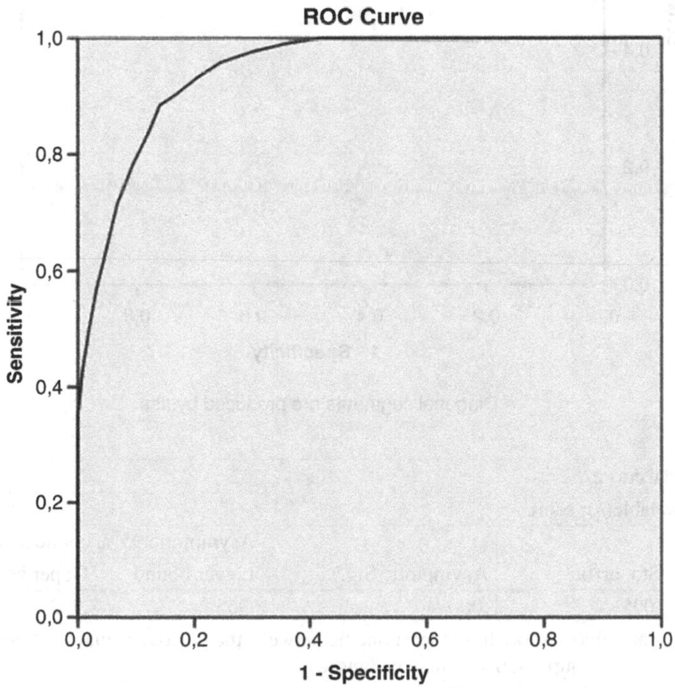

Diagonal segments are produced by ties.

Area under the curve

Test result variable(s): score

			Asymptotic 95 % confidence interval	
Area	Std. error[a]	Asymptotic Sig.[b]	Lower bound	Upper bound
,945	,009	,000	,928	,961

The test result variable(s): score has at least one tie between the positive actual state group and the negative actual state group. Statistics may be biased

[a]Under the nonparametric assumption

[b]Null hypothesis: true area = 0.5

Subsequently the same procedure is followed for data file 2.

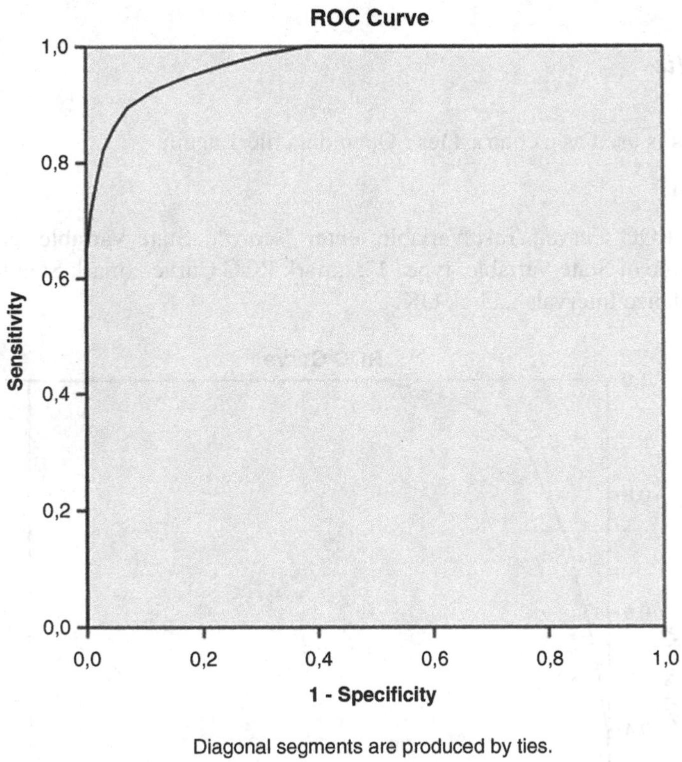

Area under the curve

Test result variable(s): score

			Asymptotic 95 % confidence interval	
Area	Std. error[a]	Asymptotic Sig.[b]	Lower bound	Upper bound
,974	,005	,000	,965	,983

The test result variable(s): score has at least one tie between the positive actual state group and the negative actual state group. Statistics may be biased

[a]Under the nonparametric assumption

[b]Null hypothesis: true area = 0.5

The Area under curve of data file 2 is larger than that of data file 1. The test 2 seems to perform better. The z-test can again be used to test for significance of difference.

$$z = (0.974 - 0.945) / \sqrt{(0.009^2 + 0.005^2)} = 2.90$$

$$p = < 0.01.$$

Conclusion

Both logistic regression with the presence of disease as outcome and test scores of as predictor and c-statistics can be used for comparing the performance of qualitative diagnostic tests. However, c-statistics may perform less well with very large areas under the curve, and it assesses relative risks while in practice absolute risk levels may be more important

Note

More background, theoretical and mathematical information of logistic regression and c-statistics is in Machine learning in medicine part two, Chap. 6, pp 45–52, Logistic regression for assessment of novel diagnostic tests against controls, Springer Heidelberg Germany, 2013, from the same authors.

Chapter 42
Quantile-Quantile Plots, a Good Start for Looking at Your Medical Data (50 Cholesterol Measurements and 58 Patients)

General Purpose

A good place to start looking at your data before analysis is a data plot, e.g., a scatter plot or histogram. It can help you decide whether the data are normal (bell shape, Gaussian), and give you a notion of outlier data and skewness. Another approach is using a normality test like the chi-square goodness of fit, the Shapiro-Wilkens, or the Kolmogorov Smirnov tests (Cleophas, Zwinderman, Chap. 42, pp 469–478, Testing clinical trials for randomness, in: Statistics applied to clinical studies 5th edition, Springer Heidelberg Germany, 2012), but these tests often have little power, and, therefore, do not adequately identify departures from normality. This chapter is to assess the performance of another and probably better method, the Q-Q (quantile-quantile) plot.

Specific Scientific Question

Are Q-Q plots of medical records capable of identifying normality and departures from normality. Random samples of hdl cholesterol and ages are used for examples.

Q-Q Plots for Assessing Departures from Normality

hdl cholesterol values (mmol/l)
3,80
4,20
4,27
3,70

(continued)

T.J. Cleophas, A.H. Zwinderman, *Machine Learning in Medicine - a Complete Overview*, DOI 10.1007/978-3-319-15195-3_42

hdl cholesterol values (mmol/l)
3,76
4,11
4,24
4,20
4,24
3,63

The above table gives the first 10 values of a 50 value data file of hdl cholesterol measurements. The entire file is in the SPSS file entitled "q-q plot", and is available on the internet at extras.springer.com. SPSS statistical software is applied. Start by opening the data file in SPSS.

Command:

click Graphs....Legacy Dialogs....Histogram....Variable: enter hdlcholesterol....click OK.

A histogram with individual hdl cholesterol values on the x-axis and "how often" on the y-axis is given in the output sheet: 50 hdl cholesterol values are classified in percentages (%) or quantiles (= frequencies = numbers of observations/50 here). E.g., one value is between 2,5 and 3,0, two values are between 3,0 and 3,5, etc. The pattern tends to be somewhat bell shape, but there is obvious outlier frequencies close to 3 mmol/l and close to 4 mmol/l. Also some skewness to the right is observed, and the values around 4 mmol/l look a little bit like Manhattan rather than Gaussian.

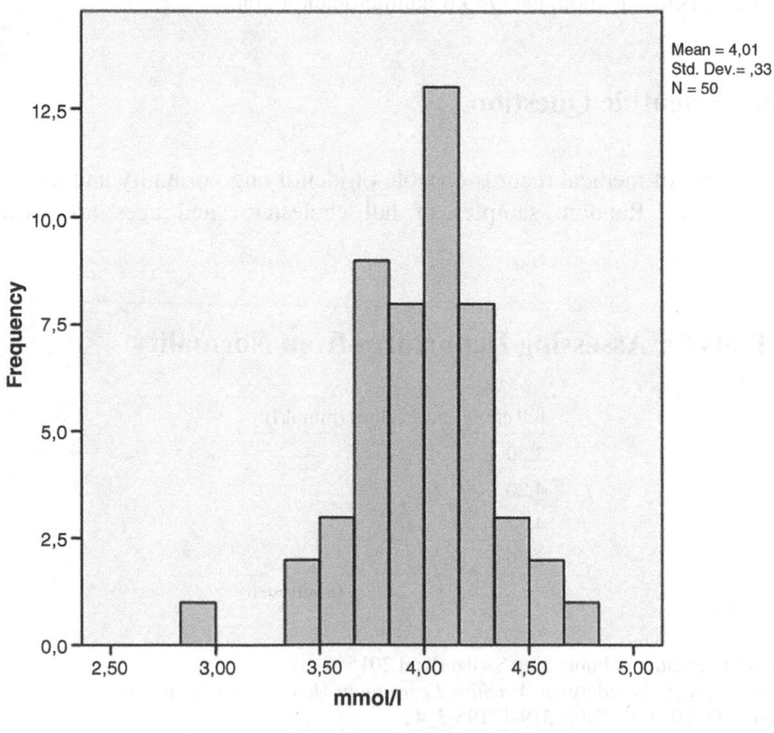

A Q-Q plot (quantile-quantile plot) can be helpful do decide what type of data we have here. First, the best fit normal curve is construed, e.g., based on the mean and standard deviation of the data. A graph of it is easy to produce in SPSS.

Command:

click Graphs....Legacy Dialogs....Histogram....Variable: enter hdlcholesterol .... mark: Display normal curve....click OK.

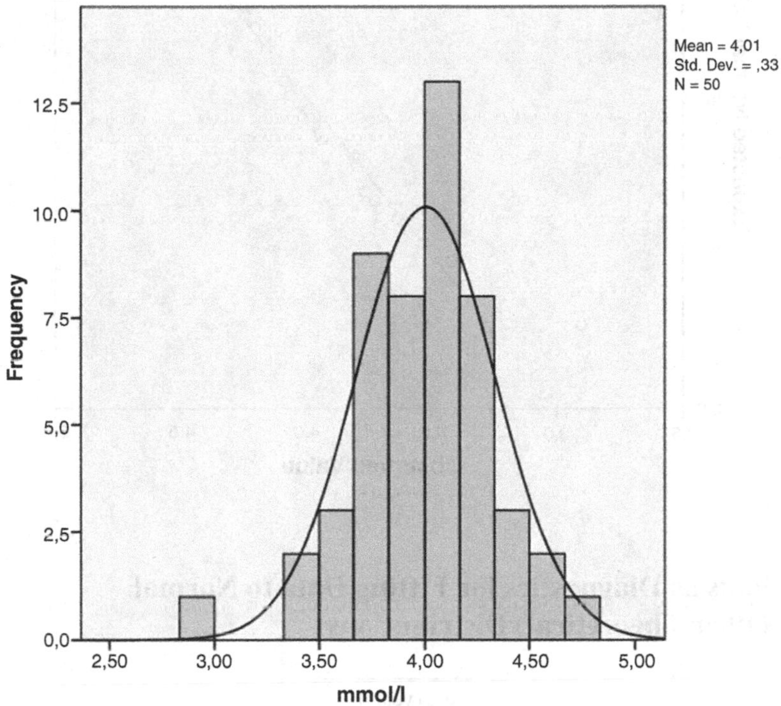

SPSS uses the curve to calculate the values for a Q-Q plot.

Command:

Analyze....Descriptive Statistics....Q-Q plots....Variables: enter hdlcholesterol.... click OK.

The underneath plot is construed of the observed x-values versus the same x-values taken from the above best fit normal curve. If our data perfectly matched the best fit Gaussian curve, then all of the x-values would be on the 45° diagonal line. However, we have outliers. The x-value close to 3 mmol/l is considerably left from the diagonal, and thus smaller than expected. The value close to 4 mmol/l is obviously on the right side of the diagonal, and thus larger than expected. Nonetheless, The remainder of the observed values vary well fit the diagonal, and it seems adequate to conclude that normal statistical test for analysis of these data will be appropriate.

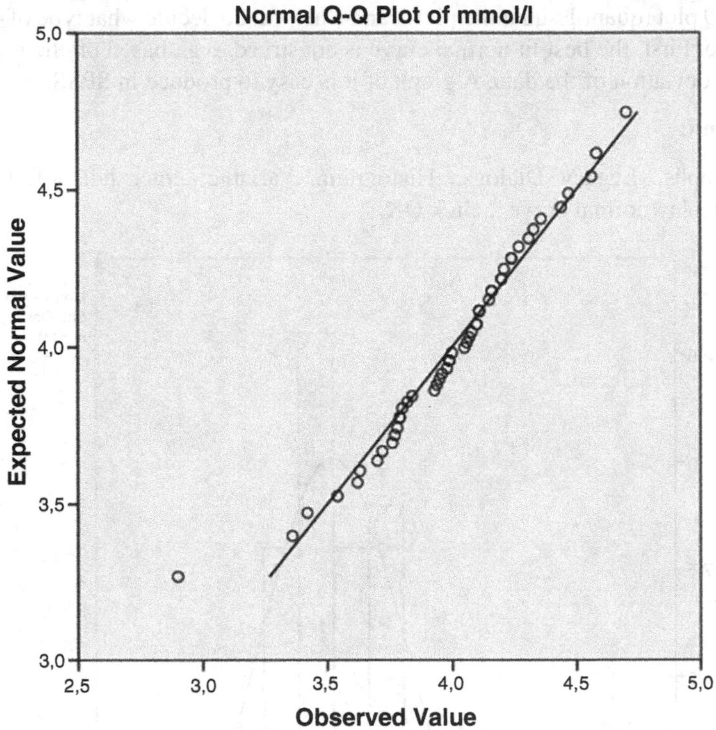

Q-Q Plots as Diagnostics for Fitting Data to Normal (and Other Theoretical) Distributions

Age (years)
85,00
89,00
50,00
63,00
76,00
57,00
86,00
56,00
76,00
66,00

The above table gives the first 10 values of a 58 value data file of patients with different ages. The entire file is in the SPSS file entitled "q-q plot", and is available on the internet at extras.springer.com. SPSS statistical software is applied. Start by opening the data file in SPSS.

Command:

Analyze....Descriptive Statistics....Q-Q plots....Variables: enter age....click OK.

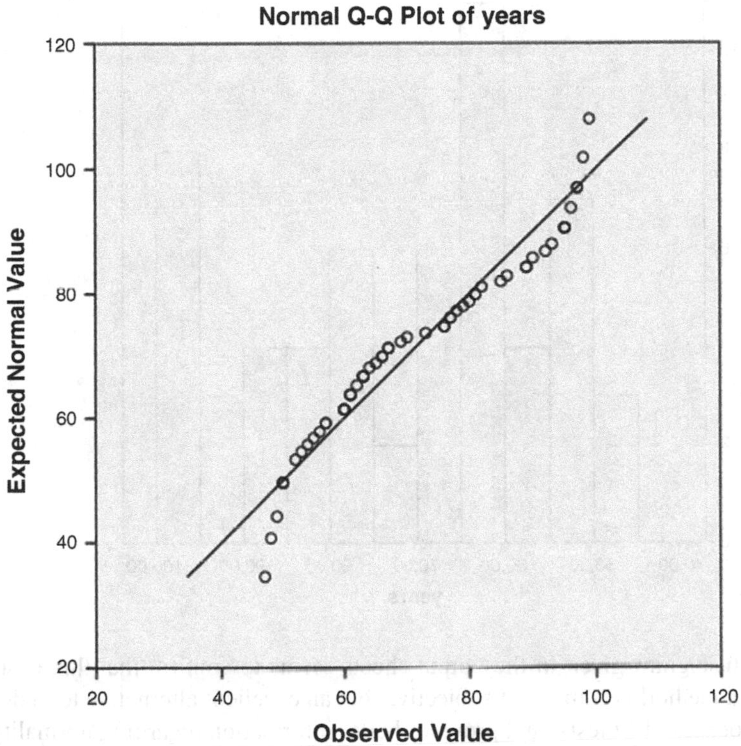

In the output sheets is the above graph. It shows a pattern with the left end below the diagonal line and the right end above it. Also the overall pattern seems to be somewhat undulating with the initially an increasing slope, and then a decreasing slope. The possible interpretations of these patterns are the following.

1. Left end below and right end above the diagonal may indicate a bells shape with long tails (overdispersion).
2. In contrast, left end above and right end below indicates short tails.
3. An increasing slope from left to right may indicate skewness to the right.
4. In contrast, a decreasing slope suggests skewness to the left.
5. The few cases with largest departures from the diagonal may of course also be interpreted as outliers.

The above Q-Q plot can hardly be assumed to indicate Gaussian data. The histogram confirms this.

Command:

click Graphs....Legacy Dialogs....Histograms....Variables: enter age....click OK.

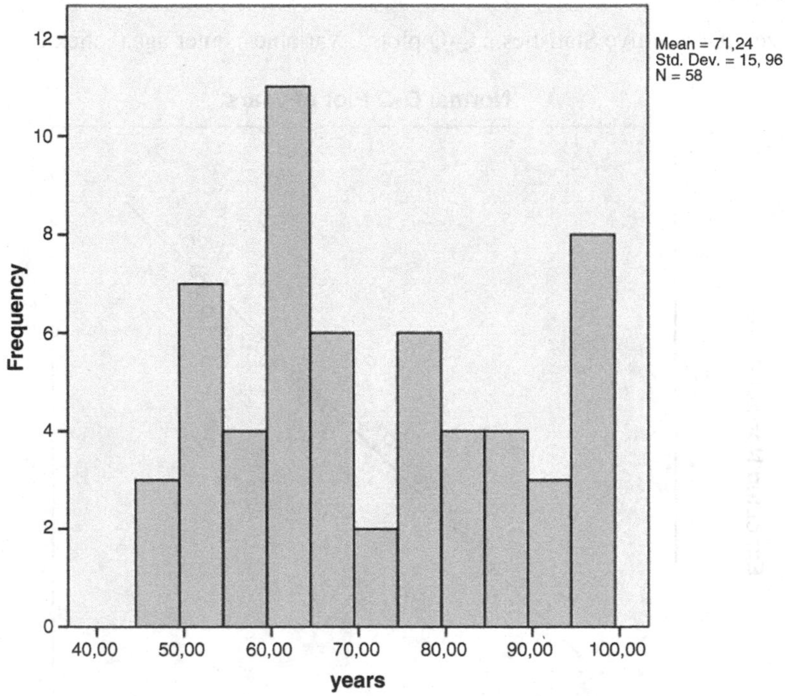

The histogram given in the output sheets seems to confirm that this is so. The Q-Q plot method is somewhat subjective, but an excellent alternative to underpowered goodness of fit tests, and provides better information regarding normality than simple data plots or histograms do, because each datum assessed against its best fit normal distribution counterpart. We should add that SPSS and other software also offer the construction of Q-Q plots using other than normal distributions.

Conclusion

Q-Q plots are adequate assess whether your data have a Gaussian-like pattern. Non-Gaussian patterns and outliers are visualized, and often an interpretation can be given of them. The Q-Q plot method is similar to the less popular P-P (probability-probability) plot method, which has cumulative probabilities (= areas under curve left from the x-value), instead of the x-values on the x-axis and their expected counterparts on the y-axis. They are a little bit harder to understand.

Note

More background, theoretical and mathematical information of frequency distributions and goodness of fit testing is in the Chap. 42, pp 469–478, Testing clinical trials for randomness, in: Statistics applied to clinical studies 5th edition, Springer Heidelberg Germany, 2012, from the same authors as the current work.

Chapter 43
Rate Analysis of Medical Data Better than Risk Analysis (52 Patients)

General Purpose

For the assessment of medical treatments clinical event analysis with logistic regression is often performed. Treatment modalities are used as predictor and the odds of the event as outcome. However, instead of the odds of event, counted rates of events can be computed and statistically tested. This may produce better sensitivity of testing, because their standard errors are smaller.

Specific Scientific Question

Does rate analysis of medical events provide better sensitivity of testing than traditional risk analysis.

Example

We will use an example also used in the Chap. 10 of SPSS for starters part two, pp 43–48, Poisson regression, Springer Heidelberg Germany, 2012, from the same authors. In a parallel-group study of 52 patients the presence of torsade de pointes was measured during two treatment modalities.

T.J. Cleophas, A.H. Zwinderman, *Machine Learning in Medicine - a Complete Overview*, DOI 10.1007/978-3-319-15195-3_43

treatment modality	Presence torsade de pointes
,00	1,00
,00	1,00
,00	1,00
,00	1,00
,00	1,00
,00	1,00
,00	1,00
,00	1,00
,00	1,00
,00	1,00

The first 10 patients are above. The entire data file is in extras.springer.com, and is entitled "rates". SPSS statistical software will be used for analysis. First, we will perform a traditional binary logistic regression with torsade de pointes as outcome and treatment modality as predictor.

Command:

Analyze….Regression….Binary Logistic….Dependent: torsade….. Covariates: treatment….OK.

Variables in the Equation

		B	S.E.	Wald	df	Sid.	Exp(B)
Step 1[a]	VAR00001	1,224	,626	3,819	1	,051	3,400
	Constant	-,125	,354	,125	1	,724	,882

[a]Variable(s) entered on step 1: VAR00001

The above table shows that the treatment modality does not significantly predict the presence of torsades de pointes. The numbers of torsades in one group is not significantly different from the other group.

A rate analysis is performed subsequently.

Command:

Generalized Linear Models ….mark Custom….Distribution: Poisson ….Link Function: Log….Response: Dependent Variable: torsade…. Predictors: Main Effect: treatment…..Estimation: mark Robust Tests….OK.

Parameter estimates							
			95 % Wald confidence interval		Hypothesis test		
Parameter	B	Std. Error	Lower	Upper	Wald Chi- Square	df	Sig.
(Intercept)	-,288	,1291	-,541	-,035	4,966	1	,026
[VAR00001=,00]	-,470	,2282	-.917	-,023	4,241	1	,039
[VAR00001=1,00]	0[a]						
(Scale)	1[b]						

Dependent Variable: torsade
Model: (Intercept), VAR00001
[a]Set to zero because this parameter is redundant
[b]Fixed at the displayed value

The predictor treatment modality is now statistically significant at p=0.039. And so, using the Poisson distribution in Generalized Linear Models, we found that treatment one performed significantly better in predicting numbers of torsades de pointe than did treatment zero at 0.039. We will check with a 3-dimensional graph of the data if this result is in agreement with the data as observed.

Command:

Graphs….Legacy Dialog….3-D Bar: X-Axis mark: Groups of Cases, Z-Axis mark: Groups of Cases…Define 3-D Bar: X Category Axis: treatment, Z Category Axis: torsade….OK.

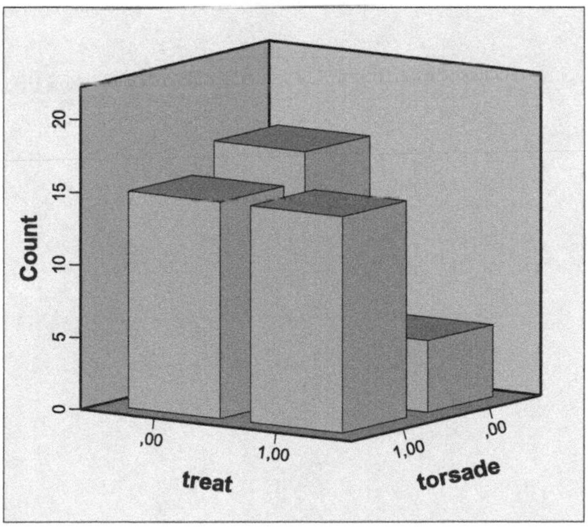

The above graph shows that in the 0-treatment (placebo) group the number of patients with torsades de pointe is virtually equal to that of the patients without. However, in the 1-treatment group it is smaller. The treatment seems to be efficacious.

Conclusion

Rate analysis using Poisson regression is different from logistic regression, because it uses a log transformed dependent variable. For the analysis of rates Poisson regression is very sensitive and, thus, better than standard logistic regression.

Note

More background, theoretical and mathematical information of rate analysis is given in Chap. 10 of SPSS for starters part two, pp 43–48, Poisson regression, Springer Heidelberg Germany, 2012, from the same authors.

Chapter 44
Trend Tests Will Be Statistically Significant if Traditional Tests Are Not (30 and 106 Patients)

General Purpose

Incremental dosages of medicines usually cause incremental treatment efficacies. This chapter is to assess whether trend tests are more sensitive than traditional ANOVAs for continuous outcome data (analyses of variance) and chi-square tests for binary outcome data to demonstrate the incremental efficacies.

Specific Scientific Questions

In patients with hypertension do incremental treatment dosages cause incremental beneficial effect on blood pressure? We will use the examples previously used in the Chaps. 9 and 12 of SPSS for starters part one, pp 33–34, and 43–46, entitled "Trend test for continuous data" and "trend tests for binary data", Springer Heidelberg Germany, 2010, from the same authors.

Example 1

In a parallel group study of 30 patients with hypertension 3 incremental antihypertensive treatment dosages are assessed. The first 13 patients of the data file is given underneath. The entire data file is in extras.springer.com, and is entitled "trend.sav".

Variable	
1	2
1,00	113,00
1,00	131,00

(continued)

T.J. Cleophas, A.H. Zwinderman, *Machine Learning in Medicine - a Complete Overview*, DOI 10.1007/978-3-319-15195-3_44

Variable	
1,00	112,00
1,00	132,00
1,00	114,00
1,00	130,00
1,00	115,00
1,00	129,00
1,00	122,00
2,00	118,00
2,00	109,00
2,00	127,00
2,00	110,00

Var 1 = treatment dosage (Var = variable)
Var 2 = treatment response (mean blood pressure after treatment)

We will first perform a one-way ANOVA (see also Chap. 8, SPSS for starters part one, entitled "One way ANOVA, Kruskall-Wallis", pp 29–31, Springer Heidelberg Germany, 2012, from the same authors) to see, if there are any significant differences in the data. If not, we will perform a trend test using simple linear regression.

Command:

Analyze....Compare Means....One-way ANOVA....dependent list: mean blood pressure after treatment - factor: treatment dosage....OK

ANOVA					
VAR00002					
	Sum of squares	df	Mean square	F	Sig.
Between groups	246,667	2	123,333	2,035	,150
Within groups	1636,000	27	60,593		
Total	1882,667	29			

The output table shows that there is no significant difference in efficacy between the treatment dosages, and so, sadly, this is a negative study. However, a trend test having just 1 degree of freedom has more sensitivity than a usual one-way ANOVA, and it could, therefore, be statistically significant even so.

Command:

Analyze....regression....linear....dependent = mean blood pressure after treatment.... independent = treatment dosage....OK

ANOVA[b]					
Model	Sum of squares	df	Mean square	F	Sig.
1 Regression	245,000	1	245,000	4,189	,050[a]
Residual	1637,667	28	58,488		
Total	1882,667	29			

[a]Predictors: (Constant), VAR00001
[b]Dependent Variable: VAR00002

The above output table shows that treatment dosage is a significant predictor of treatment response wit a p-value of 0.050. There is, thus, a significantly incremental response with incremental dosages.

Example 2

In a parallel group study of 106 patients with hypertension 3 incremental antihypertensive treatment dosages are assessed. The first 13 patients of the data file is given underneath. The entire data file is in extras.springer.com, and is entitled "trend.sav".

responder (1 = yes, 0 = no)	Treatment (1 = low, 2 = medium, 3 = high dosage)
1,00	1,00
1,00	1,00
1,00	1,00
1,00	1,00
1,00	1,00
1,00	1,00
1,00	1,00
1,00	1,00
1,00	1,00
1,00	1,00
1,00	2,00
1,00	2,00
1,00	2,00

Command:

Analyze....Descriptive Statistics....Crosstabs....Row(s): enter responders.... Column(s): enter treatment....click Cell(s)....Counts: mark Observed..... Percentage: mark Columns....click continue....click OK

The underneath contingency table shows that with incremental dosages the % of responders incrementally rises from 40 % to 51.3 % and then to 64.3 %.

			Treatment			
			1,00	2,00	3,00	Total
Responder	,00	Count	15	19	15	49
		% within treatment	60,0 %	48,7 %	35,7 %	46,2 %
	1,00	Count	10	20	27	57
		% within treatment	40,0 %	51,3 %	64,3 %	53,8 %
Total		Count	25	39	42	106
		% within treatment	100,0 %	100,0 %	100,0 %	100,0 %

Subsequently, a chi-square test will be performed to assess whether the cells are significantly different from one another.

Command:

Analyze....Descriptive Statistics....Crosstabs.... Row(s): enter responders.... Column(s): enter treatment....click Statistics....Chi-square....OK

Chi-square tests

	Value	df	Asy mp. Sig. (2-sided)
Pearson chi-square	3,872[a]	2	,144
Likelihood ratio	3,905	2	,142
Linear-by-linear association	3,829	1	,050
N of valid cases	106		

[a]0 cells (,0 %) have expected court less than 5. The minimum expected count is 11,56

The output table shows that the Pearson chi-square value for multiple groups testing is not significant with a value of 3.872 and a p-value of 0.144, and we need to conclude that there is no significant difference between the cells. Subsequently, a chi-square test for trends is required for that purpose. Actually, the "linear-by-linear association" from the same table is appropriate. It has approximately the same chi-square value, but it has only 1 degree of freedom, and, therefore it reaches statistical significance with a p-value of 0.050. There is, thus, a significant incremental trend of responding with incremental dosages. As an alternative the trend in this example can also be tested using logistic regression with responding as outcome variable and treatment as independent variable.

Command:

Analyze....Regression....Binary Logistic Regression....Dependent: enter responder.... Covariates: enter treatment....click OK

Variables in the equation

		B	S.E.	Wald	df	Sig.	Exp(B)
Step 1[a]	Treatment	,500	,257	3,783	1	,052	1,649
	Constant	-,925	,587	2,489	1	,115	,396

[a]Variable(s) entered on step 1: treatment.

The output sheet shows that the p-value of the logistic model is virtually identical to the p-value of chi-square test for trends, 0.052 and 0.050.

Conclusion

The examples in this chapter show that both with continuous and binary outcome variables trend tests are more sensitive to demonstrate significant effects in dose response studies than traditional statistical tests.

Note

More background, theoretical and mathematical information of trend tests are given in the Chap. 27, Trend-testing, pp 313–318, in: Statistics applied to clinical studies 5th edition, Springer Heidelberg Germany, 2012, from the same authors.

Chapter 45
Doubly Multivariate Analysis of Variance for Multiple Observations from Multiple Outcome Variables (16 Patients)

General Purpose

One way analysis of variance (ANOVA) is for analysis of studies with multiple unpaired observations (i.e. 1 subject is observed once) and a single outcome variable (see Chap. 8, One way anova and Kruskall-Wallis, pp 29–31, in: SPSS for starters part one, Springer Heidelberg Germany, 2010, from the same authors).

Repeated measures ANOVA is for studies with multiple paired observations (i.e. more than a single observation per subject) and also with a single outcome variable (see Chap. 6, Repeated measures anova, pp 21–24, in: SPSS for starters part one, Springer Heidelberg Germany, 2010, from the same authors).

Multivariate ANOVA is for studies with multiple unpaired observations and more than a single outcome variable (see Chap. 4, Multivariate anova, pp 13–20, in: SPSS for starters part two, Springer Heidelberg Germany, 2012, from the same authors).

Finally, doubly multivariate ANOVA is for studies with multiple paired observations and more than a single outcome variable.

An example of the latter is given in the SPSS tutorial case studies: in a diet study of overweight patients the triglyceride and weight values were the outcome variables and they were measured repeatedly during several months of follow up.

Primary Scientific Question

Can doubly multivariate analysis be used to simultaneously assess the effects of three different sleeping pills on two outcome variables, (1) hours of sleep and (2) morning body temperatures (in patients with sleep deprivation morning body temperature is higher than in those without sleep deprivation).

T.J. Cleophas, A.H. Zwinderman, *Machine Learning in Medicine - a Complete Overview*, DOI 10.1007/978-3-319-15195-3_45

Example

In 16 patients a three period crossover study of three sleeping pills (treatment levels) were studied. The underneath table give the data of the first 8 patients. The entire data file is entitled "doubly.sav", and is in extras.springer.com. Two outcome variables are measured at three levels each. This study would qualify for a doubly multivariate analysis, because we have multiple paired outcomes and multiple measures of each of the outcomes.

hours			age	gen	temp		
a	b	c		a	b	c	
6,10	6,80	5,20	55,00	0,00	35,90	35,30	36,80
7,00	7,00	7,90	65,00	0,00	37,10	37,80	37,00
8,20	9,00	3,90	74,00	0,00	38,30	34,00	39,10
7,60	7,80	4,70	56,00	1,00	37,50	34,60	37,70
6,50	6,60	5,30	44,00	1,00	36,40	35,30	36,70
8,40	8,00	5,40	49,00	1,00	38,30	35,50	38,00
6,90	7,30	4,20	53,00	0,00	37,00	34,10	37,40
6,70	7,00	6,10	76,00	0,00	36,80	36,10	36,90

hours = hours of sleep on sleeping pill
a, b, c = different sleeping pills (levels of treatment)
age = patient age
gen = gender
temp = different morning body temperatures on sleeping pill

SPSS statistical software will be used for data analysis. We will start by opening the data file in SPSS.

Then Command:

Analyze....General Linear Models....Repeated Measures....Within-Subject Factor Name: type treatment....Number of Levels: type 3....click Add....Measure Name: type hours....click Add....Measure Name: type temp....click Add....click Define.... Within-Subjects Variables(treatment): enter hours a, b, c, and temp a, b, c.... Between-Subjects Factor(s): enter gender....click Contrast....Change Contrast.... Contrast....select Repeated....click Change....click Continue....click Plots.... Horizontal Axis: enter treatment....Separate Lines: enter gender....click Add....click Continue....click Options....Display Means for: enter gender*treatment....mark Estimates of effect size....mark SSCP matrices....click Continue....click OK.

The underneath table is in the output sheets.

Multivariate tests[b]

Effect			Value	F	Hypothesis df	Error df	Sig.	Partial Eta Squared
Between subjects	Intercept	Pillai's Trace	1,000	3,271 E6	2,000	13,000	,000	1,000
		Wilks' Lambda	,000	3,271 E6	2,000	13,000	,000	1,000
		Hotelling's Trace	503211,785	3,271 E6	2,000	13,000	,000	1,000
		Roy's Largest Root	503211,785	3,271 E6	2,000	13,000	,000	1,000
	Gender	Pillai's Trace	,197	1,595[a]	2,000	13,000	,240	,197
		Wilks' Lambda	,803	1,595[a]	2,000	13,000	,240	,197
		Hotelling's Trace	,245	1,595[a]	2,000	13,000	,240	,197
		Roy's Largest Root	,245	1,595[a]	2,000	13,000	,240	,197
Within subjects	Treatment	Pillai's Trace	,562	3,525[a]	4,000	11,000	,044	,562
		Wilks' Lambda	,438	3,525[a]	4,000	11,000	,044	,562
		Hotelling's Trace	1,282	3,525[a]	4,000	11,000	,044	,562
		Roy's Largest Root	1,282	3,525[a]	4,000	11,000	,044	,562
	Treatment * gender	Pillai's Trace	,762	8,822[a]	4,000	11,000	,002	,762
		Wilks' Lambda	,238	8,822[a]	4,000	11,000	,002	,762
		Hotelling's Trace	3,208	8,822[a]	4,000	11,000	,002	,762
		Roy's Largest Root	3,208	8,822[a]	4,000	11,000	,002	,762

[a]Exactstatistic
[b]Design: Intercept + gender
Within Subjects Design: treatment

Doubly multivariate analysis has multiple paired outcomes and multiple measures of these outcomes. For analysis of such data both between and within subjects tests are performed. We are mostly interested in the within subject effects of the treatment levels, but the above table starts by showing the not so interesting gender effect on hours of sleep and morning temperatures. They are not significantly different between the genders. More important is the treatment effects. The hours of sleep and the morning temperature are significantly different between the different treatment levels at p=0.044. Also these significant effects are different between males and females at p=0.002.

Tests of within-subjects contrasts

Source	Measure	Treatment	Type III sum of squares	df	Mean square	F	Sia.	Partial eta squared
Treatment	Hours	Level 1 vs. Level 2	,523	1	,523	6,215	,026	,307
		Level 2 w. Level 3	62,833	1	62,833	16,712	,001	,544
	Temp	Level 1 vs. Level 2	49,323	1	49,323	15,788	,001	,530
		Level 2 vs. Level 3	62,424	1	62,424	16,912	,001	,547
Treatment* gender	Hours	Level 1 vs. Level 2	,963	1	,963	11,447	,004	,450
		Level 2 vs. Level 3	,113	1	,113	,030	,865	,002
	Temp	Level 1 vs. Level 2	,963	1	,963	,308	,588	,022
		Level 2 w. Level 3	,054	1	,054	,015	,905	,001
Error(treatment)	Hours	Level 1 vs. Level 2	1,177	14	,084			
		Level 2 vs. Level 3	52,637	14	3,760			
	Temp	Level 1 w. Level 2	43,737	14	3,124			
		Level 2 vs. Level 3	51,676	14	3,691			

The above table shows, whether differences between levels of treatment were significantly different from one another by comparison with the subsequent levels (contrast tests). The effects of treatment levels 1 versus (vs) 2 on hours of sleep were different at p=0.026, levels 2 vs 3 at p=0.001. The effects of treatments levels 1 vs 2 on morning temperatures were different at p=0.001, levels 2 vs 3 on morning temperatures were also different at p=0.001. The effects on hours of sleep of treatment levels 1 vs 2 accounted for the differences in gender remained very significant at p=0.004.

Gender * treatment						
					95 % Confidence interval	
Measure	Gender	Treatment	Mean	Std. Error	Lower bound	Upper bound
Hours	,00	1	6,980	,268	6,404	7,556
		2	7,420	,274	6,833	8,007
		3	5,460	,417	4,565	6,355
	1,00	1	7,350	,347	6,607	8,093
		2	7,283	,354	6,525	8,042
		3	5,150	,539	3,994	6,306
Temp	,00	1	37,020	,284	36,411	37,629
		2	35,460	,407	34,586	36,334
		3	37,440	,277	36,845	38,035
	1,00	1	37,250	,367	36,464	38,036
		2	35,183	,526	34,055	36,311
		3	37,283	,358	36,515	38,051

The above table shows the mean hours of sleep and mean morning temperatures for the different subsets of observations. Particularly, we observe the few hours of sleep on treatment level 3, and the highest morning temperatures at the same level. The treatment level 2, in contrast, causes pretty many hours of sleep and, at the same time, the lowest morning temperatures (consistent with longer periods of sleep). The underneath figures show the same.

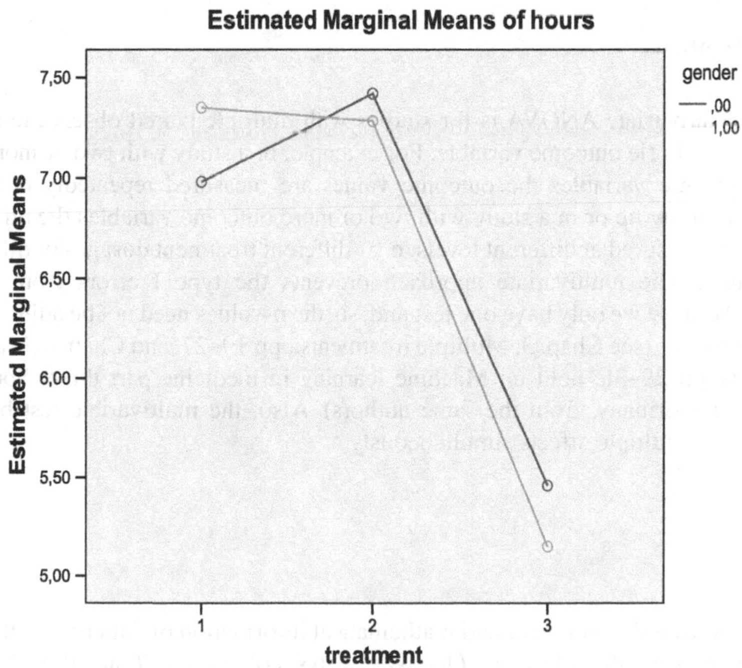

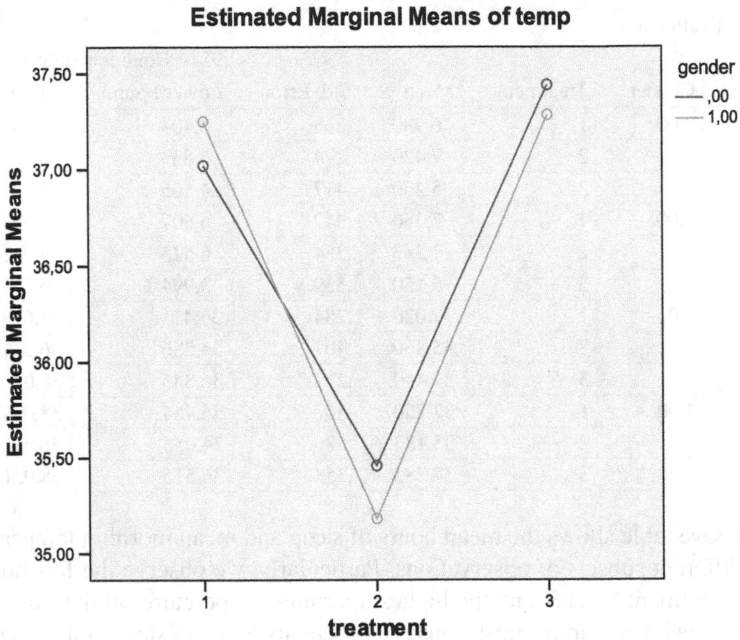

Conclusion

Doubly multivariate ANOVA is for studies with multiple paired observations and more than a single outcome variable. For example, in a study with two or more different outcome variables the outcome values are measured repeatedly during a period of follow up or in a study with two or more outcome variables the outcome values are measured at different levels, e.g., different treatment dosages or different compounds. The multivariate approach prevents the type I errors from being inflated, because we only have one test and, so, the p-values need not be adjusted for multiple testing (see Chap. 3, Multiple treatments,, pp 19–27, and Chap. 4, Multiple endpoints, pp 29–36, both in: Machine learning in medicine part three, Springer Heidelberg Germany, from the same authors). Also, the multivariate test battery accounts for multiple effects simultaneously.

Note

More background, theoretical and mathematical information of data files with multiple variables are the following. One way analysis of variance (anova) analysis of studies with multiple unpaired observations (i.e. 1 subject is observed once) and a single outcome variable (see Chap. 8, One way anova and Kruskall-Wallis, pp 29–31, in: SPSS for starters part one, Springer Heidelberg Germany, 2010, from the same authors), repeated measures ANOVA for studies with multiple paired observations (i.e. more than a single observation per subject) and also with a single outcome variable (see Chap. 6, Repeated measures anova, pp 21–24, in: SPSS for starters part one, Springer Heidelberg Germany, 2010, from the same authors), and multivariate ANOVA is for studies with multiple unpaired observations and more than a single outcome variable (see Chap. 4, Multivariate anova, pp 13–20, in: SPSS for starters part two, Springer Heidelberg Germany, 2012, from the same authors). The advantages of multivariate analyses as compared to univariate analyses are discussed in the Chap. 3, Multiple treatments, pp 19–27, and the Chap. 4, Multiple endpoints, pp 29–36, both in: Machine learning in medicine part three, Springer Heidelberg Germany, 2013, from the same authors.

Chapter 46
Probit Models for Estimating Effective Pharmacological Treatment Dosages (14 Tests)

General Purpose

Probit regression is, just like logistic regression, for estimating the effect of predictors on yes/no outcomes. If your predictor is multiple pharmacological treatment dosages, then probit regression may be more convenient than logistic regression, because your results will be reported in the form of response rates instead of odds ratios. The dependent variable of the two methods log odds (otherwise called logit) and log prob (otherwise called probit) are closely related to one another. Log prob (probability), is the z-value corresponding to its area under the curve value of the normal distribution. It can be shown that the log odds of responding $\approx (\pi/\sqrt{3})$ x log prob of responding (see Chap. 7, Machine learning in medicine part three, Probit regression, pp 63–68, 2013, Springer Heidelberg Germany, from the same authors).

Primary Scientific Question

This chapter will assess whether probit regression is able to find response rates of different dosages of mosquito repellents.

Example

Simple Probit Regression

repellent nonchem	repellent chem	mosquitos gone	n mosquitos
1	,02	1000	18000
1	,03	1000	18500

(continued)

T.J. Cleophas, A.H. Zwinderman, *Machine Learning in Medicine - a Complete Overview*, DOI 10.1007/978-3-319-15195-3_46

repellent nonchem	repellent chem	mosquitos gone	n mosquitos
1	,03	3500	19500
1	,04	4500	18000
1	,07	9500	16500
1	,09	17000	22500
1	,10	20500	24000

In 14 test sessions the effect measured as the numbers of mosquitos gone after administration of different dosages of a chemical repellent was assessed. The first 7 sessions are in the above table. The entire data file is entitled probit.sav, and is in extras.springer.com. Start by opening the data file in SPSS statistical software.

Command:

Analyze....Regression....Probit Regression....Response Frequency: enter "mosquitos gone"....Total Observed: enter "n mosquitos"....Covariate(s): enter "chemical".... Transform: select "natural log"....click OK.

Chi-Square tests

		Chi-Square	df[a]	Sig.
PROBIT	Pearson Goodness-of-Fit Test	7706,816	12	,000[b]

[a]Statistics based on individual cases differ from statistics based on aggregated cases
[b]Since the significance level is less than, 150, a heterogeneity factor is used in the calculation of confidence limits

In the output sheets the above table shows that the goodness of fit tests of the data is significant, and, thus, the data do not fit the probit model very well. However, SPSS is going to produce a heterogeneity correction factor and we can proceed. The underneath shows that chemical dilution levels are a very significant predictor of proportions of mosquitos gone.

Parameter estimates

Parameter		Estimate	Std. Error	Z	Sig.	95 % Confidence interval Lower bound	95 % Confidence interval Upper bound
PROBIT[a]	Chemical (dilution)	1,649	,006	286,098	,000	1,638	1,660
	Intercept	4,489	,017	267,094	,000	4,472	4,506

[a]PROBIT model: PROBIT(p) = Intercept + BX (Covariates X are transformed using the base 2.718 logarithm.)

Cell counts and residuals

Number		Chemical (dilution)	Number of subjects	Observed responses	Expected responses	Residual	Probability
PROBIT	1	-3,912	18000	1000	448,194	551,806	,025
	2	-3,624	18500	1000	1266,672	-266,672	,068
	3	-3,401	19500	3500	2564,259	935,741	,132
	4	-3,124	18000	4500	4574,575	-74,575	,254
	5	-2,708	16500	9500	8405,866	1094,134	,509
	6	-2,430	22500	17000	15410,676	1589,324	,685
	7	-2,303	24000	20500	18134,992	2365,008	,756
	8	-3,912	22500	500	560,243	-60,243	,025
	9	-3,624	18500	1500	1266,672	233,328	,068
	10	-3,401	19000	1000	2498,508	-1498,508	,132
	11	-3,124	20000	5000	5082,861	-82,861	,254
	12	-2,708	22000	10000	11207,821	-1207,821	,509
	13	-2,430	16500	8000	11301,162	-3301,162	,685
	14	-2,303	18500	13500	13979,056	-479,056	,756

The above table shows that according to chi-square tests the differences between observed and expected proportions of mosquitos gone is several times statistically significant.

It does, therefore, make sense to make some inferences using the underneath confidence limits table.

Confidence limits

Probability		95 % Confidence limits for chemical (dilution)			95 % Confidence limits for log (chemical (dilution)[b]		
		Estimate	Lower bound	Upper bound	Estimate	Lower bound	Upper bound
PROBIT[a]	,010	,016	,012	,020	-4,133	-4,453	-3,911
	,020	,019	,014	,023	-3,968	-4,250	-3,770
	,030	,021	,016	,025	-3,863	-4,122	-3,680
	,040	,023	,018	,027	-3,784	-4,026	-3,612
	,050	,024	,019	,029	-3,720	-3,949	-3,557
	,060	,026	,021	,030	-3,665	-3,882	-3,509
	,070	,027	,022	,031	-3,617	-3,825	-3,468
	,080	,028	,023	,032	-3,574	-3,773	-3,430
	,090	,029	,024	,034	-3,535	-3,726	-3,396
	,100	,030	,025	,035	-3,500	-3,683	-3,365
	,150	,035	,030	,039	-3,351	-3,506	-3,232
	,200	,039	,034	,044	-3,233	-3,368	-3,125
	,250	,044	,039	,048	-3,131	-3,252	-3,031

(continued)

Confidence limits

Probability		95 % Confidence limits for chemical (dilution)			95 % Confidence limits for log (chemical (dilution)[b]		
		Estimate	Lower bound	Upper bound	Estimate	Lower bound	Upper bound
	,300	,048	,043	,053	−3,040	−3,150	−2,943
	,350	,052	,047	,057	−2,956	−3,059	−2,860
	,400	,056	,051	,062	−2,876	−2,974	−2,778
	,450	,061	,055	,067	−2,799	−2,895	−2,697
	,500	,066	,060	,073	−2,722	−2,819	−2,614
	,550	,071	,064	,080	−2,646	−2,745	−2,529
	,600	,077	,069	,087	−2,569	−2,672	−2/442
	,650	,083	,074	,095	−2,489	−2,598	−2,349
	,700	,090	,080	,105	−2,404	−2,522	−2,251
	,750	,099	,087	,117	−2,313	−2/441	−2,143
	,800	,109	,095	,132	−2,212	−2,351	−2,022
	,850	,123	,106	,153	−2,094	−2,248	−1,879
	,900	,143	,120	,183	−1,945	−2,120	−1,699
	,910	,148	,124	,191	−1,909	−2,089	−1,655
	,920	,154	,128	,200	−1,870	−2,055	−1,608
	,930	,161	,133	,211	−1,827	−2,018	−1,556
	,940	,169	,138	,224	−1,780	−1,977	−1/497
	,950	,178	,145	,239	−1,725	−1,931	−1/430
	,960	,190	,153	,259	−1,661	−1,876	−1,352
	,970	,206	,164	,285	−1,582	−1,809	−1,255
	,980	,228	,179	,324	−1,477	−1,719	−1,126
	,990	,269	,206	,397	−1,312	−1,579	−,923

[a]A heterogeneity factor is used
[b]Logarithm base=2.718

E.g., one might conclude that a 0,143 dilution of the chemical repellent causes 0,900 (=90 %) of the mosquitos to have gone. And 0,066 dilution would mean that 0,500 (=50 %) of the mosquitos disappeared.

Multiple Probit Regression

Like multiple logistic regression using multiple predictors, probit regression can also be applied with multiple predictors. We will add as second predictor to the above example the nonchemical repellents ultrasound (=1) and burning candles (=2) (see uppermost table of this chapter).

Command:

Analyze....Regression....Probit Regression....Response Frequency: enter "mosquitos gone"....Total Observed: enter "n mosquitos"....Covariate(s): enter "chemical"....Transform: select "natural log"....click OK.

Chi-Square tests				
		Chi-Square	df[a]	Sig.
PROBIT	Pearson Goodness-of-Fit Test	3863,489	11	,000[b]

[a]Statistics based on individual cases differ from statistics based on aggregated cases
[b]Since the significance level is less than, 150, a heterogeneity factor is used in the calculation of confidence limits

Again, the goodness of fit is not what it should be, but SPSS adds a correction factor for heterogeneity. The underneath shows the regression coefficients for the multiple model. The no chemical repellents have significantly different effects on the outcome.

Parameter estimates

Parameter			Estimate	Std. Error	Z	Sig.	95 % Confidence interval Lower bound	Upper bound
PROBIT[a]	Chemical (dilution)		1,654	,006	284,386	,000	1,643	1,665
	Intercept[b]	Ultrasound	4,678	,017	269,650	,000	4,661	4,696
		Burning candles	4,321	,017	253,076	,000	4,304	4,338

[a]PROBIT model: PROBIT(p) = Intercept + BX(Covariates X are transformed using the base 2.718 logarithm.)
[b]Corresponds to the grouping variable repellentnonchemical

Cell counts and residuals

Number		Repellent non chemical	chemical (dilution)	Number of subjects	Observed responses	Expected responses	Residual	Probability
PROBIT	1	1	-3,912	18000	1000	658,233	341,767	,037
	2	1	-3,624	18500	1000	1740,139	-740,139	,094
	3	1	-3,401	19500	3500	3350,108	149,892	,172
	4	1	-3,124	18000	4500	5630,750	-1130,750	,313
	5	1	-2,708	16500	9500	9553,811	-53,811	,579
	6	1	-2,430	22500	17000	16760,668	239,332	,745
	7	1	-2,303	24000	20500	19388,521	1111,479	,808
	8	2	-3,912	22500	500	355,534	144,466	,016
	9	2	-3,624	18500	1500	871,485	628,515	,047
	10	2	-3,401	19000	1000	1824,614	-824,614	,096
	11	2	-3,124	20000	5000	3979,458	1020,542	,199
	12	2	-2,708	22000	10000	9618,701	381,299	,437
	13	2	-2,430	16500	8000	10202,854	-2202,654	,618
	14	2	-2,303	18500	13500	12873,848	626,152	,696

In the above Cell Counts table, it is shown that according to the chi-square tests the differences of observed and expected proportions of mosquitos gone were statistically significant several times. The next page table gives interesting results. E.g., a 0,128 dilution of the chemical repellent causes 0,900 (=90 %) of the mosquitos to have gone in the ultrasound tests. And 0,059 dilution would mean that 0,500 (=50 %) of the mosquitos disappeared. The results of burning candles were less impressive. 0,159 dilution caused 90 % of the mosquitos to disappear, 0,073 dilution 50 %.

Confidence limits

			95 % Confidence limits for chemical (dilution)			95 % Confidence limits for log (chemical (dilution)[b]		
Nonchemical		Probability	Estimate	Lower bound	Upper bound	Estimate	Lower bound	Upper bound
PROBIT[a]	Ultrasound	,010	,014	,011	,018	–4,235	–4,486	–4,042
		,020	,017	,014	,020	–4,070	–4,296	–3,895
		,030	,019	,015	,022	–3,966	–4,176	–3,801
		,040	,021	,017	,024	–3,887	–4,086	–3,731
		,050	,022	,018	,025	–3,823	–4,013	–3,673
		,060	,023	,019	,027	–3,769	–3,951	–3,624
		,070	,024	,020	,028	–3,721	–3,896	–3,581
		,080	,025	,021	,029	–3,678	–3,848	–3,542
		,090	,026	,022	,030	–3,639	–3,804	–3,506
		,100	,027	,023	,031	–3,603	–3,763	–3,473
		,150	,032	,027	,036	–3,455	–3,597	–3,337
		,200	,036	,031	,040	–3,337	–3,467	–3,227
		,250	,039	,035	,044	–3,236	–3,356	–3,131
		,300	,043	,038	,048	–3,146	–3,258	–3,043
		,350	,047	,042	,052	–3,062	–3,169	–2,961
		,400	,051	,046	,056	–2,982	–3,085	–2,882
		,450	,055	,049	,061	–2,905	–3,006	–2,803
		,500	,059	,053	,066	–2,829	–2,929	–2,725
		,550	,064	,058	,071	–2,753	–2,853	–2,646
		,600	,069	,062	,077	–2,675	–2,777	–2,564
		,650	,075	,067	,084	–2,596	–2,700	–2,478
		,700	,081	,073	,092	–2,512	–2,620	–2,387
		,750	,089	,079	,102	–2,421	–2,534	–2,287
		,800	,098	,087	,114	–2,320	–2,440	–2,174
		,850	,111	,097	,130	–2,202	–2,332	–2,042
		,900	,128	,111	,153	–2,054	–2,197	–1,874
		,910	,133	,115	,160	–2,018	–2,165	–1,833
		,920	,138	,119	,167	–1,979	–2,129	–1,789
		,930	,144	,124	,175	–1,936	–2,091	–1,740
		,940	,151	,129	,185	–1,889	–2,048	–1,686
		,950	,160	,135	,197	–1,834	–1,999	–1,623
		,960	,170	,143	,212	–1,770	–1,942	–1,550
		,970	,184	,154	,232	–1,691	–1,871	–1,459
		,980	,205	,169	,262	–1,587	–1,778	–1,339
		,990	,241	,196	,317	–1,422	–1,632	–1,149

(continued)

Confidence limits

Nonchemical		Probability	95 % Confidence limits for chemical (dilution) Estimate	Lower bound	Upper bound	95 % Confidence limits for log (chemical (dilution)[b] Estimate	Lower bound	Upper bound
	Burning candles	,010	,018	,014	,021	–4,019	–4,247	–3,841
		,020	,021	,017	,025	–3,854	–4,058	–3,693
		,030	,024	,019	,027	–3,750	–3,939	–3,599
		,040	,025	,021	,029	–3,671	–3,850	–3,528
		,050	,027	,023	,031	–3,607	–3,777	–3,469
		,060	,029	,024	,033	–3,553	–3,716	–3,420
		,070	,030	,026	,034	–3,505	–3,662	–3,376
		,080	,031	,027	,036	–3,462	–3,614	–3,336
		,090	,033	,028	,037	–3,423	–3,571	–3,300
		,100	,034	,029	,038	–3,387	–3,531	–3,267
		,150	,039	,034	,044	–3,239	–3,367	–3,128
		,200	,044	,039	,049	–3,121	–3,240	–3,015
		,250	,049	,044	,054	–3,020	–3,132	–2,916
		,300	,053	,048	,059	–2,930	–3,037	–2,826
		,350	,058	,052	,065	–2,845	–2,950	–2,741
		,400	,063	,057	,070	–2,766	–2,869	–2,658
		,450	,068	,061	,076	–2,688	–2,793	–2,578
		,500	,073	,066	,082	–2,613	–2,718	–2,497
		,550	,079	,071	,089	–2,537	–2,644	–2,415
		,600	,085	,076	,097	–2,459	–2,571	–2,331
		,650	,093	,082	,106	–2,380	–2,495	–2,244
		,700	,101	,089	,116	–2,295	–2,417	–2,151
		,750	,110	,097	,129	–2,205	–2,333	–2,049
		,800	,122	,106	,144	–2,104	–2,240	–1,936
		,850	,137	,119	,165	–1,986	–2,133	–1,802
		,900	,159	,136	,195	–1,838	–1,999	–1,633
		,910	,165	,140	,203	–1,802	–1,966	–1,592
		,920	,172	,145	,213	–1,763	–1,932	–1,548
		,930	,179	,151	,223	–1,720	–1,893	–1,499
		,940	,188	,157	,236	–1,672	–1,850	–1,444
		,950	,198	,165	,251	–1,618	–1,802	–1,381
		,960	,211	,175	,270	–1,554	–1,745	–1,308
		,970	,229	,187	,296	–1,475	–1,675	–1,217
		,980	,254	,206	,334	–1,371	–1,582	–1,096
		,990	,299	,238	,404	–1,206	–1,436	–,906

[a]A heterogenelty factor is used
[b]Logarithm base = 2.718

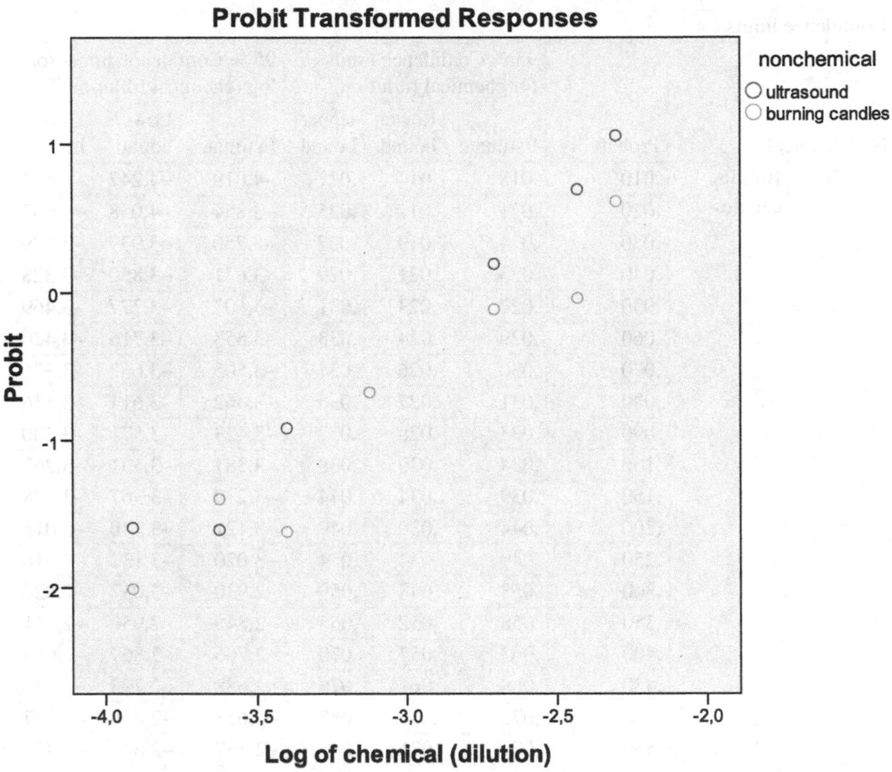

The above figure supports the adequacy of the multiple variables probit model, with two similarly sloped linear patterns (the blue and the green one) of "chemical repellent levels" versus "mosquitos gone levels" regressions.

Conclusion

Probit regression is, just like logistic regression, for estimating the effect of predictors on yes/no outcomes. If your predictor is multiple pharmacological treatment dosages, then probit regression may be more convenient than logistic regression, because your results will be reported in the form of response rates instead of odds ratios.

This chapter shows that probit regression is able to find response rates of different dosages of mosquito repellents.

Note

More background, theoretical and mathematical information of probit regression is given in the Chap. 7, Machine learning in medicine part three, Probit regression, pp 63–68, 2013, Springer Heidelberg Germany, (from the same authors).

Chapter 47
Interval Censored Data Analysis for Assessing Mean Time to Cancer Relapse (51 Patients)

General Purpose

In survival studies often time to first outpatient clinic check instead of time to event is measured. Somewhere in the interval between the last and current visit an event may have taken place. For simplicity such data are often analyzed using the proportional hazard model of Cox (Chap. 17, Cox regression, pp. 209–212, in: Statistics applied to clinical studies 5th edition, Springer Heidelberg Germany, 2012, from the same authors). However, this analysis is not entirely appropriate. It assumes that time to first outpatient check is equal to time to relapse. However, instead of a time to relapse an interval is given, in which the relapse has occurred, and so this variable is somewhat more loose than the usual variable time to event. An appropriate statistic for the current variable would be the mean time to relapse inferenced from a generalized linear model with an interval censored link function, rather than the proportional hazard method of Cox.

Primary Scientific Question

This chapter is to assess whether an appropriate statistic for the variable "time to first check" in survival studies would be the mean time to relapse, as inferenced from a generalized linear model with an interval censored link function.

T.J. Cleophas, A.H. Zwinderman, *Machine Learning in Medicine - a Complete Overview*, DOI 10.1007/978-3-319-15195-3_47

Example

In 51 patients in remission their status at the time-to-first-outpatient-clinic-control was checked (mths = months).

treatment (0 and 1)	time to first check (mths)	result (0 = remission 1 = relapse)
1	11	0
0	12	1
0	9	1
1	12	0
0	12	0
1	12	0
1	5	1
1	12	0
1	12	0
0	12	0

The first 10 patients are above. The entire data file is entitled "intervalcensored.sav", and is in extras.springer.com. Cox regression was applied. Start by opening the data file in SPSS statistical software.

Command:

Analyze….Survival….Cox Regression….Time : time to first check….Status : result….Define Event….Single value: type 1….click Continue….Covariates: enter treatment….click Categorical….Categorical Covariates: enter treatment….click Continue….click Plots….mark Survival….Separate Lines for: enter treatment….click Continue….click OK.

Variables in the Equation

	B	SE	Wald	df	Sig.	Exp(B)
Treatment	.919	.477	3.720	1	.054	2.507

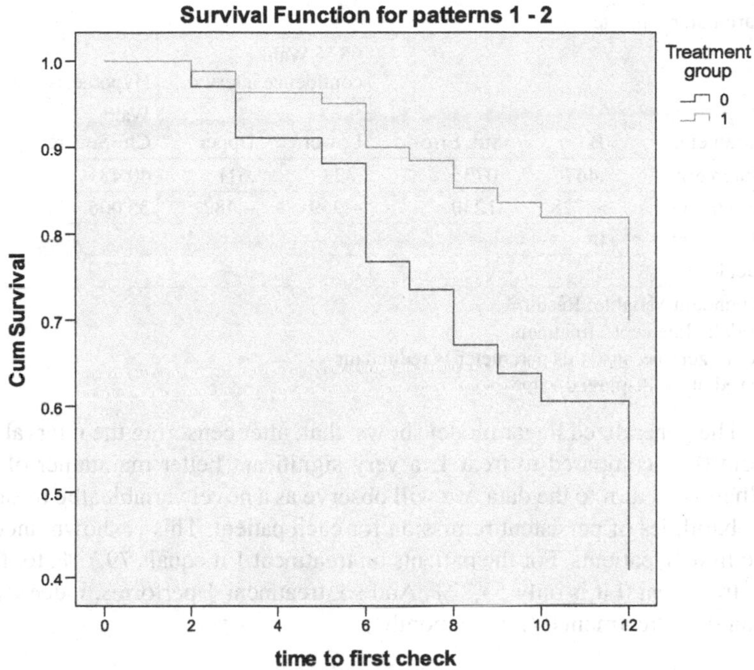

The above table is in the output. It shows that treatment is not a significant predictor for relapse. In spite of the above Kaplan-Meier curves, suggesting the opposite, the treatments are not significantly different from one another because $p>0.05$. However, the analysis so far is not entirely appropriate. It assumes that time to first outpatient check is equal to time to relapse. However, instead of a time to relapse an interval is given between 2 and 12 months in which the relapse has occurred, and so this variables is somewhat more loose than the usual variable time to event. An appropriate statistic for the current variable would be the mean time to relapse inferenced from a generalized linear model with an interval censored link function, rather than the proportional hazard method of Cox.

Command:

Analyze….click Generalized Linear Models….click once again Generalized Linear Models….Type of Model….mark Interval censored survival….click Response…. Dependent Variable: enter Result….Scale Weight Variable: enter "time to first check"….click Predictors….Factors: enter "treatment"….click Model….click once again Model: enter once again "treatment"….click Save….mark Predicted value of mean of response….click OK.

Parameter estimates

Parameter	B	Std. Error	95 % Wald confidence interval		Hypothesis test		
			Lower	Upper	Wald Chi-Square	df	Sig.
(Intercept)	.467	.0735	.323	.611	40.431	1	.000
[treatments]	–.728	.1230	–.969	–.487	35.006	1	.000
[treatments]	0[a]						
(Scale)	1[b]						

Dependent Variable: Result
Model: (Intercept), treatment
[a]Set to zero because this parameter Is redundant
[b]Fixed at the displayed value

The generalized linear model shows, that, after censoring the intervals, the treatment 0 is, compared to treat 1, a very significant better maintainer of remission. When we return to the data, we will observe as a novel variable, the mean predicted probabilities of persistent remission for each patient. This is shown underneath for the first 10 patients. For the patients on treatment 1 it equals 79,7 %, for the patients on treatment 0 it is only 53,7 %. And so, treatment 1 performs, indeed, a lot better than does treatment 0 (mths = months).

treatment (0 and 1)	time to first check (mths)	result (0 = remission)	Mean Predicted_ 1 1 = relapse)
1	11	0	.797
0	12	1	.537
0	9	1	.537
1	12	0	.797
0	12	0	.537
1	12	0	.797
1	5	1	.797
1	12	0	.797
1	12	0	.797
0	12	0	.537

Conclusion

This chapter assesses whether an appropriate statistic for the variable "time to first check" in survival studies is the mean time to relapse, as inferenced from a generalized linear model with an interval censored link function. The current example shows that, in addition, more sensitivity of testing is obtained with p-values of 0.054

versus 0.0001. Also, predicted probabilities of persistent remission or risk of relapse for different treatment modalities are given. This method is an important tool for analyzing such data.

Note

More background, theoretical and mathematical information of survival analyses is given in Chap. 17, Cox regression, pp. 209–212, in: Statistics applied to clinical studies 5th edition, Springer Heidelberg Germany, 2012, from the same authors.

Chapter 48
Structural Equation Modeling (SEM) with SPSS Analysis of Moment Structures (Amos) for Cause Effect Relationships I (35 Patients)

General Purpose

In clinical efficacy studies the outcome is often influenced by multiple causal factors, like drug - noncompliance, frequency of counseling, and many more factors. Structural equation modeling (SEM) was only recently formally defined by Pearl (In: Causality, reason, and inference, Cambridge University Press, Cambridge UK 2000). This statistical methodology includes

1. factor analysis (see also Chap.14, Factor analysis, pp 167–181, in: Machine learning in medicine part one, Springer Heidelberg Germany, 2013, from the same authors),
2. path analysis (see also Chap. 2, Multistage regression, in: SPSS for starters part two, pp 3–6, Springer Heidelberg Germany, 2012 from the same authors),
3. regression analysis (see also Chap. 14, Linear regression, basic approach, in: Statistics applied to clinical studies 5th edition, pp 161–176, Springer Heidelberg Germany, 2012, from the same authors).

An SEM model looks like a complex regression model, but it is more. It extends the prior hypothesis of correlation to that of causality, and this is accomplished by a network of variables tested versus one another with standardized rather than unstandardized regression coefficients.

The network is commonly named a Bayesian network, otherwise called a DAG (directed acyclic graph), (see also Chap. 16, Bayesian networks, pp 163–170, in: Machine learning in medicine part 2, Springer Heidelberg Germany, 2013, from the same authors), which is a probabilistic graphical model of nodes (the variables) and connecting arrows presenting the conditional dependencies of the nodes.

This chapter is to assess whether the Amos (analysis of moment structures) add-on module of SPSS statistical software, frequently used in econo-/sociometry, but little used in medicine, is able to perform an SEM analysis of pharmacodynamic data.

T.J. Cleophas, A.H. Zwinderman, *Machine Learning in Medicine - a Complete Overview*, DOI 10.1007/978-3-319-15195-3_48

Primary Scientific Question

Can SEM modeling in Amos (Analysis of Moment Structures) demonstrate direct and indirect effects of non-compliance and counseling on treatment efficacy.

Example

We will use the same example as the one used in Chap. 2, Multistage regression, in: SPSS for starters part two, pp 3–6, Springer Heidelberg Germany, 2012 from the same authors.

stool	counseling	noncompliance
stools/month	counselings/month	drug noncompliances/month
24,00	8,00	25,00
30,00	13,00	30,00
25,00	15,00	25,00
35,00	10,00	31,00
39,00	9,00	36,00
30,00	10,00	33,00
27,00	8,00	22,00
14,00	5,00	18,00
39,00	13,00	14,00
42,00	15,00	30,00

The first 10 patients of the 35 patient data file is above. The entire data file is in extras.springer.com, and is entitled "amos1.sav". We will first perform traditional linear regressions. Start by opening the data file.

Command:

Analyze....Regression....Linear....Dependent: enter "stool"....Independent(s): enter "counseling and non-compliance"....click OK.

Coefficients[a]

Model		Unstandardized coefficients		Standardized coefficients	t	Sig.
		B	Std. Error	Beta		
1	(Constant)	2,270	4,823		,471	,641
	Counseling	1,876	,290	,721	6,469	,000
	Non-compliance	,285	,167	,190	1,705	,098

[a]Dependent variable: ther eff

The above table is given on the output sheet, and shows that, with p=0.10 as cut-off for statistical significance both variables are significant.

Command:

Analyze....Regression....Linear....Dependent: enter "counseling"....Independent(s): enter "non-compliance"....click OK.

Coefficients[a]

Model		Unstandardized coefficients		Standardized coefficients		
		B	Std. Error	Beta	t	Sig.
1	(Constant)	4,228	2,800		1,510	,141
	Non-compliance	,220	,093	,382	2,373	,024

[a]Dependent variable: counseling

The above table shows that non-compliance is also a significant predictor of counseling. This would mean that non-compliance works two ways: it predicts therapeutic efficacy directly and indirectly through counseling. However, the indirect way is not taken into account in the one step linear regression. We will now use the Amos add-on module for further analysis.

Command:

Analyze....click IBM SPSS Amos

The work area of Amos appears. The menu is in the second upper row. The toolbar is on the left. In the empty area on the right you can draw your networks.

click File....click Save as....Browse the folder you selected in your personal computer, and enter Amos1....click Save.

In the first upper row the title Amos1 has appeared, in the bottom rectangle left from the empty area the title Amos1 has also appeared.

click Diagram....left click "Draw Observed" and drag to empty area....click the green rectangle and a colorless rectangle appears....left click it and a red rectangle appears.... do this 2 more times and have the rectangles at different places....click Diagram again.... left click "Draw Unobserved" and drag to right part of empty area....click the green ellipse.....a colorless ellipse appears, and later a red and finally black ellipse.

The underneath figure shows how your screen will look by now. There are three rectangle nodes for observed variables, and one oval node for an unobserved, otherwise called latent, variable.

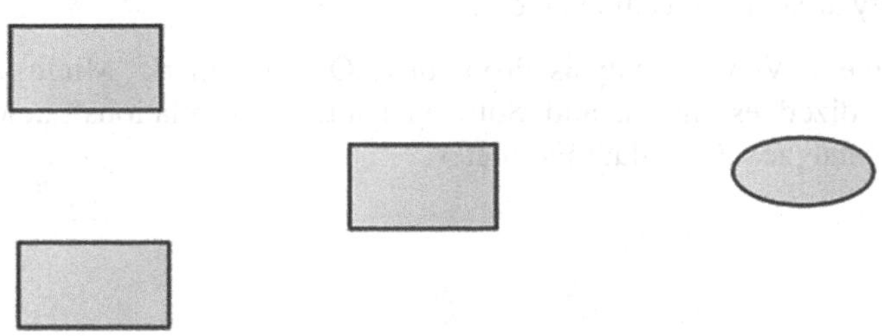

Next we will have to enter the names of the variables.

Command:

right click in the left upper rectangle....click Object Properties....Variable name: type "noncompliance"....close dialog box....the name is now in the rectangle....do the same for the other two rectangles and type in the ellipse the term others (it indicates the remainder of variables not taken into account in the current model, together with the variables present the outcome is explained by 100 %).
Next arrows have to be added to the diagram.

Command:

click Diagram....click Draw Path for arrows....click Draw Covariance for double-headed arrow.

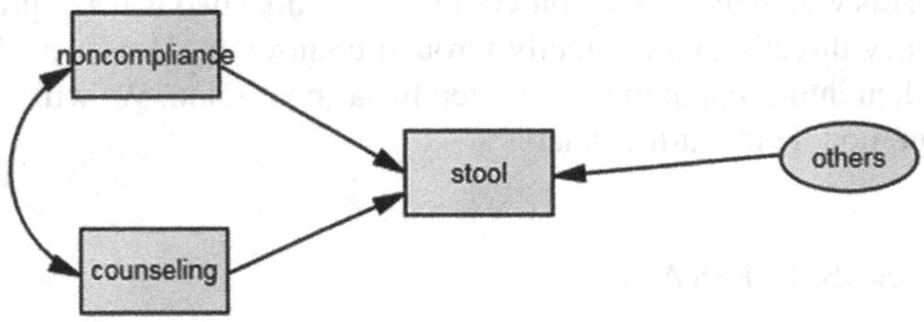

The above figure is now in the empty area. In order to match the "others" variables in the ellipse with the three other variables of the model, they a regression weight, like the value 1, has to be added.

right click at the arrow of the ellipse....click Object Properties....click Parameters.... Regression weights: enter 1....close dialog box.

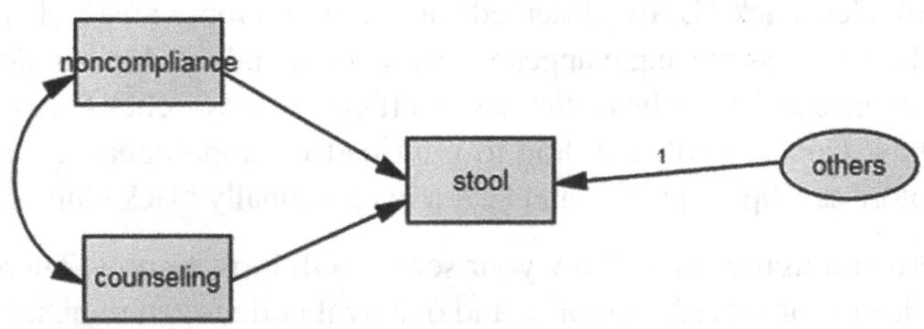

The empty area now has the value 1.

click from menu View....Analysis Properties....Output....mark "Minimization history, Standardized estimates, and Squared multiple correlations"....close dialog box....click Analyze....Calculate Estimates.

A new path diagram button has appeared in the upper white rectangle left from the empty area. Click it

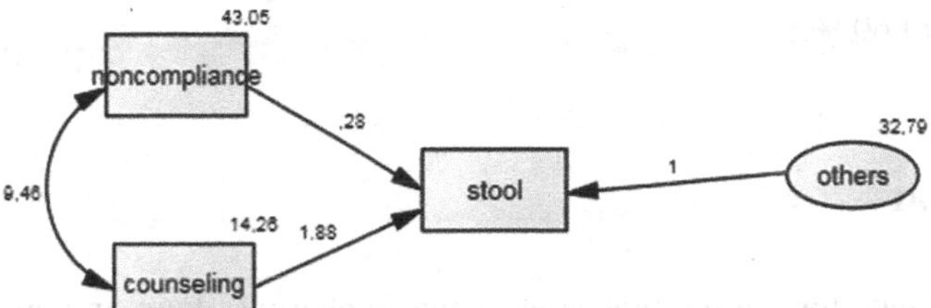

Unstandardized regression coefficients are now in the model, that of counseling versus stool equals 1.88, that of noncompliance versus stool equals 0.28. These values are identical to the values obtained by ordinary multiple linear regression as shown in the previous tabs. However, for path analysis standardized values are more important.

In order to view the standardized values, click in the third white rectangle left from the empty area "Standardized estimates".

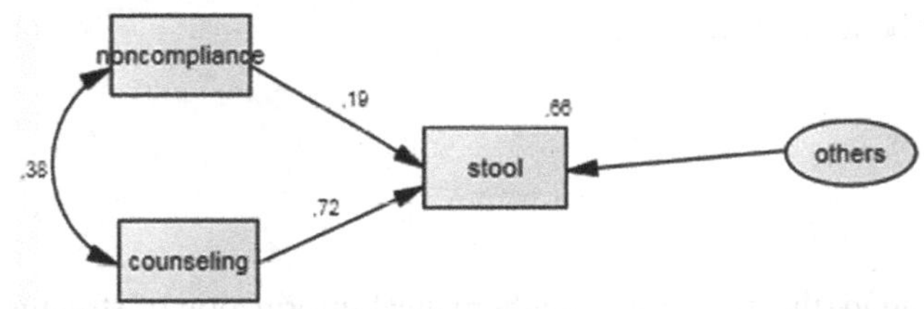

Now we observe the standardized regression coefficients. They are identical to the standardized regression coefficients as computed by the ordinary linear regression models as shown in the previous tabs:

0.19 noncompliance versus stool
0.72 counseling versus stool
0.38 noncompliance versus counseling.

What advantage does this path analysis give us as compared to traditional regression modeling. The advantage is that multiple regression coefficients, as they are standardized, can be simply added up after weighting in order to estimate the entire strength of prediction. Single path analysis gives a standardized regression coefficient of 0.19. This underestimates the real effect of non-compliance. Two step path analysis is more realistic and shows that the add-up path statistic is larger and equals

$$0.19 + 0.38 \times 0.72 = 0.46$$

The two-path statistic of 0.46 is a lot better than the single path statistic of 0.19 with an increase of 60 %.

Conclusion

SEM is adequate for cause effect assessments in pharmacology, and, in addition, it is very easy to use. Arbuckle, the author of IBM SPSS Amos 19 User's Guide noted, that it may open the way to data analysis to nonstatisticians, because it avoids mathematics, and, like other machine learning software, e.g., SPSS modeler (see the Chaps. 61, 64, 65), Knime (see the Chaps. 7, 8, 70, 71, 74), and Weka (see the Chap. 70), it makes extensively use of beautiful graphs to visualize procedures and results instead.

The current chapter gives only the simplest applications of SEM modeling. SEM modeling can also handle binary data using chi-square tests, include multiple models in a single analysis, replace more complex multivariate analysis of variance with similar if not better power.

Note

More background, theoretical and mathematical information of structural equation models like path analysis, factor analysis, and regression models are in (1) the Chap. 14, Factor analysis, pp 167–181, in: Machine learning in medicine part 1, Springer Heidelberg Germany, 2013, (2) the Chap. 2, Multistage regression, in: SPSS for starters part 2, pp 3–6, Springer Heidelberg Germany, 2012, (3) the Chap. 14, Linear regression, basic approach, in: Statistics applied to clinical studies 5th edition, pp 161–176, Springer Heidelberg Germany, 2012, all from the same authors.

Chapter 49
Structural Equation Modeling (SEM) with SPSS Analysis of Moment Structures (Amos) for Cause Effect Relationships in Pharmacodynamic Studies II (35 Patients)

General Purpose

In clinical efficacy studies the outcome is often influenced by multiple causal factors, like drug - noncompliance, frequency of counseling, and many more factors. Structural equation modeling (SEM) was only recently formally defined by Pearl (In: Causality, reason, and inference, Cambridge University Press, Cambridge UK 2000). This statistical methodology includes

1. factor analysis (see also Chap. 14, Factor analysis, pp 167–181, in: Machine learning in medicine part one, Springer Heidelberg Germany, 2013, from the same authors),
2. path analysis (see also Chap. 2, Multistage regression, in: SPSS for starters part two, pp 3–6, Springer Heidelberg Germany, 2012 from the same authors),
3. regression analysis (see also Chap. 14, Linear regression, basic approach, in: Statistics applied to clinical studies 5th edition, pp 161–176, Springer Heidelberg Germany, 2012, from the same authors).

An SEM model looks like a complex regression model, but it is more. It extends the prior hypothesis of correlation to that of causality, and this is accomplished by a network of variables tested versus one another with standardized rather than unstandardized regression coefficients.

The network is commonly named a Bayesian network, otherwise called a DAG (directed acyclic graph), (see also Chap.16, Bayesian networks, pp 163–170, in: Machine learning in medicine part 2, Springer Heidelberg Germany, 2013, from the same authors), which is a probabilistic graphical model of nodes (the variables) and connecting arrows presenting the conditional dependencies of the nodes.

This chapter is to assess whether the Amos (analysis of moment structures) add-on module of SPSS statistical software, frequently used in econo-/sociometry but little used in medicine, is able to perform an SEM analysis of pharmacodynamic data.

T.J. Cleophas, A.H. Zwinderman, *Machine Learning in Medicine - a Complete Overview*, DOI 10.1007/978-3-319-15195-3_49

Primary Scientific Question

Can SEM modeling in Amos (analysis of moment structures) demonstrate direct and indirect effects of non-compliance and counseling on treatment efficacy and quality of life.

Example

We will use the same example as the one used in Chap.3, Multivariate analysis using path statistics, in: SPSS for starters part 2, pp 7–11, Springer Heidelberg Germany, 2012 from the same authors.

stool	counseling	noncompliance	qol
stools/month	counselings/month	drug noncompliances/month	quality of life score
24,00	8,00	25,00	69,00
30,00	13,00	30,00	110,00
25,00	15,00	25,00	78,00
35,00	10,00	31,00	103,00
39,00	9,00	36,00	103,00
30,00	10,00	33,00	102,00
27,00	8,00	22,00	76,00
14,00	5,00	18,00	75,00
39,00	13,00	14,00	99,00
42,00	15,00	30,00	107,00

The first 10 patients of the 35 patient data file is above. The entire data file is in extras.springer.com, and is entitled "amos2.sav".

We will use SEM modeling for estimating variances and covariances in these data.

$$\text{Variance} = \Sigma\ [(x - x_{mean})^2].$$

It is a measure for the spread of the data of the variable x.

$$\text{Covariance} = \Sigma\ [(x_1 - x_{1mean})\ (x_2 - x_{2mean})].$$

It is a measure for the strength of association between the two variables x_1 and x_2. If the covariances are significantly larger than zero, this would mean that there is a significant association between them.

Command:

Analyze....click IBM SPSS Amos

The work area of Amos appears. The menu is in the second upper row. The toolbar is on the left. In the empty area on the right you can draw your networks.

click File....click Save as....Browse the folder you selected in your personal computer, and enter amos2....click Save.

In the first upper row the title amos2 has appeared, in the bottom rectangle left from the empty area the title amos2 has also appeared.

click Diagram....left click "Draw Observed" and drag to empty area....click the green rectangle and a colorless rectangle appears....left click it and a red rectangle appears....do this 3 more times and have the rectangles at different places

The underneath figure shows how your screen will look by now. There are four rectangle nodes for observed variables.

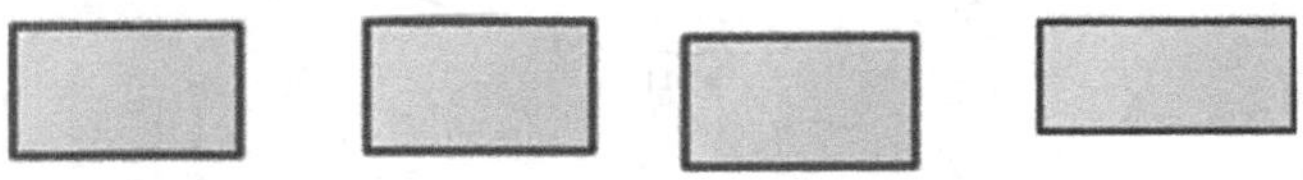

Next we will have to enter the names of the variables.

Command:

right click in the left upper rectangle....click Object Properties....Variable name: type "noncompliance"....close dialog box....the name is now in the rectangle....do the same for the other three rectangles.

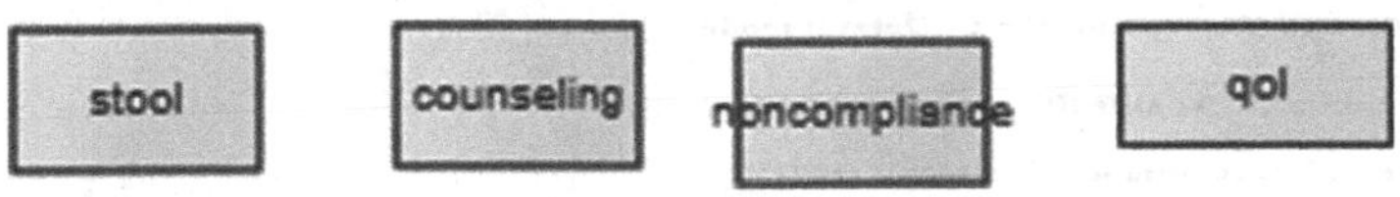

Next arrows have to be added to the diagram.

Command:

click Diagram....click Draw Covariances.

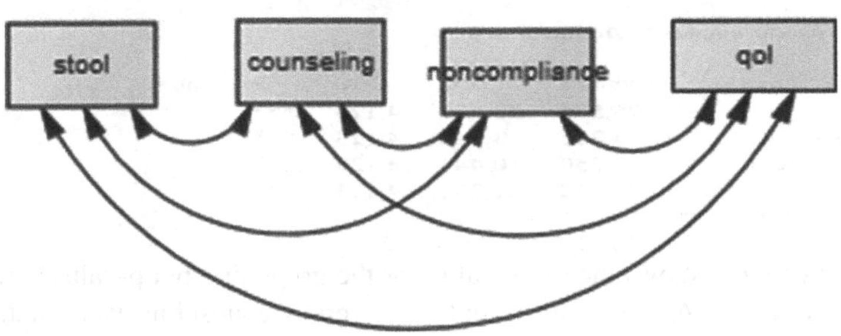

The above figure is now in the empty area. We will subsequently perform the analysis.

Command:

Analyze....Calculate Estimates....click File....click Save as....Browse for the folder of your choice and enter a name....click Save....click the new path diagram button that has appeared in the upper white rectangle left from the empty area.

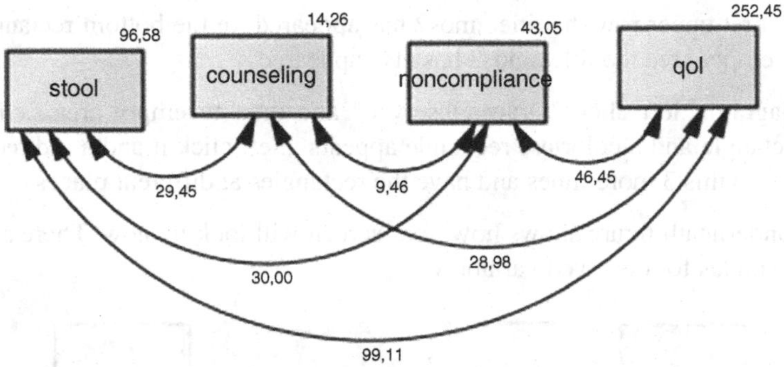

Unstandardized covariances of the variables are now in the graph and variances of the variables are in the right upper corner of the nodes.

We will also view the text output.

Command:

click View....click Text output.

Estimates (Group number 1 - Default model)

Scalar Estimates (Group number 1 - Default model)

Maximum Likelihood Estimates

Covariances: (Group number 1 - Default model)

			Estimate	S.E.	C.R.	P	Label
stool	<-->	counseling	29,449	8,125	3,624	***	
counseling	<-->	noncompliance	9,461	4,549	2,080	,038	
noncompliance	<-->	qol	46,454	19,574	2,373	,018	
stool	<-->	noncompliance	30,003	12,197	2,460	,014	
counseling	<-->	qol	28,980	11,428	2,536	,011	
stool	<-->	qol	99,109	31,718	3,125	,002	

Variances: (Group number 1 - Default model)

	Estimate	S.E.	C.R.	P	Label
stool	96,576	23,423	4,123	***	
counseling	14,261	3,459	4,123	***	
noncompliance	43,050	10,441	4,123	***	
qol	252,462	61,231	4,123	***	

The above table shows the same values as the graph did, but p-values are added to the covariances. All of them except stool versus counseling were statistically significant with p-values from 0.002 to 0.038, meaning that all of these variables were closer associated with one another than could happen by chance.

Unstandardized covariances of variables with different units are not appropriate, and, therefore, Amos also produces standardized values (= unstandardized divided by their own standard errors).

click View....click Analysis Properties....click Output tab....mark Standardized estimates....close dialog box....choose Analyze....click Calculate Estimates....click the path diagram button....click standardized estimates in third white rectangle left from the empty area.

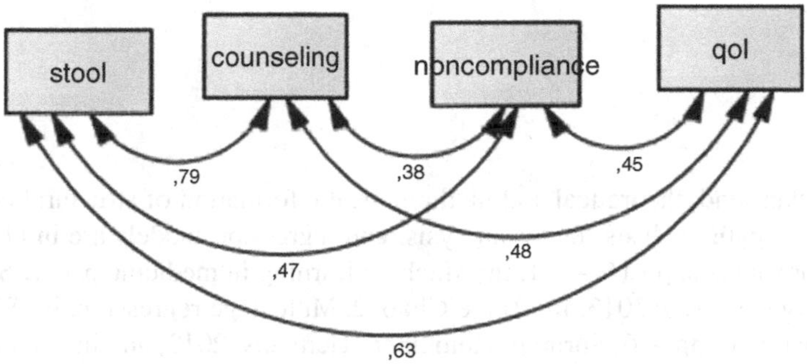

The standardized covariances is given.

Finally, we will view the standardized results as table.

click View....click Text Output.

Variables

Name	Label	Observed	Variance Estimate	SE
stool		☑	96,58	23,42
counseling		☑	14,26	3,46
noncompliance		☑	43,05	10,44
qol		☑	252,46	61,23

Regression weights

Dependent	Independent	Estimate	SE	Standardized

Covariances

Variable 1	Variable 2	Estimate	SE	Correlation
stool	counseling	29,45	8,13	,79
counseling	noncompliance	9,46	4,55	,38
noncompliance	qol	46,45	19,57	,45
stool	noncompliance	30,00	12,20	,47
counseling	qol	28,98	11,43	,48
stool	qol	99,11	31,72	,63

The standardized covariances are in the column entitled Correlation.

Conclusion

SEM modeling can estimate covariances with their standard error and p-values. Significant p-values mean that the association of the variables is statistically significant and that the paired data are thus closer to one another than could happen by chance. The analyses of covariances is a basic methodology of SEM modeling used for testing and making clinical inferences like the presence of meaningful cause effect relationships like pharmacodynamic relationships.

Note

More background, theoretical and mathematical information of structural equation models like path analysis, factor analysis, and regression models are in (1) Chap. 14, Factor analysis, pp 167–181, in: Machine learning in medicine part 1, Springer Heidelberg Germany, 2013, in (2) the Chap. 2, Multistage regression, in: SPSS for starters part two, pp 3–6, Springer Heidelberg Germany, 2012, and in (3) the Chap. 14, Linear regression, basic approach, in: Statistics applied to clinical studies 5th edition, pp 161–176, Springer Heidelberg Germany, 2012, all from the same authors.

Part III
Rules Models

Chapter 50
Neural Networks for Assessing Relationships That Are Typically Nonlinear (90 Patients)

General Purpose

Unlike regression analysis which uses algebraic functions for data fitting, neural networks uses a stepwise method called the steepest decent method for the purpose. To asses whether typically nonlinear relationships can be adequately fit by this method.

Specific Scientific Question

Body surface is a better indicator for drug dosage than body weight. The relationship between body weight, length and surface are typically nonlinear. Can a neural network be trained to predict body surface of individual patients.

This chapter was previously published in "Machine learning in medicine-cookbook 1" as Chap. 13, 2013.

T.J. Cleophas, A.H. Zwinderman, *Machine Learning in Medicine - a Complete Overview*, DOI 10.1007/978-3-319-15195-3_50

Var 1	Var 2	Var 3
30,50	138,50	10072,90
15,00	101,00	6189,00
2,50	51,50	1906,20
30,00	141,00	10290,60
40,50	154,00	13221,60
27,00	136,00	9654,50
15,00	106,00	6768,20
15,00	103,00	6194,10
13,50	96,00	5830,20
36,00	150,00	11759,00
12,00	92,00	5299,40
2,50	51,00	2094,50
19,00	121,00	7490,80
28,00	130,50	9521,70

Var 1 weight (kg)
Var 2 height (m)
Var 3 body surface measured photometrically (cm^2)

The first 14 patients are shown only, the entire data file is entitled "neuralnetworks" and is in extras.springer.com.

The Computer Teaches Itself to Make Predictions

SPSS 19.0 is used for training and outcome prediction. It uses XML (eXtended Markup Language) files to store data. MLP stands for multilayer perceptron, and indicates the neural network methodology used.

Command:

Click Transform....click Random Number Generators....click Set Starting Point....click Fixed Value (2,000,000)....click OK....click Analyze....Neural Networks.... Multilayer Perceptron....Dependent Variable: select body surface ....Factors: select weight and height....click Partitioning: set the training sample (7), test sample (3), hold out sample (0)....click Architecture: click Custom Architecture....set the numbers of hidden layers (2)....click Activation Function: click hyperbolic tangens....click Save: click Save predicted values or category for each dependent variable....click Export: click Export synaptic weight estimates to XML file....click Browse....File name: enter "exportnn"....click Save....Options: click Maximum training time Minutes (15)....click OK.

The output warns that in the testing sample some cases have been excluded from analysis because of values not occurring in the training sample. Minimizing the output sheets shows the data file with predicted values (MLP_PredictedValue).

They are pretty much similar to the measured body surface values. We will use linear regression to estimate the association between the two.

Command:

Analyze....Regresssion....Linear....Dependent: bodysurface ....Independent: MLP_PredictedValue....OK.

The output sheets show that the r-value is 0.998, r-square 0.995, p<0.0001. The saved XML file will now be used to compute the body surface in five individual patients.

patient no	weight	height
1	36,00	130,50
2	28,00	150,00
3	12,00	121,00
4	19,00	92,00
5	2,50	51,00

Enter the above data in a new SPSS data file.

Command:

Utilities....click Scoring Wizard....click Browse....click Select....Folder: enter the exportnn.xml file....click Select....in Scoring Wizard click Next....click Use value substitution....click Next....click Finish.

The above data file now gives the body surfaces computed by the neural network with the help of the XML file.

Patient no	weight	height	computed body surfaces
1	36,00	130,50	10290,23
2	28,00	150,00	11754,33
3	12,00	121,00	7635,97
4	19,00	92,00	4733,40
5	2,50	51,00	2109,32

Conclusion

Multilayer perceptron neural networks can be readily trained to provide accurate body surface values of individual patients, and other nonlinear clinical outcomes.

Note

More background, theoretical and mathematical information of neural networks is available in Machine learning in medicine part one, Chaps. 12 and 13, entitled "Artificial intelligence, multilayer perceptron" and "Artificial intelligence, radial basis functions", pp 145–156 and 157–166, Springer Heidelberg Germany 2013, and the Chap. 63.

Chapter 51
Complex Samples Methodologies for Unbiased Sampling (9,678 Persons)

General Purpose

The research of entire populations is costly and obtaining information from selected samples instead is generally biased by selection bias. Complex sampling produces weighted, and, therefore, unbiased population estimates. This chapter is to assess whether this method can be trained for predicting health outcomes.

Specific Scientific Question

Can complex samples be trained to predict unbiased current health outcomes from previous health outcomes in individual members of an entire population.

This chapter was previously published in "Machine learning in medicine-cookbook 1" as Chap. 14, 2013.

T.J. Cleophas, A.H. Zwinderman, *Machine Learning in Medicine - a Complete Overview*, DOI 10.1007/978-3-319-15195-3_51

Var 1	Var 2	Var 3	Var 4	Var 5	Var 6
1	1	1	9	19,26	3,00
1	1	1	7	21,11	6,00
1	1	1	9	22,42	9,00
1	1	1	7	20,13	12,00
1	1	1	5	16,37	15,00
1	1	1	8	20,49	18,00
1	1	1	7	20,79	21,00
1	1	1	7	17,52	24,00
1	1	1	7	18,12	27,00
1	1	1	6	18,60	30,00

Var 1 neighborhood
Var 2 town
Var 3 county
Var 4 time (years)
Var 5 last health score
Var 6 case identity number (defined as property ID)

Prior health scores of a 9,768 member population recorded some 5–10 years ago were available as well as topographical information (the data file is entitled "complexsamples" and is in extras.springer.com). We wish to obtain information of individual current health scores. For that purpose the information of the entire data plus additional information on the current health scores from a random sample of 1,000 from this population were used. First, a *sampling plan* was designed with different counties, townships and neighborhoods weighted differently. A *random sample* of 1,000 was taken, and additional information was obtained from this random sample, and included.

The latter data file plus the *sampling plan* were, then, used for analysis. The SPSS modules complex samples (cs) "general linear model" and "ratios" modules were applied for analyses. A *sampling plan* of the above population data was designed using SPSS. Open in extras.springer.com the database entitled "complexsamples".

Command:

click Analyze….Complex Samples…. Select a sample…. click Design a sample, click Browse: select a map and enter a name, e.g., complexsamplesplan….click Next….Stratify by: select county….Clusters: select township….click Next…Type: Simple Random Sampling….click Without replacement….click Next….Units: enter Counts….click Value: enter 4….click Next….click Next….click (Yes, add stage 2 now)….click Next…Stratify by: enter neighbourhood….next…Type: Simple random sampling….click Without replacement….click Next….Units: enter proportions….click Value: enter 0,25….click Next….click Next….click (No, do not add another stage now)….click Next…Do you want to draw a sample: click Yes….Click Custom value….enter 123….click Next….click External file, click Browse: select a map and enter a name, e.g., complexsamplessample ….click Save….click Next….click Finish.

In the original data file the weights of 1,006 randomly sampled individuals are now given. In the maps selected above we find two new files,

1. entitled "complexsamplesplan" (this map can not be opened, but it can in closed form be entered whenever needed during further complex samples analyses of these data), and
2. entitled "complexsamplessample" containing 1,006 randomly selected individuals from the main data file.

The latter data file is first completed with current health scores before the definitive analysis. Only of 974 individuals the current information could be obtained, and these data were added as a new variable (see "complexsamplessample" at extras.springer.com). Also "complexsamplesplan" has for convenience been made available at extras.springer.com.

The Computer Teaches Itself to Predict Current Health Scores from Previous Health Scores

We now use the above data files "complexsamplessample" and "complexsamplesplan" for predicting individual current health scores and odds ratios of current versus previous health scores. Also, an XML (eXtended Markup Language) file will be designed for analyzing future data. First, open "complexsamplessample".

Command:

Click Transform....click Random Number Generators....click Set Starting Point.... click Fixed Value (2000000)....click OK....click Analyze....Complex Samples.... General Linear Model....click Browse: select the appropriate map and enter complexsamplesplan....click Continue...Dependent variable: enter curhealthscore .... Covariates: enter last healthscores....click Statistics: mark Estimates, 95 % Confidence interval, t-test....click Save....mark Predicted Values....in Export Model as XML click Browse....in appropriate folder enter File name: "exportcslin"....click Save....click Continue....click OK.

The underneath table gives the correlation coefficient and the 95 % confidence intervals. The lower part gives the data obtained through the usual commands (Analyze, Regression, Linear, Dependent (curhealthscore), Independent (s) (last healthscore), OK). It is remarkable to observe the differences between the two analyses. The correlation coefficients are largely the same but their standard errors are respectively 0.158 and 0.044. The t-value of the complex sampling analysis equals 5.315, while that of the traditional analysis equals no less than 19.635. Nonetheless, the reduced precision of the complex sampling analysis did not produce a statistically insignificant result, and, in addition, it was, of course, again adjusted for inappropriate probability estimates.

Parameter estimates[a]

Parameter	Estimate	Std. error	95 % confidence interval		Hypothesis test		
			Lower	Upper	t	df	Sig.
(Intercept)	8,151	2,262	3,222	13,079	3,603	12,000	,004
Lasthealthscore	,838	,158	,494	1,182	5,315	12,000	,000

[a]Model: curhealthscore = (Intercept) + lasthealthscore

Coefficients[a]

Model		Unstandardized coefficients		Standardized coefficients	t	Sig.
		B	Std. error	Beta		
1	(Constant)	7,353	,677		10,856	,000
	Last healthscore	,864	,044	,533	19,635	,000

[a]Dependent Variable: curhealthscore

The saved XML file will now be used to compute the predicted current health score in five individual patients from this population.

	Var 5
1	19,46
2	19,77
3	16,75
4	16,37
5	18,35

Var 5 Last health score

Enter the above data in a new SPSS data file.

Command:

Utilities….click Scoring Wizard….click Browse….click Select….Folder: enter the exportcslin.xml file….click Select….in Scoring Wizard click Next….mark Predicted Value….click Next….click Finish.

The above data file now gives the predicted current health scores with the help of the XML file.

	Var 5	Var 6
1	19,46	24,46
2	19,77	24,72
3	16,75	22,19
4	16,37	21,87
5	18,35	23,53

Var 5 last health score
Var 6 predicted value of current health score

The Computer Teaches Itself to Predict Individual Odds Ratios of Current Health Scores Versus Previous Health Scores

Open again the data file "complexsamplessample".

Command:

Click Transform....click Random Number Generators....click Set Starting Point.... click Fixed Value (2000000)....click OK....click Analyze....Complex Samples ....Ratios....click Browse: select the appropriate map and enter "complexsamples-plan"....click Continue...Numerators: enter curhealthscore.... Denominator: enter last healthscore ....Subpopulations: enter County....click Statistics: mark Standard error, Confidence interval (enter 95 %), Design effect....click Continue....click OK.

The underneath table (upper part) gives the overall ratio and the ratios per county plus 95 % confidence intervals. The design effects are the ratios of the variances of the complex sampling method versus that of the traditional, otherwise called simple random sampling (srs), method. In the given example the ratios are mostly 3–4, which means that the uncertainty of the complex samples methodology is 3–4 times larger than that of the traditional method. However, this reduction in precision is compensated for by the removal of biases due to the use of inappropriate probabilities used in the srs method.

The lower part of the table gives the srs data obtained through the usual commands (Analyze, Descriptive Statistics, Ratio, Numerator (curhealthscore), Denominator (lasthealthscore), Group Variable (County), Statistics (means, confidence intervals etc)). Again the ratios of the complex samples and traditional analyses are rather similar, but the confidence intervals are very different. E.g., the 95 % confidence intervals of the Northern County went from 1.172 to 1.914 in the complex samples, and from 1.525 to 1.702 in the traditional analysis, and was thus over 3 times wider.

Ratios 1

Numerator	Denominator	Ratio estimate	Standard error	95 % confidence interval Lower	95 % confidence interval Upper	Design effect
Curhealthscore	Last healthscore	1,371	,059	1,244	1,499	17,566

Ratios 1

Country	Numerator	Denominator	Ratio estimate	Standard error	95 % confidence interval Lower	Upper	Design effect
Eastern	Curhealthscore	Last healthscore	1,273	,076	1,107	1,438	12,338
"Southern	Curhealthscore	Last healthscore	1,391	,100	1,174	1,608	21,895
"Western	Curhealthscore	Last healthscore	1,278	,039	1,194	1,362	1,518
Northern	Curhealthscore	Last healthscore	1,543	,170	1,172	1,914	15,806

Ratio statistics for curhealthscore/last healthscore

Group	Mean	95 % confidence interval tor mean Lower bound	Upper bound	Price related differential	Coefficient of dispersion	Coefficient of variation Median centered
Eastern	1,282	1,241	1,323	1,007	,184	24,3 %
"Southern	1,436	1,380	1,492	1,031	,266	33,4 %
"Western	1,342	1,279	1,406	1,051	,271	37,7 %
Northern	1,613	1,525	1,702	1,044	,374	55,7 %
Overall	1,429	1,395	1,463	1,047	,285	41,8 %

The confidence intends are constructed by assuming a Normal distribution for the ratios

In addition to the statistics given above, other complex samples statistics are possible, and they can be equally well executed in SPSS, that is if the data are appropriate. If you have a binary outcome variable (dichotomous) available, then logistic regression modeling is possible, if an ordinal outcome variable is available, complex samples ordinal regression, if time to event information is in the data, complex samples Cox regression can be performed.

Conclusion

Complex samples is a cost-efficient method for analyzing target populations that are large and heterogeneously distributed. Also it is time-efficient, and offers greater scope and deeper insight, because specialized equipments are feasible.

Traditional analysis of limited samples from heterogeneous target populations is a biased methodology, because each individual selected is given the same probability, and the spread in the data is, therefore, generally underestimated. In complex sampling this bias is adjusted for by assigning appropriate weights to each individual included.

Note

More background, theoretical and mathematical information of complex samples methodologies is given in Machine learning in medicine part three, Chap. 12, Complex samples, pp 127–139, Springer Heidelberg Germany 2013.

Chapter 52
Correspondence Analysis for Identifying the Best of Multiple Treatments in Multiple Groups (217 Patients)

General Purpose

Multiple treatments for one condition are increasingly available, and a systematic assessment would serve optimal care. Research in this field to date is problematic.

This chapter is to propose a novel method based on cross-tables, correspondence analysis.

Specific Scientific Question

Can correspondence analysis avoid the bias of multiple testing, and identify the best of multiple treatments in multiple groups

---

This chapter was previously published in "Machine learning in medicine-cookbook 1" as Chap. 15, 2013.

T.J. Cleophas, A.H. Zwinderman, *Machine Learning in Medicine - a Complete Overview*, DOI 10.1007/978-3-319-15195-3_52

Var 1	Var 2
1	1
1	1
1	1
1	1
1	1
1	1
1	1
1	1
1	1
1	1
1	1
1	1

Var 1 treatment modality (1–3)
Var 2 response (1 = complete remission, 2 = partial remission, 3 = no response)
Only the first 12 patients are given, the entire data file entitled "correspondenceanalysis" is in extras.springer.com. 217 patients were randomly treated with one of three treatments (treat = treatment) and produced one of three responses (1 = complete remission, 2 = partial remission, 3 = no response). We will use SPSS statistical software 19.0

Correspondence Analysis

First, a multiple groups chi-square test is performed. Start by opening the data file.

Command:

Analyze....Descriptive Statistics....Crosstabs....Row(s): enter treatment.... Column(s): enter remission, partial, no [Var 2]....click Statistics....mark Chi-square....click Continue....click Cell Display ....mark Observed....mark Expected ....click Continue....OK.

Treatment * remission, partial, no Crosstabulation

			Remission, partial, no			
			1,00	2,00	3,00	Total
Treatment	1,00	Count	19	21	18	58
		Expected count	21,6	10,7	25,7	58,0
	2,00	Count	41	9	39	89
		Expected count	33,2	16,4	39,4	89,0
	3,00	Count	21	10	39	70
		Expected count	26,1	12,9	31,0	70,0
Total		Count	81	40	96	217
		Expected count	81,0	40,0	96,0	217,0

The output file compares the observed counts (patients) per cell with the expected count, if no significant difference existed. Also, a chi-square value is given, 21.462 with 4° of freedom, p-value<0.0001. There is a significantly different pattern in numbers of responders between the different treatment groups. To find out what treatment is best a correspondence analysis is performed. For that purpose the individual chi-square values are calculated from the values of the above table according to the underneath equation.

$$\left[(\text{observed count} - \text{expected count})^2 / \text{expected count}\right]$$

Then, the individual chi-square values are converted to similarity measures. With these values the software program creates a two-dimensional quantitative distance measure that is used to interpret the level of nearness between the treatment groups and response groups. We will use again SPSS 19.0 statistical software for the analysis.

Command:

Analyze....Dimension Reduction....Correspondence Analysis ....Row: enter treatment....click Define Range....Minimum value: enter1....Maximum value: enter 3....click Update....Column: enter remission, partial, no [Var 2] ....click Define Range....Minimum value: enter1....Maximum value: enter 3....click Update.... click Continue ....click Model....Distance Measure: click Chi square....click Continue....click Plots....mark Biplot....OK.

		Remission		
Treatment		yes	partial	no
1	residual	–2,6	10,3	–7,7
	$(o\text{-}e)^2/e$	0,31	9,91	2,31
	similarity	–0,31	9,91	–2,31
2	residual	7,9	–7,4	–0,4
	$(o\text{-}e)^2/e$	1,88	3,34	0,004
	similarity	1,88	–3,34	–0.004
3	residual	–4,1	–2,9	8,0
	$(o\text{-}e)^2/e$	0,64	0.65	2,65
	similarity	–0,64	–0,65	2,65

The above table of similarity values is given in the output. Also the underneath plot of the coordinates of both the treatment groups and the response groups in a one two-dimensional plane is shown in the output. This plot is meaningful. As treatment group 2 and response group 1 tend to join, and treatment group 1 and response group 2 do, equally, so, we have reason to believe that treatment group 2 has the best treatment and treatment group 1 the second best. This is, because response group 1 has a complete remission, and response group 2 has a partial remission. If a 2×2 table of the treatment groups 1 and 2 versus the response groups 1 and 2 shows a significant difference between the treatments, then we can argue, that the best treatment is, indeed, significantly better than the second best treatment.

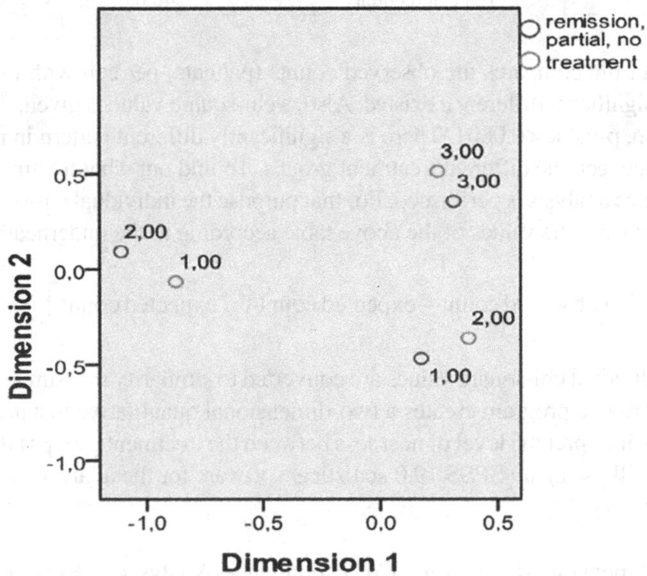

For statistical testing response 1 and 2 versus treatment 1 and 2 recoding of the variables is required, but a simpler solution is to use a pocket calculator method for computing the chi-square value.

	response		
treatment	1	2	total
1	19	21	40
2	41	9	50
	60	30	90

$$\text{Chi-square} = \frac{\left[(9\times19)-(21\times41)\right]^2\times90}{60\times30\times50\times40} = 11.9 \text{ with 1 degree of freedom, } p < 0.0001$$

Treatment 2, indeed, produced significantly more complete remissions than did treatment 1, as compared to the partial remissions.

Conclusion

In our example correspondence analysis was able to demonstrate which one of three treatments was best, and it needed, instead of *multiple* 2×2 tables, only a single 2×2 table for that purpose. The advantage of this procedure will be even more obvious, if larger sets of categorical data have to be assessed. A nine cells data file would require only nine 2×2 tables to be tested, a sixteen cells data file would require thirty-six of them. This procedure will almost certainly produce significant effects by chance rather than true effects, and is, therefore, rather meaningless. In contrast, very few tests are needed, when a correspondence analysis is used to identify the proximities in the data, and the risk of type I errors is virtually negligible.

Note

We should add that, instead of a two-dimensional analysis as used in the current chapter, correspondence analysis can also be applied for multidimensional analyses. More background, theoretical and mathematical information of correspondence analysis is given in Machine learning in medicine part two, Chap. 13, Correspondence analysis, pp 129–137, Springer Heidelberg Germany 2013.

Chapter 53
Decision Trees for Decision Analysis (1,004 and 953 Patients)

General Purpose

Decision trees are, so-called, non-metric or non-algorithmic methods adequate for fitting nominal and interval data (the latter either categorical or continuous). Better accuracy from decision trees is sometimes obtained by the use of a training sample (Chap. 8). This chapter is to assess whether decision trees can be appropriately applied to predict health risks and improvements.

Specific Scientific Question

Can decision trees be trained to predict in individual future patients risk of infarction and ldl (low density lipoprotein) cholesterol decrease.

Decision Trees with a Binary Outcome

Var 1	Var 2	Var 3	Var 4	Var 5	Var 6
,00	44,86	1,00	,00	1,00	2,00
,00	42,71	2,00	,00	1,00	2,00
,00	43,34	3,00	,00	2,00	2,00

(continued)

This chapter was previously published in "Machine learning in medicine-cookbook 1" as Chap. 16, 2013.

T.J. Cleophas, A.H. Zwinderman, *Machine Learning in Medicine - a Complete Overview*, DOI 10.1007/978-3-319-15195-3_53

Var 1	Var 2	Var 3	Var 4	Var 5	Var 6
,00	44,02	3,00	,00	1,00	2,00
,00	67,97	1,00	,00	2,00	2,00
,00	40,31	2,00	,00	2,00	2,00
,00	66,56	1,00	,00	2,00	2,00
,00	45,95	1,00	,00	2,00	2,00
,00	52,27	1,00	,00	1,00	2,00
,00	43,86	1,00	,00	1,00	2,00
,00	46,58	3,00	,00	2,00	1,00
,00	53,83	2,00	,00	2,00	2,00
,00	49,48	1,00	,00	2,00	1,00

Var 1 infarct_rating (,00 no, 1,00 yes)
Var 2 age (years)
Var 3 cholesterol_level (1,00-3,00)
Var 4 smoking (,00 no, 1,00 yes)
Var 5 education (levels 1,00 and 2,00)
Var 6 weight_level (levels 1,00 and 2,00)

The data from the first 13 patients are shown only. See extra.springer.com for the entire data file entitled "decisiontreebinary": in a 1,004 patient data file of risk factors for myocardial infarct a so-called chi-squared automatic interaction (CHAID) model is used for analysis. Also an XML (eXtended Markup Language) will be exported for the analysis of future data. Start by opening the data file.

Command:

Click Transform….click Random Number Generators….click Set Starting Point…. click Fixed Value (2000000)….click OK….click Classify….Tree…. Dependent Variable: enter infarct rating….Independent Variables: enter age, cholesterol level, smoking, education, weight level….Growing Method: select CHAID….click Categories: Target mark yes….Continue….click Output: mark Tree in table format….Criteria: Parent Node type 200, Child Node type 100…. click Continue…. click Save: mark Terminal node number, Predicted probabilities…. in Export Tree Model as XML mark Training sample….click Browse… …..in File name enter "exportdecisiontreebinary" ….in Look in: enter the appropriate map in your computer for storage….click Save….click OK.

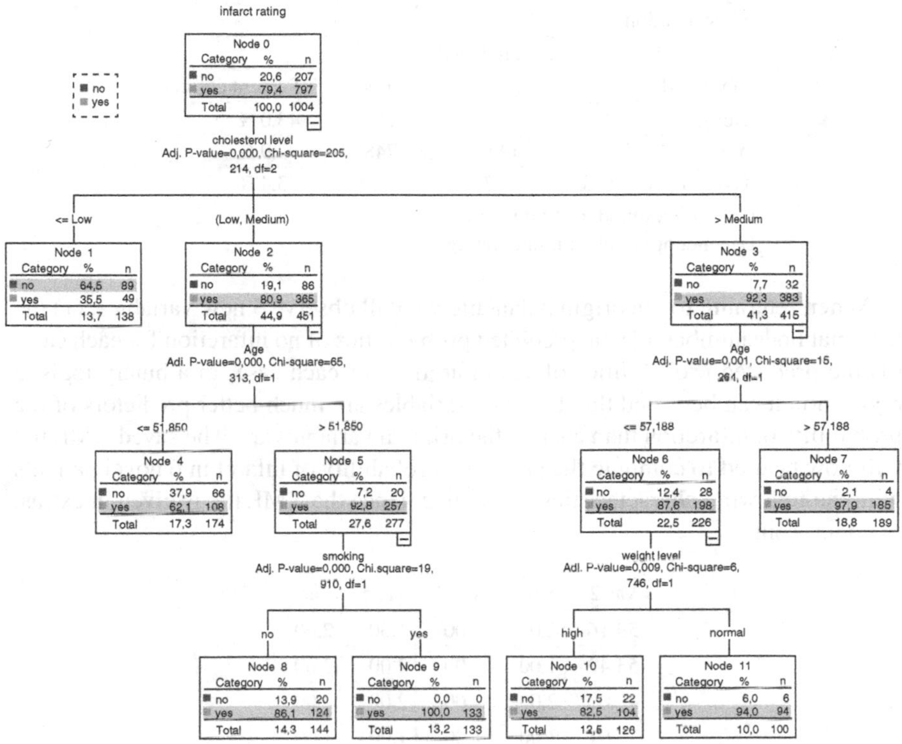

The output sheets show the decision tree and various tables. The Cholesterol level is the best predictor of the infarct rating. For low cholesterol the cholesterol level is the only significant predictor of infarction: only 35.5 % will have an infarction. In the medium and high cholesterol groups age is the next best predictor. In the elderly with medium cholesterol smoking contributes considerably to the risk of infarction. In contrast, in the younger with high cholesterol those with normal weight are slightly more at risk of infarction than those with high weights. For each node (subgroup) the number of cases, the chi-square value, and level of significance is given. A p-value<0.05 indicates that the difference between the 2×2 or 3×2 tables of the paired nodes are significantly different from one another. All of the p-values were very significant.

The risk and classification tables indicate that the category infarction predicted by the model is wrong in 0.166 = 16.6 % of the cases (underneath table). A correct prediction of 83.4 % is fine. However, in those without an infarction no infarction is predicted in only 43.0 % of the cases (underneath table).

Risk	
Estimate	Std. error
,166	,012

Growing Method: CHAID
Dependent Variable: infarct rating

Classification

	Predicted		
Observed	No	Yes	Percent correct
No	89	118	43,0 %
Yes	49	748	93,9 %
Overall percentage	13,7 %	86,3 %	83,4 %

Growing Method: CHAID
Dependent Variable: infarct rating

When returning to the original data file we will observe 3 new variables, (1) the terminal node number, (2) the predicted probabilities of no infarction for each case, (3) the predicted probabilities of yes infarction for each case. In a binary logistic regression it can be tested that the later variables are much better predictors of the probability of infarction than each of the original variables are. The saved XML file will now be used to compute the predicted probability of infarct in 6 novel patients with the following characteristics. For convenience the XML file is given in extras. springer. com.

Var 2	Var 3	Var 4	Var 5	Var 6
59,16	2,00	,00	1,00	2,00
53,42	1,00	,00	2,00	2,00
43,02	2,00	,00	2,00	2,00
76,91	3,00	1,00	1,00	1,00
70,53	2,00	,00	1,00	2,00
47,02	3,00	1,00	1,00	1,00

Var 2 age (years)
Var 3 cholesterol_level (1,00-3,00)
Var 4 smoking (,00 no, 1,00 yes)
Var 5 education (level 1,00 and 2,00)
Var 6 weight_level (1,00 and 2,00)

Enter the above data in a new SPSS data file.

Command:

Utilities....click Scoring Wizard....click Browse....click Select....Folder: enter the exportdecisiontreebinary.xml file....click Select....in Scoring Wizard click Next.... mark Node Number....mark Probability of Predicted Category....click Next.... click Finish.

The above data file now gives the individual predicted nodes numbers and probabilities of infarct for the six novel patients as computed by the linear model with the help of the XML file. Enter the above data in a new SPSS data file.

Var 2	Var 3	Var 4	Var 5	Var 6	Var 7	Var 8
59,16	2,00	,00	1,00	2,00	8,00	,86
53,42	1,00	,00	2,00	2,00	1,00	,64
43,02	2,00	,00	2,00	2,00	4,00	,62
76,91	3,00	1,00	1,00	1,00	7,00	,98
70,53	2,00	,00	1,00	2,00	8,00	,86
47,02	3,00	1,00	1,00	1,00	11,00	,94

Var 2 age
Var 3 cholesterol_level
Var 4 smoking
Var 5 education
Var 6 weight_level
Var 7 predicted node number
Var 8 predicted probability of infarct

Decision Trees with a Continuous Outcome

Var 1	Var 2	Var 3	Var 4	Var 5	Var 6
3,41	0	1	3,00	3	0
1,86	−1	1	2,00	3	1
,85	−2	1	1,00	4	1
1,63	−1	1	2,00	3	1
6,84	4	0	4,00	2	0
1,00	−2	0	1,00	3	0
1,14	−2	1	1,00	3	1
2,97	0	1	3,00	4	0
1,05	−2	1	1,00	4	1
,63	−2	0	1,00	3	0
1,18	−2	0	1,00	2	0
,96	−2	1	1,00	2	0
8,28	5	0	4,00	2	1

Var 1 ldl_reduction
Var 2 weight_redcution
Var 3 gender
Var 4 sport
Var 5 treatment_level
Var 6 diet

For the decision tree with continuous outcome the classification and regression tree (CRT) model is applied. A 953 patient data file is used of various predictors of ldl (low-density-lipoprotein)-cholesterol reduction including weight reduction, gender, sport, treatment level, diet. The file is in extras.springer.com and is entitled "decisiontreecontinuous". The file is opened.

Command:

Click Transform….click Random Number Generators….click Set Starting Point…. click Fixed Value (2000000)….click OK….click Analyze….Classify…Tree….

Dependent Variable: enter ldl_reduction.... Independent Variables: enter weight reduction, gender, sport, treatment level, diet....Growing Methods: select CRT ....click Criteria: enter Parent Node 300, Child Node 100....click Output: Tree mark Tree in table format....click Continue....click Save....mark Terminal node number....mark Predicted value....in Export Tree Model as XML mark Training sample....click Browse........in File name enter "exportdecisiontreecontinuous" ....in Look in: enter the appropriate map in your computer for storage....click Save....click OK.

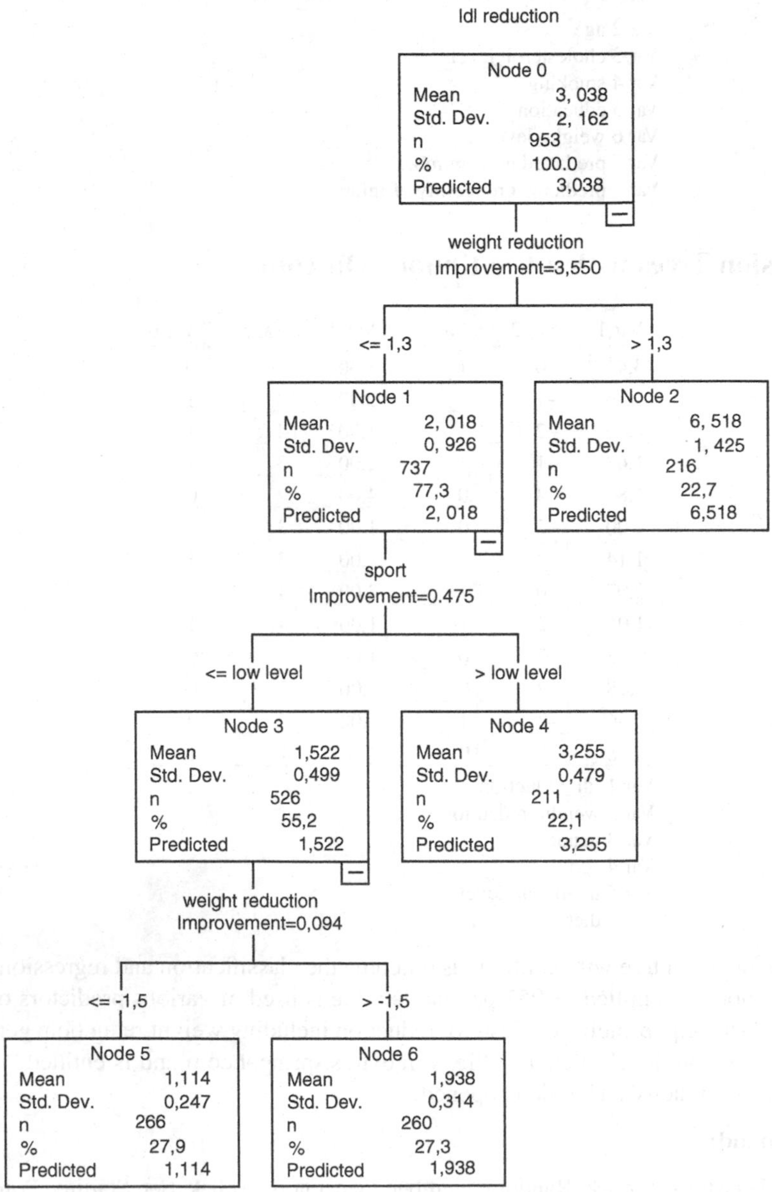

The output sheets show the classification tree. Only weight reduction and sport significantly contributed to the model, with the overall mean and standard deviation dependent variable ldl cholesterol in the parent (root) node. Weight reduction with a cut-off level of 1.3 units is the best predictor of ldl reduction. In the little weight reduction group sport is the best predictor. In the low sport level subgroup again weight reduction is a predictor, but here there is a large difference between weight gain (≤1.5 units) and weight loss (≥1.5 units). Minimizing the output shows the original data file. It now contains two novel variables, the npde classification and the predicted value of ldl cholesterol reduction. They are entitled NodeId and PredictedValue. The saved XML (eXtended Markup Language) file will now be used to compute the predicted node classification and value of ldl cholesterol reduction in 5 novel patients with the following characteristics. For convenience the XML file is given in extras.springer.com.

Var 2	Var 3	Var 4	Var 5	Var 6
–,63	1,00	2,00	1,00	,00
2,10	,00	4,00	4,00	1,00
–1,16	1,00	2,00	1,00	1,00
4,22	,00	4,00	1,00	,00
–,59	,00	3,00	4,00	1,00

Var 2 weight_reduction
Var 3 gender
Var 4 sport
Var 5 treatment_level
Var 6 diet

Enter the above data in a new SPSS data file.

Command:

Utilities....click Scoring Wizard....click Browse....click Select....Folder: enter the exportdecisiontreecontinuous.xml file....click Select....in Scoring Wizard click Next....mark Node Number....mark Predicted Value....click Next....click Finish.

The above data file now gives individually predicted node classifications and predicted ldl cholesterol reductions as computed by the linear model with the help of the XML file.

Var 2	Var 3	Var 4	Var 5	Var 6	Var 7	Var 8
–,63	1,00	2,00	1,00	,00	6,00	1,94
2,10	,00	4,00	4,00	1,00	2,00	6,52
–1,16	1,00	2,00	1,00	1,00	6,00	1,94
4,22	,00	4,00	1,00	,00	2,00	6,52
–,59	,00	3,00	4,00	1,00	4,00	3,25

Var 2 weight_reduction
Var 3 gender
Var 4 sport
Var 5 treatment_level
Var 6 diet
Var 7 predicted node classification
Var 8 predicted ldl cholesterol reduction

Conclusion

The module decision trees can be readily trained to predict in individual future patients risk of infarction and ldl (low density lipoprotein) cholesterol decrease. Instead of trained XML files for predicting about future patients, also syntax files are possible for the purpose. They perform better if predictions from multiple instead of single future patients are requested.

Note

More background, theoretical and mathematical information of decision trees as well as the steps for utilizing syntax files is available in Machine learning in medicine part three, Chap. 14, entitled "Decision trees", pp 153–168, Springer Heidelberg, Germany 2013. Better accuracy from decision trees is sometimes obtained by the use of a training sample (Chap. 8).

Chapter 54
Multidimensional Scaling for Visualizing Experienced Drug Efficacies (14 Pain-Killers and 42 Patients)

General Purpose

To individual patients, objective criteria of drug efficacy, like pharmaco-dynamic/-kinetic and safety measures may not mean too much, and patients' personal opinions are important too. This chapter is to assess whether multidimensional scaling can visualize subgroup differences in experienced drug efficacies, and whether data-based dimensions can be used to match dimensions as expected from pharmacological properties.

Specific Scientific Question

Can proximity and preference scores of pain-killers as judged by patient samples be used for obtaining insight in the real priorities both in populations and in individual patients. Can the data-based dimensions as obtained by this procedure be used to match dimensions as expected from pharmacological properties.

This chapter was previously published in "Machine learning in medicine-cookbook 1" as Chap. 17, 2013.

T.J. Cleophas, A.H. Zwinderman, *Machine Learning in Medicine - a Complete Overview*, DOI 10.1007/978-3-319-15195-3_54

Proximity Scaling

Var	Var 1	Var 2	Var 3	Var 4	Var 5	Var 6	Var 7	Var 8	Var 9	Var 10	Var 11	Var 12	Var 13	Var 14
1	0													
2	8	0												
3	7	2	0											
4	5	4	5	0										
5	8	5	4	6	0									
6	7	5	6	6	8	0								
7	4	5	6	3	7	4	0							
8	8	5	4	6	3	8	7	0						
9	3	7	9	4	8	7	5	8	0					
10	5	6	7	6	9	4	4	9	6	0				
11	9	5	4	6	3	8	7	3	8	9	0			
12	9	4	3	7	5	7	7	5	8	9	5	0		
13	4	6	6	3	7	5	4	8	4	5	7	7	0	
14	6	6	7	6	8	2	4	9	7	3	9	7	5	0

Var 1–14 one by one distance scores of the pain-killers 1–14, mean estimates of 20 patients (scale 0–10). The 14 pain-killers are also given in the first column. The data file is entitled "proxscal" and is in extras.springer.com

The above matrix mean scores can be considered as one by one distances between all of the medicines connected with one another by straight lines in 14 different ways. Along an x- and y-axis they are subsequently modeled using the equation: the distance between drug i and drug j = $\sqrt{[(x_i - x_j)^2 + (y_i - y_j)^2]}$. SPSS statistical software 19.0 will be used for analysis. Start by opening the data file.

Command:

Analyze….Scale….Multidimensional scaling (PROXSCAL)….Data Format: click The data are proximities….Number of Sources: click One matrix source….One Source: click The proximities are in a matrix across columns….click Define…. enter all variables (medicines) into "Proximities"….Model: Shape: click Lower-triangular matrix….Proximity Transformation: click Interval….Dimensions: Minimum: enter 2….Maximum: enter 2….click Continue….click Plots….mark Common space….mark Transformed proximities vs distances….click Continue ….click: Output….mark Common space coordinates….mark Multiple stress measures….click Continue….click OK.

Stress and fit measures	
Normalized raw stress	,00819
Stress-I	,09051[a]
Stress-II	,21640[a]
S-stress	,02301[b]
Dispersion accounted for (DAF.)	,99181
Tucker's coefficient of congruence	,99590

PROXSCAL minimizes Normalized Raw Stress
[a]Optimal scaling factor = 1,008
[b]Optimal scaling factor = ,995

The output sheets gives the uncertainty of the model (stress = standard error) and dispersion values. The model is assumed to appropriately describe the data if they are respectively < 0.20 and approximately 1.0.

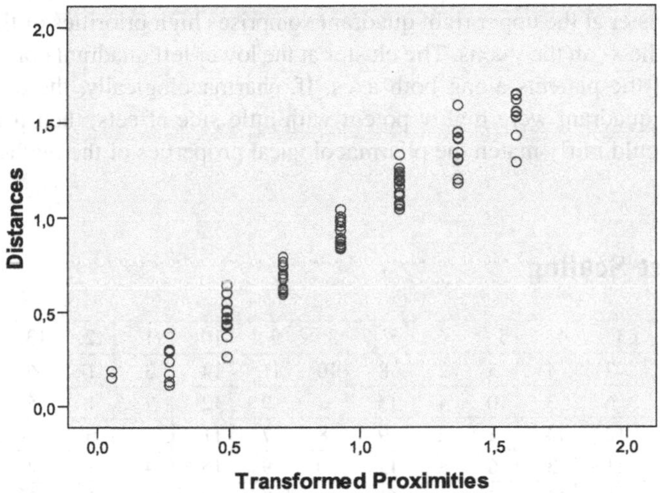

Also, a plot of the actual distances as observed versus the distances fitted by the statistical program is given. A perfect fit should produce a straight line, a poor fit produces a lot of spread around a line or even no line at all. The figure is not perfect but it shows a very good fit as expected from the stress and fit measures.

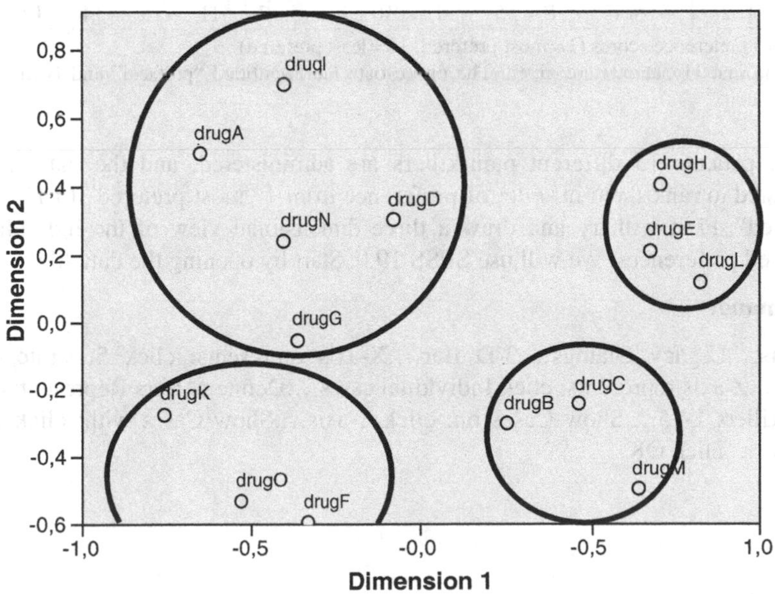

Finally, the above figure shows the most important part of the outcome. The standardized x- and y-axes values give some insight in the relative position of the medicines according to perception of our study population. Four clusters are identified. Using Microsoft's drawing commands we can encircle the clusters as identified. The cluster at the upper right quadrant comprises high priorities of the patients along both the x- an the y-axis. The cluster at the lower left quadrant comprises low priorities of the patients along both axes. If, pharmacologically, the drugs in the right upper quadrant were highly potent with little side effects, then the patients' priorities would fairly match the pharmacological properties of the medicines.

Preference Scaling

Var 1	2	3	4	5	6	7	8	9	10	11	12	13	14	15
12	13	7	4	5	2	8	10	11	14	3	1	6	9	15
14	11	6	3	10	4	15	8	9	12	7	1	5	2	13
13	10	12	14	3	2	9	8	7	11	1	6	4	5	15
7	14	11	3	6	8	12	10	9	15	4	1	2	5	13
14	9	6	15	13	2	11	8	7	10	12	1	3	4	5
9	11	15	4	7	6	14	10	8	12	5	2	3	1	13
9	14	5	6	8	4	13	11	12	15	7	2	1	3	10
15	10	12	6	8	2	13	9	7	11	3	1	5	4	14
13	12	2	4	5	8	10	11	3	15	7	9	6	1	14
15	13	10	7	6	4	9	11	12	14	5	2	8	1	3
9	2	4	13	8	5	1	10	6	7	11	15	14	12	3

Var 1–15 preference scores (1 = most prefered, 15 = least prefered)
Only the first 11 patients are given. The entire data file is entitled "prefscal" and is in extras.springer.com.

To 42 patients 15 different pain-killers are administered, and the patients are requested to rank them in order of preference from 1 "most prefered" to 15 "least prefered". First will try and draw a three dimensional view of the individually assigned preferences. We will use SPSS 19.0. Start by opening the data file.

Command:

Graphs....Legacy Dialogs....3-D Bar....X-axis represents: click Separate variables....Z-axis represents: click Individual cases....Define....Bars Represent: enter pain-killers 1-15....Show Cases on: click Y-axis....Show Cases with: click Case number....click OK.

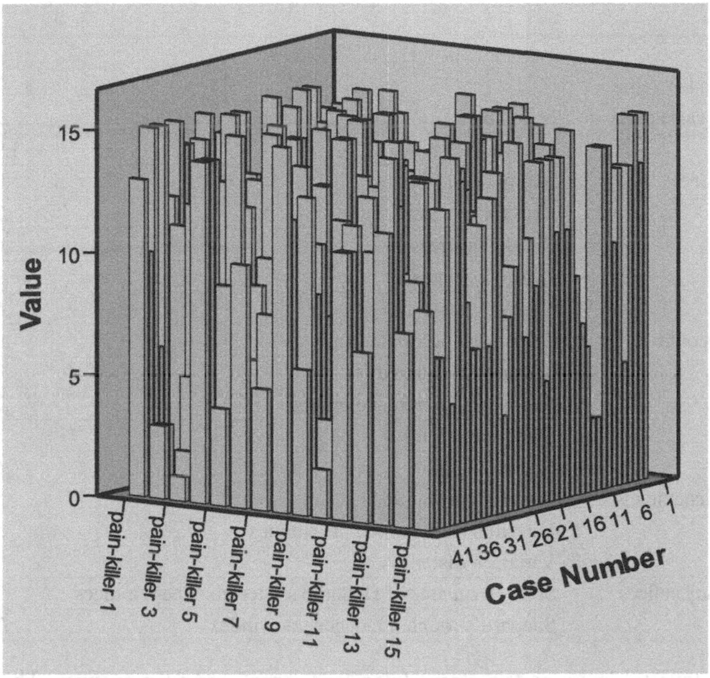

The above figure shows the result: a very irregular pattern consisting of multiple areas with either high or low preference is observed. We will now perform a preference scaling analysis. Like with proximity scaling, preference assessments is mapped in a 2 dimensional plane with the rank orders of the medicines as measures of distance between the medicines. Two types of maps are constructed: an aggregate map giving average distances of the entire population or individual maps of single patients, and an ideal point map where ideal points have to be interpreted as a map with ideal medicines, one for each patient. SPSS 19.0 is used once more.

Command:

Analyze....Scale....Multidimensional Unfolding (PREFSCAL)....enter all variables (medicines) into "Proximities"....click Model....click Dissimilarities.... Dimensions: Minimum enter 2 ....Maximum enter 2....Proximity Transformations: click Ordinal ....click Within each row separately....click Continue....click Options: imputation by: enter Spearman....click Continue....click Plots: mark Final common space....click Continue....click Output: mark Fit measures ....mark Final common space....click Continue....click OK.

Measures		
Iterations		115
Final function value		,7104127
Function value parts	Stress part	,2563298
	Penalty part	1,9688939
Badness of fit	Normalized stress	,0651568
	Kruskal's stress-I	,2552582
	Kruskal's stress-II	,6430926
	Young's S-stress-I	,3653360
	Young's S-stress-II	,5405226
Goodness of fit	Dispersion accounted for	,9348432
	Variance accounted for	,7375011
	Recovered preference orders	,7804989
	Spearman's Rho	,8109694
	Kendall's Tau-b	,6816390
Variation coefficients	Variation proximities	,5690984
	Variation transformed proximities	,5995274
	Variation distances	,4674236
Degeneracy indices	Sum-of-squares of DeSarbo's intermixedness indices	,2677061
	Shepard's rough nondegeneracy index	,7859410

The above table gives the stress (standard error) and fit measures. The best fit distances as estimated by the model are adequate: measures of stress including normalized stress and Kruskal's stress-I are close to 0.20 or less, the value of dispersion measures (Dispersion Accounted For) is close to 1.0. The table also shows whether there is a risk of a *degenerate* solution, otherwise called loss function. The individual proximities have a tendency to form circles, and when averaged for obtaining average proximities, there is a tendency for the average treatment places to center in the middle of the map. The solution is a penalty term, but in our example we need not worry. The DeSarbo's and Shepard criteria are close to respectively 0 and 80 %, and no penalty adjustment is required.

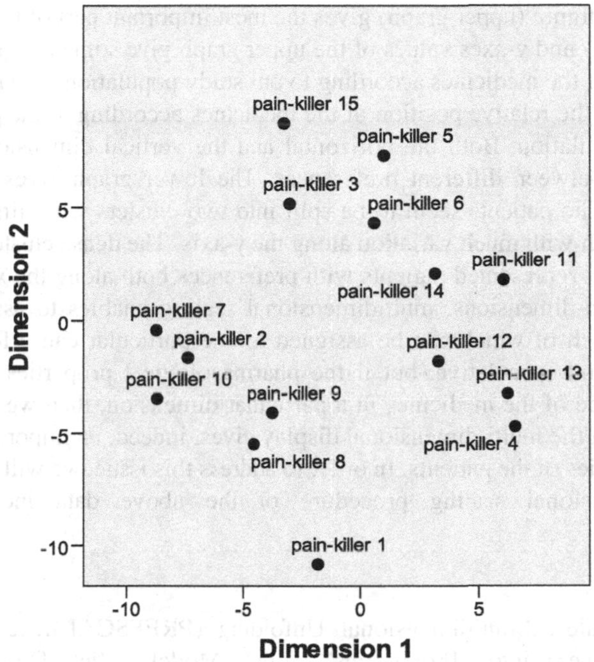
pain-killer 15
pain-killer 5
pain-killer 3
pain-killer 6
pain-killer 11
pain-killer 14
pain-killer 7
pain-killer 2
pain-killer 12
pain-killer 10
pain-killer 9
pain-killer 13
pain-killer 4
pain-killer 8
pain-killer 1
Dimension 2
5
0
-5
-10
-10
-5
0
5
Dimension 1

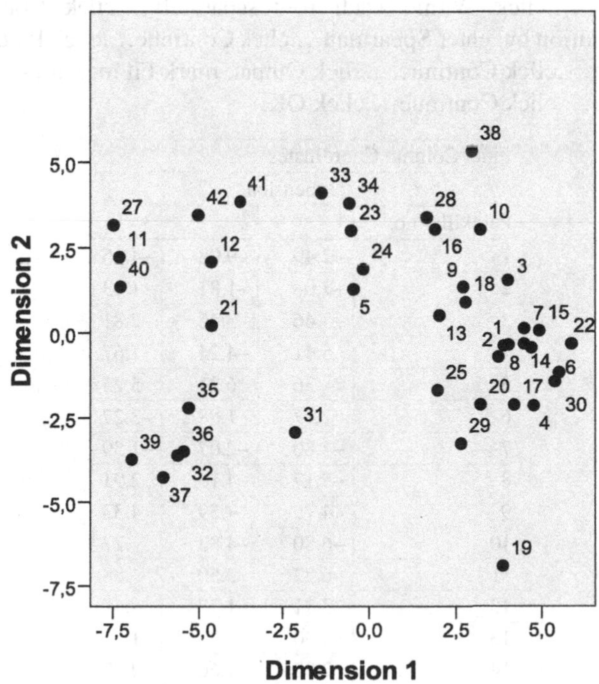
38
41
33
34
42
27
28
23
10
11
12
24
16
40
3
9
18
5
21
7
15
22
13
2
1
8
14
6
25
20
17
30
35
4
31
29
36
39
32
37
19
Dimension 2
5,0
2,5
0,0
-2,5
-5,0
-7,5
-7,5
-5,0
-2,5
0,0
2,5
5,0
Dimension 1

The above figure (upper graph) gives the most important part of the output. The standardized x- and y-axes values of the upper graph give some insight in the relative position of the medicines according to our study population. The results can be understood as the relative position of the medicines according to the perception of our study population. Both the horizontal and the vertical dimension appears to discriminate between different preferences. The lower graph gives the patients' *ideal points*. The patients seem to be split into two clusters with different preferences, although with much variation along the y-axis. The dense cluster in the right lower quadrant represented patients with preferences both along the x- and y-axis. Instead of two-dimensions, multidimensional scaling enables to assess multiple dimensions each of which can be assigned to one particular cause for proximity. This may sound speculative, but if the pharmacological properties of the drugs match the place of the medicines in a particular dimension, then we will be more convinced that the multi-dimensional display gives, indeed, an important insight in the real priorities of the patients. In order to address this issue, we will now perform a multidimensional scaling procedure of the above data including three dimensions.

Command:

Analyze….Scale….Multidimensional Unfolding (PREFSCAL)….enter all variables (medicines) into "Proximities"….click Model….click Dissimilarities…. Dimensions: Minimum enter 3 ….Maximum enter 3….Proximity Transformations: click Ordinal ….click Within each row separately….click Continue….click Options: imputation by: enter Spearman….click Continue….click Plots: mark Final common space….click Continue….click Output: mark Fit measures ….mark Final common space….click Continue….click OK.

Final Column Coordinates			
	Dimension		
Painkiller no.	1	2	3
1	−2.49	−9.08	−4.55
2	−7.08	−1.81	1.43
3	−3.46	3.46	−2.81
4	5.41	−4.24	1.67
5	−.36	6.21	5.25
6	.17	1.88	−3.27
7	−7.80	−2.07	−1.59
8	−5.17	−4.18	2.91
9	4.75	−.59	4.33
10	−6.80	−4.83	.27
11	6.22	2.50	.88
12	3.71	−1.27	−.49
13	5.30	−2.95	1.51
14	2.82	1.66	−2.09
15	−4.35	2.76	−6.72

The output sheets shows the standardized mean preference values of the different pain-killers as x- y-, and z-axis coordinates. The best fit outcome of the three-dimensional (3-D) model can be visualized in a 3-D figure. SPSS 19.0 is used. First cut and paste the data from the above table to the preference scaling file or another file. Then proceed.

Command:

Graphs....Legacy Dialogs....Scatter/Dot....click 3-D Scatter....click Define....Y-Axis: enter dimension 1....X-Axis: enter dimension 2....Z-Axis: enter dimension 3....click OK.

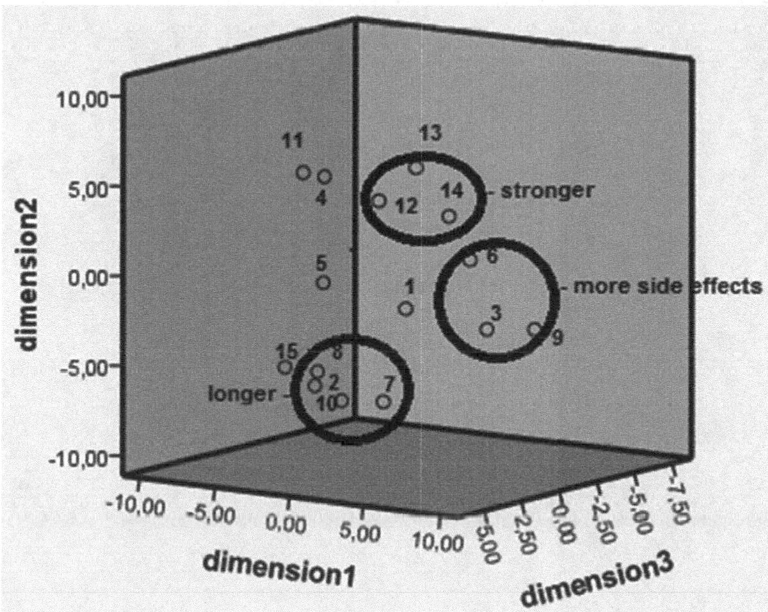

The above figure gives the best fit outcome of a 3-dimensional scaling model. Three clusters were identified, consistent with patients' preferences along an x-, y-, and z-axis. Using Microsoft's drawing commands we can encircle the clusters as identified. In the figure an example is given of how pharmacological properties could be used to explain the cluster pattern.

Conclusion

Multidimensional scaling is helpful both to underscore the pharmacological properties of the medicines under studies, and to identify what effects are really important to patients, and uses for these purposes estimated proximities as surrogates for counted estimates of patients' opinions. Multidimensional scaling can, like regression analysis, be used two ways, (1) for estimating preferences of treatment modalities in a population, (2) for assessing the preferred treatment modalities in individual patients.

Note

More background, theoretical and mathematical information of multidimensional scaling is given in Machine learning in medicine part two, Chap. 12, Multidimensional scaling, pp 115–127, Springer Heidelberg Germany 2013.

Chapter 55
Stochastic Processes for Long Term Predictions from Short Term Observations

General Purpose

Markov modeling, otherwise called stochastic processes, assumes that per time unit the same % of a population will have an event, and it is used for long term predictions from short term observations. This chapter is to assess whether the method can be applied by non-mathematicians using an online matrix-calculator.

Specific Scientific Questions

If per time unit the same % of patients will have an event like surgery, medical treatment, a complication like a co-morbidity or death, what will be the average time before such events take place.

Example 1

Patients with three states of treatment for a disease are checked every 4 months. The underneath matrix is a so-called transition matrix. The states 1–3 indicate the chances of treatment: 1 = no treatment, 2 = surgery, 3 = medicine. If you are in state 1 today, there will be a 0.3 = 30 % chance that you will receive no treatment in the next 4 months, a 0.2 = 20 % chance of surgery, and a 0.5 = 50 % chance of medicine treatment. If you are still in state 1 (no treatment) after 4 months, there

---

This chapter was previously published in "Machine learning in medicine-cookbook 1" as Chap. 18, 2013.

T.J. Cleophas, A.H. Zwinderman, *Machine Learning in Medicine - a Complete Overview*, DOI 10.1007/978-3-319-15195-3_55

will again be a 0.3 chance that this will be the same in the second 4 month period etc. So, after 5 periods the chance of being in state 1 equals 0.3 × 0.3 × 0.3 × 0.3 × 0.3 = 0.00243. The chance that you will be in the states 2 or 3 is much larger, and there is something special about these states. Once you are in these states you will never leave them anymore, because the patients who were treated with either surgery or medicine are no longer followed in this study. That this happens can be observed from the matrix: if you are in state 2, you will have a chance of 1 = 100 % to stay in state 2 and a chance of 0 = 0 % not to do so. The same is true for the state 3.

	State in next period (4 months)		
	1	2	3
State in current time			
1	0.3	0.2	0.5
2	0	1	0
3	0	0	1

Now we will compute what will happen with the chances of a patient in the state 1 after several 4 month periods.

	chances of being in state:		
	state 1	state 2	state 3
4 month period			
1st	30 %	20 %	50 %
2nd	30 × 0.3 = 9 %	20 + 0.3 × 20 = 26 %	50 + 0.3 × 50 = 65 %
3rd	9 × 0.3 = 3 %	26 + 9 × 0.2 = 27.8 %	65 + 9 × 0.5 = 69.5 %
4th	3 × 0.3 = 0.9 %	27.8 + 3 × 0.2 = 28.4 %	69.5 + 3 × 0.5 = 71.0 %
5th	0.9 × 0.3 = 0.27 %	28.4 + 0.9 × 0.2 = 28.6 %	71.0 + 0.9 × 0.5 = 71.5

Obviously, the chances of being in the states 2 or 3 will increase, though increasingly slowly, and the chance of being in state 1 is, ultimately, going to approximate zero. In clinical terms: postponing the treatment does not make much sense, because everyone in the no treatment group will eventually receive a treatment and the ultimate chances of surgery and medicine treatment are approximately 29 and 71 %. With larger matrices this method for calculating the ultimate chances is rather laborious. Matrix algebra offers a rapid method.

	State in next period (4 months)			
	1	2	3	
State in current time				
1	[0.3]	[0.2 0.5]	matrix Q	matrix R
2	[0]	[1 0]	matrix O	matrix I
3	[0]	[0 1]		

The states are called transient, if they can change (the state 1), and absorbing if not (the states 2 and 3). The original matrix is partitioned into four submatrices, otherwise called the canonical form:

[0.3]	Upper left corner:
	This square matrix Q can be sometimes very large with rows and columns respectively presenting the transient states.
[0.2 0.5]	Upper right corner:
	This R matrix presents in rows the chance of being absorbed from the transient state.
[1 0]	Lower right corner:
[0 1]	This identity matrix I presents rows and columns with chances of
	being in the absorbing states, the I matrix must be adjusted to the
	size of the Q matrix (here it will look like [1] instead of [1 0]
[0]	Lower left corner.
[0]	This is a matrix of zeros (0 matrix).

From the above matrices a fundamental matrix (F) is constructed.

$$\left[(\text{matrix I})-(\text{matrix R})\right]^{-1}=\left[0.7\right]^{-1}=10/7.$$

With larger matrices a matrix calculator, like the Bluebit Online Matrix Calculator can be used to compute the matrix to the −1 power by clicking "Inverse".

The fundamental matrix F equals 10/7. It can be interpreted as the average time, before someone goes into the absorbing state (10/7 × 4 months = 5.714 months). The product of the fundamental matrix F and the R matrix gives more exact chances of a person in state 1 ending up in the states 2 and 3.

$$F\times R=(10/7)\times\begin{bmatrix}0.2 & 0.5\end{bmatrix}=\begin{bmatrix}2/7 & 5/7\end{bmatrix}=\begin{bmatrix}0.285714 & 0.714286\end{bmatrix}.$$

The two latter values add up to 1.00, which indicates a combined chance of ending up in an absorbing state equal to 100 %.

Example 2

Patients with three states of treatment for a chronic disease are checked every 4 months.

	State in next period (4 months)		
	1	2	3
State in current time			
1	0.3	0.6	0.1
2	0.45	0.5	0.05
3	0	0	1

The above matrix of three states and second periods of time gives again the chances of different treatment for a particular disease, but it is slightly different from the first example. Here state 1 = no treatment state, state 2 = medicine treatment, state 3 = surgery state. We assume that medicine can be stopped while surgery is irretrievable, and, thus, an absorbing state. We first partition the matrix.

	State in next period (4 months)			
	1	2	3	
State in current time				
1	[0.3 0.6]	[0.1]	matrix Q	matrix R
2	[0.45 0.5]	[0.05]		
3	[0 0]	[1]	matrix O	matrix I

The R matrix	[0.1] is in the upper right corner.
	[0.05]
The Q matrix	[0.3 0.6] is in the left upper corner.
	[0.45 0.5]
The I matrix	[1] is in the lower right corner, and must be adjusted,
	before it can be subtracted from the Q matrix according
	to $\begin{bmatrix} 1 & 0 \\ 0 & 1 \end{bmatrix}$
The 0 matrix	[0 0] is in the lower left corner

$$I - Q = \begin{bmatrix} 1 & 0 \\ 0 & 1 \end{bmatrix} - \begin{bmatrix} 0.3 & 0.6 \\ 0.45 & 0.5 \end{bmatrix} = \begin{bmatrix} 0.7 & -0.6 \\ 0.45 & -0.5 \end{bmatrix}.$$

The inverse of [I – Q] is obtained by marking "Inverse" at the online Bluebit Matrix Calculator and equals

$$[I - Q]^{-1} = \begin{bmatrix} 6.25 & 7.5 \\ 5.625 & 8.75 \end{bmatrix} = \text{fundamental matrix F.}$$

It is interpreted as the average periods of time before some transient state goes into the absorbing state:

(6.25 + 7.5 = 13.75) × 4 months for the patients in state 1 first and state 2 second,
(5.625 + 8.75 = 14.375) × 4 months for the patients in state 2 first and state 1 second.

Finally, the product of matrix F times matrix R is calculated. It gives the chances of ending up in the absorbing state for those starting in the states 1 and 2.

$$\begin{bmatrix} 6.25 & 7.5 \\ 5.625 & 8.75 \end{bmatrix} \times \begin{bmatrix} 0.1 \\ 0.05 \end{bmatrix} = \begin{bmatrix} 1.00 \\ 1.00 \end{bmatrix}.$$

Obviously the chance of both the transient states for ending up in the absorbing state is 1.00 = 100 %.

Example 3

State 1 = stable coronary artery disease (CAD),
state 2 = complications,
state 3 = recovery state,
state 4 = death state.

	State in next period (4 months)			
	1	2	3	4
State in current time				
1	0.95	0.04	0	0.01
2	0	0	0.9	0.1
3	0	0.3	0.3	0.4
4	0	0	0	1

If you take higher powers of this transition matrix (P), you will observe long-term trends of this model. For that purpose use the matrix calculator and square the transition matrix (P^2 gives the chances in the 2nd 4 month period etc) and compute also higher powers (P^3,P^4,P^5, etc).

P^2

0.903 0.038 0.036 0.024
0.000 0.270 0.270 0.460
0.000 0.090 0.360 0.550
0.000 0.000 0.000 1.000

P^6

0.698 0.048 0.063 0.191
0.000 0.026 0.064 0.910
0.000 0.021 0.047 0.931
0.000 0.000 0.000 1.000

The above higher order transition matrices suggest that with rising powers, and, thus, after multiple 4 month periods, there is a general trend towards the absorbing state: in each row the state 4 value continually rises. In the end we all will die, but in order to be more specific about the time, a special matrix like the one described in the previous examples is required. In order to calculate the precise time before the transient states go into the absorbing state, we need to partition the initial transition matrix.

	State in next period (4 months)			
	1	2	3	4
State in current time				
1	$\begin{bmatrix} 0.95 & 0.04 & 0.0 \\ 0.0 & 0.0 & 0.9 \\ 0.0 & 0.3 & 0.3 \end{bmatrix}$	$\begin{bmatrix} 0.01 \\ 0.1 \\ 0.4 \end{bmatrix}$	matrix Q	matrix R
2				
3				
4	[0 0 0]	[1]	matrix O	matrix I

$$F = (I-Q)^{-1}$$

$$I-Q=\begin{bmatrix} 1 & 0 & 0 \\ 0 & 1 & 0 \\ 0 & 0 & 1 \end{bmatrix}-\begin{bmatrix} 0.95 & 0.04 & 0.0 \\ 0.0 & 0.0 & 0.9 \\ 0.0 & 0.3 & 0.3 \end{bmatrix}$$

$$F=\begin{bmatrix} 0.5 & -0.04 & 0 \\ 0.0 & 1.0 & -0.9 \\ 0.0 & -0.3 & 0.7 \end{bmatrix}^{-1}$$

The online Bluebit Matrix calculator (mark inverse) produces the underneath result.

$$F=\begin{bmatrix} 20.0 & 1.302 & 1.674 \\ 0.0 & 1.628 & 2.093 \\ 0.0 & 0.698 & 2.326 \end{bmatrix}$$

The average time before various transient states turn into the absorbing state (dying in this example) is given.

$$\text{State 1: } (20+1.302+1.674)\times 4\,\text{months} = 91.904\,\text{months.}$$
$$\text{State 2: } (0.0+1.628+2.093)\times 4\,\text{months} = 14.884\,\text{months.}$$
$$\text{State 3: } (0.0+0.698+2.326)\times 4\,\text{months} = 12.098\,\text{months.}$$

The chance of dying for each state is computed from matrix F times matrix R (click multiplication, enter the data in the appropriate fields and click calculate).

$$F.R=\begin{bmatrix} 20.0 & 1.302 & 1.672 \\ 0.0 & 1.628 & 2.093 \\ 0.0 & 0.698 & 2.326 \end{bmatrix}\times\begin{bmatrix} 0.01 \\ 0.1 \\ 0.4 \end{bmatrix}=\begin{bmatrix} 1.0 \\ 1.0 \\ 1.0 \end{bmatrix}.$$

Like in the previous examples again the products of the matrices F and R show that all of the states end up with death. However, in the state 1 this takes more time than it does in the other states.

Conclusion

Markov chains are used to analyze the long-term risks of reversible and irreversible complications including death. The future is not shown, but it is shown, what will happen, if everything remains the same. Markov chains assume, that the chance of an event is not independent, but depends on events in the past.

Note

More background, theoretical and mathematical information of Markov chains (stochastic modeling) is given in Machine learning in medicine part three, Chaps. 17 and 18, "Stochastic processes: stationary Markov chains" and "Stochastic processes: absorbing Markov chains", pp 195–204 and 205–216, Springer Heidelberg Germany 2013.

Chapter 56
Optimal Binning for Finding High Risk Cut-offs (1,445 Families)

General Purpose

Optimal binning is a so-called non-metric method for describing a continuous predictor variable in the form of best fit categories for making predictions. Like binary partitioning (Machine Learning in Medicine Part One, Chap. 7, Binary partitioning, pp 79–86, Springer Heidelberg Germany, 2013) it uses an exact test called the entropy method, which is based on log likelihoods. It may, therefore, produce better statistics than traditional tests. In addition, unnecessary noise due to continuous scaling is deleted, and categories for identifying patients at high risk of particular outcomes can be identified. This chapter is to assess its efficiency in medical research.

Specific Scientific Question

Unhealthy lifestyles cause increasingly high risks of overweight children. We are, particularly, interested in the best fit cut-off values of unhealthy lifestyle estimators to maximize the difference between low and high risk.

This chapter was previously published in "Machine learning in medicine-cookbook 1" as Chap. 19, 2013.

T.J. Cleophas, A.H. Zwinderman, *Machine Learning in Medicine - a Complete Overview*, DOI 10.1007/978-3-319-15195-3_56

Var 1	Var 2	Var 3	Var 4	Var 5
0	11	1	8	0
0	7	1	9	0
1	25	7	0	1
0	11	4	5	0
1	5	1	8	1
0	10	2	8	0
0	11	1	6	0
0	7	1	8	0
0	7	0	9	0
0	15	3	0	0

Var 1fruitvegetables (0=no, 1=yes)
Var 2 unhealthysnacks (times per week)
Var 3 fastfoodmeal (times per week)
Var 4 physicalactivities (times per week)
Var 5 overweightchildren (0=no, 1=yes)

Only the first 10 families are given, the entire data file is entitled "optimalbinning" and is in extras.springer.com.

Optimal Binning

SPSS 19.0 is used for analysis. Start by opening the data file.

Command:

Transform....Optimal Binning....Variables into Bins: enter fruitvegetables, unhealthysnacks, fastfoodmeal, physicalactivities....Optimize Bins with Respect to: enter "overweightchildren"....click Output....Display: mark Endpoints....mark Descriptive statistics....mark Model Entropy....click Save: mark Create variables that contain binned data....click OK.

Descriptive statistics

	N	Minimum	Maximum	Number of distinct values	Number of bins
Fruitvegetables/wk	1,445	0	34	33	2
Unhealthysnacks/wk	1,445	0	42	1,050	3
Fastfoodmeal/wk	1,445	0	21	1,445	2
Physicalactivities/wk	1,445	0	10	1,385	2

In the output the above table is given. N=the number of adults in the analysis, Minimum/Maximum=the range of the original continuous variables, Number of Distinct Values=the separate values of the continuous variables as used in the binning process, Number of Bins=the number of bins (= categories) generated and is smaller than the initials separate values of the same variables.

Model entropy	
	Model entropy
Fruitvegetables/wk	,790
Unhealthysnacks/wk	,720
Fastfoodmeal/wk	,786
Physicalactivities/wk	,805

Smaller model entropy Indicates higher predictive accuracy of the binned variable on guide variable overweight children

Model Entropy gives estimates of the usefulness of the bin models as predictor models for probability of overweight: the smaller the entropy, the better the model.

Values under 0,820 indicate adequate usefulness.

Fruitvegetables/wk					
	End point		Number of cases by level of overweight children		
Bin	Lower	Upper	No	Yes	Total
1	a	14	802	340	1,142
2	14	a	274	29	303
Total			1,076	369	1,445

Unhealthysnacks/wk					
	End point		Number of cases by level of overweight children		
Bin	Lower	Upper	No	Yes	Total
1	a	12	830	143	973
2	12	19	188	126	314
3	19	a	58	100	158
Total			1,076	369	1,445

Fastfoodmeal/wk					
	End point		Number of cases by level of overweight children		
Bin	Lower	Upper	No	Yes	Total
1	a	2	896	229	1,125
2	2	a	180	140	320
Total			1,076	369	1,445

Physicalactivities/wk

Bin	End point Lower	Upper	Number of cases by level of overweight children No	Yes	Total
1	[a]	8	469	221	690
2	8	[a]	607	148	755
Total			1,076	369	1,445

Each bin is computed as Lower<= physicalactivities/wk<Upper
[a]Unbounded

The above tables show the high risk cut-offs for overweight children of the four predicting factors. E.g., in 1,142 adults scoring under 14 units of fruit/vegetable per week, are put into bin 1 and 303 scoring over 14 units per week, are put into bin 2. The proportion of overweight children in bin 1 is much larger than it is in bin 2: 340/1,142=0.298 (30 %) and 29/303=0.096 (10 %). Similarly high risk cut-offs are found for

unhealthy snacks less than 12, 12–19, and over 19 per week
fastfood meals less than 2, and over 2 per week
physical activities less than 8 and over 8 per week.

These cut-offs can be used as meaningful recommendation limits to future families.

When we return to the dataview page, we will observe that the four variables have been added in the form of bin variables (with suffix _bin). They can be used as outcome variables for making predictions from other variables like personal characteristics of parents. Also they can be used, instead of the original variable, as predictors in regression modeling. A binary logistic regression with overweight children as dependent variable will be performed to assess their predictive strength as compared to that of the original variables. SPSS 19.0 will again be used.

Command:

Analyze….Regression….Binary Logistic….Dependent: enter overweight children ….Covariates: enter fruitvegetables, unhealthysnack, fastfoodmeal, physicalactivities….click OK.

Variables in the equation

		B	S.E.	Wald	df	Sig.	Exp(B)
Step 1[a]	Fruitvegetables	–,092	,012	58,775	1	,000	,912
	Unhealthysnacks	,161	,014	127,319	1	,000	1,175
	Fastfoodmeal	,194	,041	22,632	1	,000	1,214
	Physicalactivities	,199	,041	23,361	1	,000	1,221
	Constant	–4,008	,446	80,734	1	,000	,018

[a]Variable(s) entered on step 1:fruitvegetables, unhealthysnacks, fastfoodmeal, physical activities

The output shows that the predictors are very significant independent predictors of overweight children. Next the bin variable will be used.

Command:

Analyze....Regression....Binary Logistic....Dependent: enter overweight children ....Covariates: enter fruitvegetables_bin, unhealthysnack_bin, fastfoodmeal_bin, physicalactivities_bin....click OK.

Variables in the equation

		B	S.E.	Wald	df	Sig.	Exp(B)
Step 1[a]	Fruitvegetables_bin	−1,694	,228	55,240	1	,000	,184
	Unhealthysnacks_bin	1,264	,118	113,886	1	,000	3,540
	Fastfbodmeal_bin	,530	,169	9,827	1	,002	1,698
	Physicalactivities_bin	,294	,167	3,086	1	,079	1,341
	Constant	−2,176	,489	19,803	1	,000	,114

[a]Variable(s) entered on step 1: fruitvegetables bin, unhealthysnacks bin, fastfoodmeal bin, physicalactivities_bin

If $p<0.10$ is used to indicate statistical significance, all of the bin variables are independent predictors, though at a somewhat lower level of significance than the original variables. Obviously, in the current example some precision is lost by the binning procedure. This is, because information may be lost if you replace a continuous variable with a binary or nominal one. Nonetheless, the method is precious for identifying high risk cut-offs for recommendation purposes.

Conclusion

Optimal binning variables instead of the original continuous variables may either produce (1) better statistics, because unnecessary noise due to the continuous scaling may be deleted, (2) worse statistics, because information may be lost if your replace a continuous variable with a binary one. It is more adequate than traditional analyses, if categories are considered clinically more relevant

Note

More background, theoretical and mathematical information of optimal binning is given in Machine learning in medicine part three, Chap. 5, Optimal binning, pp 37–48, Springer Heidelberg Germany 2013. See also the Chap. 5 of this book for bin membership assessment in future families.

Chapter 57
Conjoint Analysis for Determining the Most Appreciated Properties of Medicines to Be Developed (15 Physicians)

General Purpose

Products like articles of use, food products, or medicines have multiple characteristics. Each characteristic can be measured in several levels, and too many combinations are possible for a single person to distinguish. Conjoint analysis models a limited, but representative and meaningful subset of combinations, which can, subsequently, be presented to persons for preference scaling. The chapter is to assess whether this method is efficient for the development of new medicines.

Specific Scientific Question

Can conjoint analysis be helpful to pharmaceutical institutions for determining the most appreciated properties of medicines they will develop.

Constructing an Analysis Plan

A novel medicine is judged by five characteristics:

1. safety expressed in 3 levels,
2. efficacy in 3,
3. price in 3,
4. pill size in 2,
5. prolonged activity in 2 levels.

This chapter was previously published in "Machine learning in medicine-cookbook 1" as Chap. 20, 2013.

T.J. Cleophas, A.H. Zwinderman, *Machine Learning in Medicine - a Complete Overview*, DOI 10.1007/978-3-319-15195-3_57

From the levels $3 \times 3 \times 3 \times 2 \times 2 = 108$ combinations can be formed, which is too large a number for physicians to distinguish. In addition, some combinations, e.g., high price and low efficacy will never be prefered and could be skipped from the listing. Instead, a limited but representative number of profiles is selected. SPSS statistical software 19.0 is used for the purpose.

Command:

Data….Orthogonal Design….Generate….Factor Name: enter safety….Factor Label: enter safety design….click Add….click ?....click Define Values: enter 1,2,3 on the left, and A,B,C on the right side….Do the same for all of the characteristics (here called factors)….click Create a new dataset….Dataset name: enter medicine_plan….click Options: Minimum number of cases: enter 18….mark Number of holdout cases: enter 4….Continue….OK.

The output sheets show a listing of 22, instead of 108, combinations with two new variables (status_ and card_) added. The variable Status_ gives a "0" to the first 18 combinations used for subsequent analyses, and "1" to holdout combinations to be used by the computer for checking the validity of the program. The variable Card_ gives identification numbers to each combination. For further use of the model designed so far, we will first need to perform the Display Design commands.

Command:

Data….Orthogonal Design….Display….Factors: transfer all of the characteristics to this window….click Listing for experimenter….click OK.

The output sheet now shows a plan card, which looks virtually identical to the above 22 profile listing. It must be saved. We will use the name medicine_plan for the file. For convenience the design file is given on the internet at extras.springer.com. The next thing is to use SPSS' syntax program to complete the preparation for real data analysis.

Command:

click File….move to Open….move to Syntax….enter the following text….

```
CONJOINT PLAN = 'g:medicine_plan.sav'
/DATA = 'g:medicine_prefs.sav'
/SEQUENCE = PREF1 TO PREF22
/SUBJECT = ID
/FACTORS = SAFETY EFFICACY (DISCRETE)
PRICE (LINEAR LESS)
PILLSIZE PROLONGEDACTIVITY (LINEAR MORE)
/PRINT = SUMMARYONLY.
```

Save this syntax file at the directory of your choice. Note: the conjoint file entitled "conjoint" only works, if both the plan file and the data file to be analyzed are correctly entered in the above text. In our example we saved both files at a USB stick (recognised by our computer under the directory "g:"). For convenience the conjoint file entitled "conjoint" is also given at extras.springer.com. Prior to use it should also be saved at the USB-stick.

The 22 combinations including the 4 holdouts, can now be used to perform a conjoint analysis with real data. For that purpose 15 physicians are requested to express their preferences of the 22 different combinations.

The preference scores are entered in the data file with the IDs of the physicians as a separate variable in addition to the 22 combinations (the columns). For convenience the data file entitled "medicine_prefs" is given at extras.springer.com, but, if you want to use it, it should first be saved at the USB stick. The conjoint analysis can now be successfully performed.

Performing the Final Analysis

Command:

Open the USB stick....click conjoint....the above syntax text is shown....click Run...select All.

Model description		
	N of levels	Relation to ranks or scores
Safety	3	Linear (more)
Efficacy	3	Linear (more)
Price	3	Linear (less)
Pillsize	2	Discrete
Prolongedactivity	2	Discrete

All factors are orthogonal

The above table gives an overview of the different characteristics (here called factors), and their levels used to construct an analysis plan of the data from our data file.

Utilities			
		Utility estimate	Std. error
Pillsize	Large	–1,250	,426
	Small	1,250	,426
Prolongedactivity	No	–,733	,426
	Yes	,733	,426
Safety	A*	1,283	,491
	B*	2,567	,983
	C*	3,850	1,474
Efficacy	High	–,178	,491
	Medium	–,356	,983
	Low	–,533	1,474
Price	$4	–1,189	,491
	$6	–2,378	,983
	$8	–3,567	1,474
(Constant)		10,328	1,761

The above table gives the utility scores, which are the overall levels of the preferences expressed by the physicians. The meaning of the levels are given:

safety level C: best safety
efficacy level high: best efficacy
pill size 2: smallest pill
prolonged activity 2: prolonged activity present
price $8: most expensive pill.

Generally, higher scores mean greater preference. There is an inverse relationship between pill size and preference, and between pill costs and preference. The safest pill and the most efficaceous pill were given the best preferences.

However, the regression coefficients for efficacy were, statistically, not very significant. Nonetheless, they were included in the overall analysis by the software program. As the utility scores are simply linear regression coefficients, the scores can be used to compute total utilities (add-up preference scores) for a medicine with known characteristic levels. An interesting thing about the methodology is that, like with linear regression modeling, the characteristic levels can be used to calculate an individual add-up utility score (preference score) for a pill with e.g., the underneath characteristics:

(1) pill size (small) + (2) prolonged activity (yes) + safety (C) + efficacy (high) + price ($4) = 1.250 + 0.733 + 3.850–0.178–1.189 + constant (10.328) = 14.974.

For the underneath pill the add-up utility score is, as expected, considerably lower.

(1) pill size (large) + (2) prolonged activity (no) + safety (A) + efficacy (low) + price ($8) = –1.250-0.733 + 1.283–0.533–3.567 + constant (10.328) = 5.528.

The above procedure is the real power of conjoint analysis. It enables to predict preferences for combinations that were not rated by the physicians. In this way you will obtain an idea about the preference to be received by a medicine with known characteristics.

Importance values	
Pillsize	15,675
Prolongedactivity	12,541
Safety	28,338
Efficacy	12,852
Price	30,594

Averaged Importance Score

The range of the utility (preference) scores for each characteristic is an indication of how important the characteristic is. Characteristics with greater ranges play a larger role than the others. As observed the safety and price are the most important preference producing characteristics, while prolonged activity, efficacy, and pill size appear to play a minor role according to the respondents' judgments. The ranges are computed such that they add-up to 100 (%).

Coefficients	
	B coefficient
	Estimate
Safety	1,283
Efficacy	–,178
Price	–1,189

The above table gives the linear regression coefficients for the factors that are specified as linear. The interpretation of the utility (preference) score for the cheapest pill equals $4 × (–1.189) = –4.756

Correlations[a]		
	Value	Sig.
Pearson's R	,819	,000
Kendall's tau	,643	,000
Kendall's tau for Holdouts	,333	,248

[a]Correlations between observed and estimated preferences

The correlation coefficients between the observed preferences and the preferences calculated from conjoint model shows that the correlations by Pearson and Kendall's method are pretty good, indicating that the conjoint methodology produced a sensitive prediction model. The regression analysis of the holdout cases is intended as a validity check, and produced a pretty large p-value of 24.8 %. Still it means that we have about 75 % to find no type I error in this procedure.

Number of reversals			
Factor	Efficacy		9
	Price		5
	Safety		4
	Prolongedactivity		0
	Pillsize		0
Subject	1	Subject 1	1
	2	Subject 2	0
	3	Subject 3	0
	4	Subject 4	1
	5	Subject5	3
	6	Subject 6	1
	7	Subject 7	3
	8	Subject 8	2
	9	Subject 9	1
	10	Subject 10	0
	11	Subject 11	1
	12	Subject 12	1
	13	Subject 13	0
	14	Subject 14	1
	15	Subject 15	3

Finally, the conjoint program reports the number of physicians whose preference was different from what was expected. Particularly in the efficacy characteristic there were 9 of the 15 physicians who chose differently from expected, underlining the limited role of this characteristic.

Conclusion

Conjoint analysis is helpful to pharmaceutical institutions for determining the most appreciated properties of medicines they will develop. Disadvantage include: (1) it is pretty complex; (2) it may be hard to respondents to express preferences; (3) other characteristics not selected may be important too, e.g., physical and pharmacological factors.

Note

More background, theoretical and mathematical information of conjoint modeling is given in Machine learning in medicine part three, Chap. 19, Conjoint analysis, pp 217–230, Springer Heidelberg Germany 2013.

Chapter 58
Item Response Modeling for Analyzing Quality of Life with Better Precision (1,000 Patients)

General Purpose

Item response tests are goodness of fit tests for analyzing the item scores of intelligence tests, and they perform better for the purpose than traditional tests, based on reproducibility measures, do. Like intelligence, quality of life is a multidimensional construct, and may, therefore, be equally suitable for item response modeling.

Primary Scientific Question

Can quality of life data be analyzed through item response modeling, and provide more sensitivity than classical linear models do?

Example

As an example we will analyze the 5-items of a mobility-domain of a quality of life (QOL) battery for patients with coronary artery disease in a group of 1,000 patients. Instead of five many more items can be included. However, for the purpose of simplicity we will use only five items: the domain mobility in a quality of life battery was assessed by answering "yes or no" to experienced difficulty (1) while climbing stair, (2) on short distances, (3) on long distances, (4) on light household work,

This chapter was previously published in "Machine learning in medicine-cookbook 2" as Chap. 12, 2014.

T.J. Cleophas, A.H. Zwinderman, *Machine Learning in Medicine - a Complete Overview*, DOI 10.1007/978-3-319-15195-3_58

(5) on heavy household work. In the underneath table the data of 1,000 patients are summarized. These data can be fitted into a standard normal Gaussian frequency distribution curve (see underneath figure). From it, it can be seen that the items used here are more adequate for demonstrating low quality of life than they are for demonstrating high quality of life, but, nonetheless, an entire Gaussian distribution can be extrapolated from the data given. The lack of histogram bars on the right side of the Gaussian curve suggests that more high quality of life items in the questionnaire would be welcome in order to improve the fit of the histogram into the Gaussian curve. Yet it is interesting to observe that, even with a limited set of items, already a fairly accurate frequency distribution pattern of all quality of life levels of the population is obtained.

No. response pattern	Response pattern (1 = yes, 2 = no) to items 1 to 5	Observed Frequencies
1	11111	4
2	11112	7
3	11121	3
4	11122	12
5	11211	2
6	11212	2
7	11221	4
8	11222	5
9	12111	2
10	12112	9
11	12121	1
12	12122	17
13	12211	1
14	12212	4
15	12221	3
16	12222	16
17	21111	11
18	21112	30
19	21121	15
20	21122	21
21	21211	4
22	21212	29
23	21221	16
24	21222	81
25	22111	17
26	22112	57
27	22121	22
28	22122	174
29	22211	12
30	22212	62
31	22221	29
32	22222	263

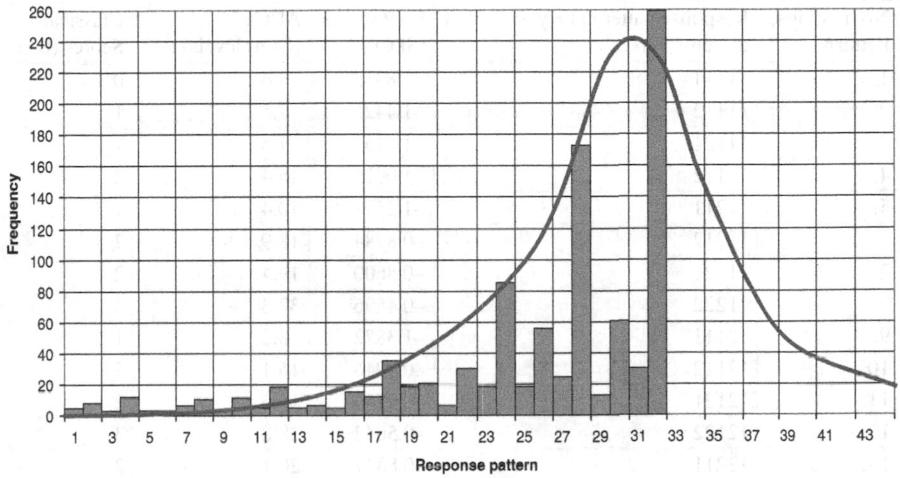

The LTA-2 (Latent Trait Analysis – 2) free software program is used (Uebersax J. Free Software LTA (latent trait analysis) -2 (with binary items), 2006, www.john-uebersax.com/stat/Ital.htm). The data file entitled "itemresponsemodeling" is available in extras.springer.com. We enter the data file by the traditional copy and paste commands.

Command:

Gaussian error model for IRF (Instrument Response Function) shape….chi-square goodness of fit for Fit Statistics…. Frequency table….EAP score table.

The software program calculates the quality of life scores of the different response patterns as EAP (Expected Ability a Posteriori) scores. These scores can be considered as the z-values of a normal Gaussian curve, meaning that the associated area under curve (AUC) of the Gaussian curve is an estimate of the level of quality of life.

There is, approximately,

a 50 % quality of life level with an EAP score of 0,
a 35 % QOL level with an EAP score of −1 (standard deviations),
a 2.5 % " " of −2
a 85 % " " of +1
a 97.5 % " " of +2

No. response Pattern	Response pattern (1 = yes, 2 = no) to items 1 to 5	EAP scores (SDs)	AUCs (QOL levels) (%)	Classical Scores (0–5)
1.	11111	–1.8315	3.4	0
2.	11112	–1.4425	7.5	1
3.	11121	–1.4153	7.8	1
4.	11122	–1.0916	15.4	2
5.	11211	–1.2578	10.4	1
6.	11212	–0.8784	18.9	2
7.	11221	–0.8600	19.4	2
8.	11222	–0.4596	32.3	3
9.	12111	–1.3872	8.2	1
10.	12112	–0.9946	16.1	2
11.	12121	–0.9740	16.6	2
12.	12122	–0.5642	28.8	3
13.	12211	–0.8377	20.1	2
14.	12212	–0.4389	33.0	3
15.	12221	–0.4247	33.4	3
16.	12222	0.0074	50.4	4
17.	21111	–1.3501	8.9	1
18.	21112	–0.9381	17.4	2
19.	21121	–0.9172	17.9	2
20.	21122	–0.4866	31.2	3
21.	21211	–0.7771	21.8	2
22.	21212	–0.3581	35.9	3
23.	21221	–0.3439	36.7	3
24.	21222	0.1120	54.4	4
25.	22111	–0.8925	18.7	2
26.	22112	–0.4641	32.3	3
27.	22121	–0.4484	32.6	3
28.	22122	0.0122	50.4	4
29.	22211	–0.3231	37.5	3
30.	22212	0.1322	55.2	4
31.	22221	0.1433	55.6	4
32.	22222	0.6568	74.5	5

EAP expected ability a posteriori, *QOL* quality of life

In the above table the EAP scores per response pattern is given as well as the AUC (= quality of life level) values as calculated by the software program are given. In the fourth column the classical score is given ranging from 0 (no yes answers) to 5 (5 yes answers). Unlike the classical scores, running from 0 to 100 %, the item scores are more precise and vary from 3.4 to 74.5 % with an overall mean score, by definition, of 50 %. The item response model produce an adequate fit for the data as demonstrated by chi-square goodness of fit values/degrees of freedom of 0.86. What is even more important, is, that we have 32 different QOL scores instead of no more than five as observed with the classical score method. With six items the numbers of scores would even rise to 64. The interpretation is: the higher the score, the better the quality of life.

Conclusion

Quality of life assessments can be analyzed through item response modeling, and provide more sensitivity than classical linear models do.

Note

More background theoretical and mathematical information of item response modeling is given in Machine learning in medicine part one, Chap. 8, Item response modeling, pp 87–98, edited by Springer Heidelberg Germany, 2012, from the same authors. In the current chapter the LTA-2 the free software program is used (Uebersax J. Free Software LTA (latent trait analysis) -2 (with binary items), 2006, www.john-uebersax.com/stat/Ital.htm).

Chapter 59
Survival Studies with Varying Risks of Dying (50 and 60 Patients)

General Purpose

Patients' predictors of survival may change across time, because people may change their lifestyles. Standard statistical methods do not allow adjustments for time-dependent predictors. Time-dependent Cox regression has been introduced as a method adequate for the purpose.

Primary Scientific Question

Predictors of survival may change across time, e.g., the effect of smoking, cholesterol, and increased blood pressure on cardiovascular disease, and patients' frailty in oncology research.

Examples

Cox Regression with a Time-Dependent Predictor

The level of LDL cholesterol is a strong predictor of cardiovascular survival. However, in a survival study virtually no one will die from elevated values in the first decade of observation. LDL cholesterol may be, particularly, a killer in the second decade of observation. The Cox regression model is not appropriate for analyzing the effect of LDL cholesterol on survival, because it assumes that the relative

---

This chapter was previously published in "Machine learning in medicine-cookbook 2" as Chap. 13, 2014.

T.J. Cleophas, A.H. Zwinderman, *Machine Learning in Medicine - a Complete Overview*, DOI 10.1007/978-3-319-15195-3_59

hazard of dying is the same in the first, second and third decade. If you want to analyze such data, an extended Cox regression model allowing for non-proportional hazards can be applied, and is available in SPSS statistical software. In the underneath example the first 10 of 60 patients are given. They were followed for 30 years for the occurrence of a cardiovascular event. Each row represents a patient, the columns are the patient characteristics, otherwise called the variables.

Variable (Var)					
1	2	3	4	5	6
1,00	1	0	65,00	0,00	2,00
1,00	1	0	66,00	0,00	2,00
2,00	1	0	73,00	0,00	2,00
2,00	1	0	54,00	0,00	2,00
2,00	1	0	46,00	0,00	2,00
2,00	1	0	37,00	0,00	2,00
2,00	1	0	54,00	0,00	2,00
2,00	1	0	66,00	0,00	2,00
2,00	1	0	44,00	0,00	2,00
3,00	0	0	62,00	0,00	2,00

Var 00001 = follow-up period (years) (Var = variable)
Var 00002 = event (0 or 1, event or lost for follow-up = censored)
Var 00003 = treatment modality (0 = treatment-1, 1 = treatment-2)
Var 00004 = age (years)
Var 00005 = gender (0 or 1, male or female)
Var 00006 = LDL-cholesterol (0 or 1, < 3.9 or >= 3.9 mmol/l)

The entire data file is in extras.springer.com, and is entitled "survivalvaryingrisks". Start by opening the file. First, a usual Cox regression is performed with LDL-cholesterol as predictor of survival (var = variable).

Command:

Analyze….survival….Cox regression….time: follow months…. status: var 2…. define event (1)….Covariates….categorical: elevated LDL-cholesterol (Var 00006) => categorical variables….continue….plots…. survival => ….hazard….continue…. OK.

Variables in the equation						
	B	SE	Wald	df	Sig.	Exp(B)
VAR00006	–,482	,307	2,462	1	,117	,618

Variables in the equation						
	B	SE	Wald	df	Siq.	Exp(B)
T_COV_	–,131	,033	15,904	1	,000	,877

The upper table shows that elevated LDL-cholesterol is not a significant predictor of survival with a p-value as large as 0.117 and a hazard ratio of 0.618. In order to assess, whether elevated LDL-cholesterol adjusted for time has an effect on survival, a time-dependent Cox regression will be performed as shown in the above lower table. For that purpose the time-dependent covariate is defined as a function of both the variable time (called "T_" in SPSS) and the LDL-cholesterol-variable, while using the product of the two. This product is applied as the "time-dependent predictor of survival", and a usual Cox model is, subsequently, performed (Cov = covariate).

Command:

Analyze....survival....Cox w/Time-Dep Cov....Compute Time-Dep Cov....Time (T_) = > in box Expression for T_Cov....add the sign * ....add the LDL-cholesterol variable....model....time: follow months....status: var 00002....?: define event:1.... continue....T_Cov = > in box covariates....OK.

The above lower table shows that elevated LDL-cholesterol after adjustment for differences in time is a highly significant predictor of survival. If we look at the actual data of the file, we will observe that, overall, the LDL-cholesterol variable is not an important factor. But, if we look at the blood pressures of the three decades separately, then it is observed that something very special is going on: in the first decade virtually no one with elevated LDL-cholesterol dies. In the second decade virtually everyone with an elevated LDL-cholesterol does: LDL cholesterol seems to be particularly a killer in the second decade. Then, in the third decade other reasons for dying seem to have occurred.

Cox Regression with a Segmented Time-Dependent Predictor

Some variables may have different values at different time periods. For example, elevated blood pressure may be, particularly, harmful not after decades but at the very time-point it is highest. The blood pressure is highest in the first and third decade of the study. However, in the second decade it is mostly low, because the patients were adequately treated at that time. For the analysis we have to use the socalled logical expressions. They take the value 1, if the time is true, and 0, if false. Using a series of logical expressions, we can create our time-dependent predictor, that can, then, be analyzed by the usual Cox model. In the underneath example 11 of 60 patients are given. The entire data file is in extras.springer.com, and is entitled "survivalvaryingrisks2" The patients were followed for 30 years for the occurrence of a cardiovascular event. Each row represents again a patient, the columns are the patient characteristics.

Var 1	2	3	4	5	6	7
7,00	1	76	,00	133,00	.	.
9,00	1	76	,00	134,00	.	.
9,00	1	65	,00	143,00	.	.
11,00	1	54	,00	134,00	110,00	.
12,00	1	34	,00	143,00	111,00	.
14,00	1	45	,00	135,00	110,00	.
16,00	1	56	1,00	123,00	103,00	.
17,00	1	67	1,00	133,00	107,00	.
18,00	1	86	1,00	134,00	108,00	.
30,00	1	75	1,00	134,00	102,00	134,00
30,00	1	65	1,00	132,00	121,00	126,00

Var 00001 = follow-up period years (Var = variable)
Var 00002 = event (0 or 1, event or lost for follow-up = censored)
Var 00003 = age (years)
Var 00004 = gender
Var 00005 = mean blood pressure in the first decade
Var 00006 = mean blood pressure in the second decade
Var 00007 = mean blood pressure in the third decade

In the second and third decade an increasing number of patients have been lost. The following time-dependent covariate must be constructed for the analysis of these data (* = sign of multiplication) using the click Transform and click Compute Variable commands:

(T_>=1&T_<11)*Var 5 + (T_>=11&T_<21)*Var 6 + (T_>=21&T_<31)*Var 7

This novel predictor variable is entered in the usual way with the commands (Cov = covariate):

Model....time: follow months....status: var 00002....?: define event:1 – continue.... T_Cov => in box covariates....OK.

The underneath table shows that, indeed, a mean blood pressure after adjustment for difference in decades is a significant predictor of survival at p = 0.040, and with a hazard ratio of 0.936 per mm Hg. In spite of the better blood pressures in the second decade, blood pressure is a significant killer in the overall analysis.

Variables in the equation

	B	SE	Wald	df	Sig.	Exp(B)
T_COV_	–,066	,032	4,238	1	,040	,936

Conclusion

Many predictors of survival change across time, e.g., the effect of smoking, cholesterol, and increased blood pressure in cardiovascular research, and patients' frailty in oncology research.

Note

More background theoretical and mathematical information is given in Machine learning in medicine part one, Chap. 9, Time-dependent predictor modeling, pp 99–111, Springer Heidelberg Germany, 2012, from the same authors.

Chapter 60
Fuzzy Logic for Improved Precision of Dose-Response Data (8 Induction Dosages)

General Purpose

Fuzzy logic can handle questions to which the answers may be "yes" at one time and "no" at the other, or may be partially true and untrue. Pharmacodynamic data deal with questions like "does a patient respond to a particular drug dose or not", or "does a drug cause the same effects at the same time in the same subject or not". Such questions are typically of a fuzzy nature, and might, therefore, benefit from an analysis based on fuzzy logic.

Specific Scientific Question

This chapter is to study whether fuzzy logic can improve the precision of predictive models for pharmacodynamic data.

This chapter was previously published in "Machine learning in medicine-cookbook 2" as Chap. 14, 2014.

T.J. Cleophas, A.H. Zwinderman, *Machine Learning in Medicine - a Complete Overview*, DOI 10.1007/978-3-319-15195-3_60

Example

Imput values	output values	fuzzy-modeled output
induction dosage of thiopental (mg/kg)	numbers of responders (n)	numbers of responders(n)
1	4	4
1.5	5	5
2	6	8
2.5	9	10
3	12	12
3.5	17	14
4	17	16
4.5	12	14
5	9	1

We will use as an example the quantal pharmacodynamic effects of different induction dosages of thiopental on numbers of responding subjects. It is usually not possible to know what type of statistical distribution the experiment is likely to follow, sometimes Gaussian, sometimes very skewed. A pleasant aspect of fuzzy modeling is that it can be applied with any type of statistical distribution and that it is particularly suitable for uncommon and unexpected non linear relationships.

Quantal response data are often presented in the literature as S-shape dose-cumulative response curves with the dose plotted on a logarithmic scale, where the log transformation has an empirical basis. We will, therefore, use a logarithmic regression model. SPSS Statistical Software is used for analysis.

Command:

Analyze...regression...curve estimation...dependent variable: data second column...independent variable: data first column...logarithmic...OK.

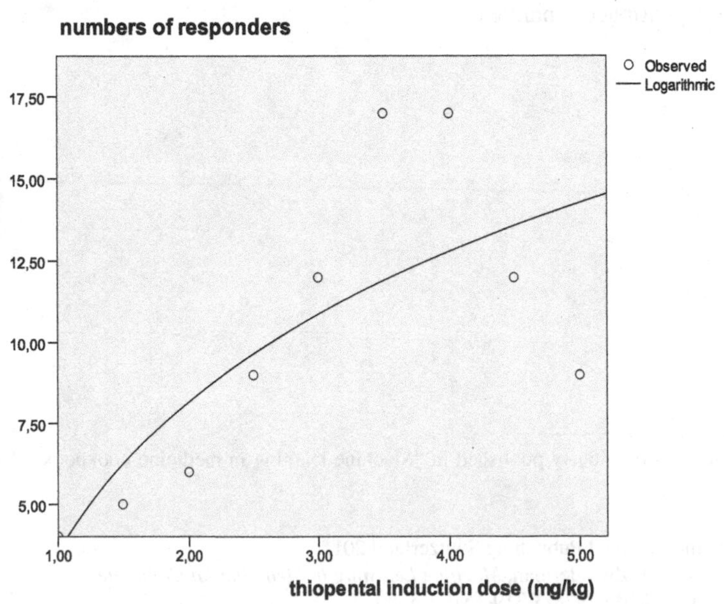

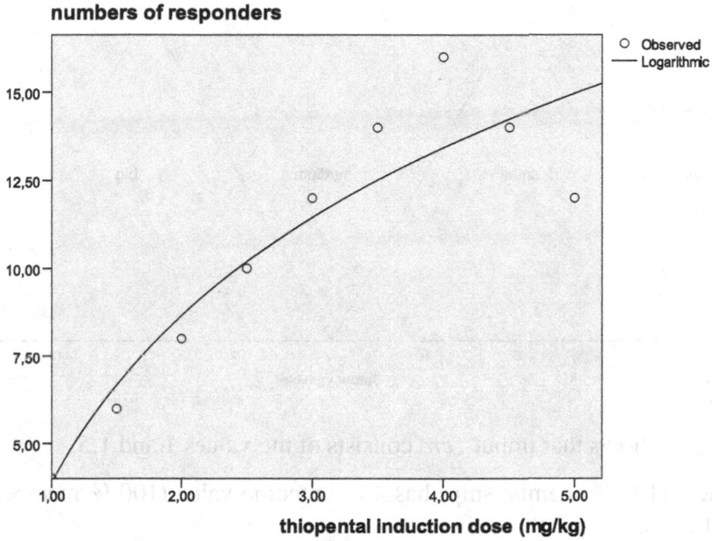

The analysis produces a moderate fit of the data (upper curve) with an r-square value of 0.555 (F-value 8.74, p-value 0.024).

We, subsequently, fuzzy-model the imput and output relationships (underneath figure). First of all, we create linguistic rules for the imput and output data.

For that purpose we divide the universal space of the imput variable into fuzzy memberships with linguistic membership names:

imput-*zero, -small, -medium, -big, -superbig.*

Then we do the same for the output variable:

output-*zero, -small, -medium, -big.*

Subsequently, we create linguistic rules.

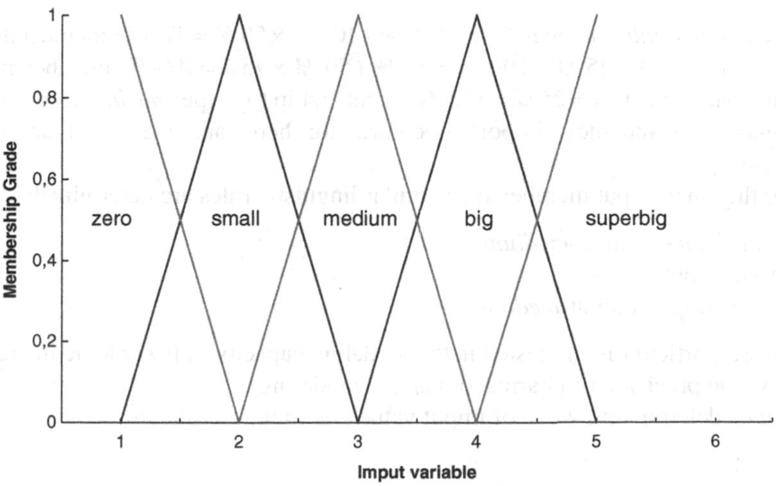

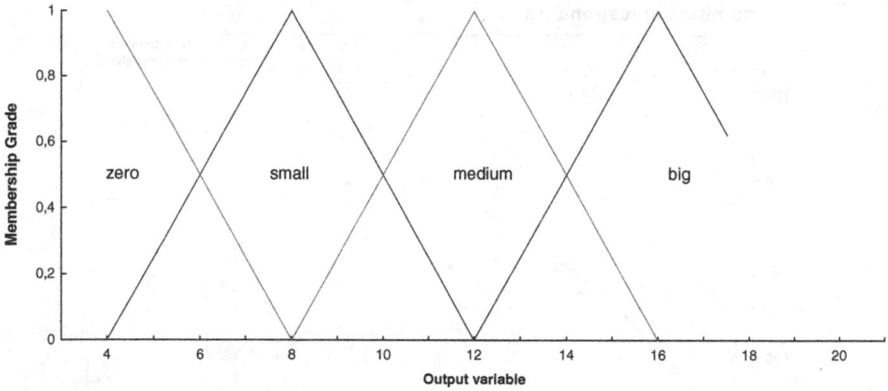

The figure shows that imput-*zero* consists of the values 1 and 1.5.

The value 1 (100 % membership) has 4 as outcome value (100 % membership of output-*zero*).
The value 1.5 (50 % membership) has 5 as outcome value (75 % membership of output-*zero*, 25 % of output-*small*).

The imput-*zero* produces 100 % × 100 % + 50 % × 75 % = 137.5 % membership to output-*zero*, and 50 % × 25 % = 12.5 % membership to output-*small*, and so, output-zero is the most important output contributor here, and we forget about the small contribution of output-*small*.

Imput-*small* is more complex, it consists of the values 1.5, and 2.0, and 2.5.

The value 1.5 (50 % membership) has 5 as outcome value (75 % membership of output-*zero*, 25 % membership of output-*small*).
The value 2.0 (100 % membership) has 6 as outcome value (50 % membership of outcome-*zero*, and 50 % membership of output-*small*).
The value 2.5 (50 % membership) has 9 as outcome value (75 % membership of output-*small* and 25 % of output-*medium*).

The imput-*small* produces 50 % × 75 % + 100 % × 50 % = 87.5 % membership to output-*zero*, 50 % × 25 % + 100 % × 50 % + 50 % × 75% = 100 % membership to output-small, and 50 % × 25 % = 12.5 % membership to output-*medium*. And so, the output-*small* is the most important contributor here, and we forget about the other two.

For the other imput memberships similar linguistic rules are determined:

Imput-*medium* → output-*medium*
Imput-*big* → output-*big*
Imput-*superbig* → output-*medium*

We are, particularly interested in the modeling capacity of fuzzy logic in order to improve the precision of pharmacodynamic modeling.

The modeled output value of imput value 1 is found as follows.

Value 1 is 100 % member of imput-*zero*, meaning that according to the above linguistic rules it is also associated with a 100 % membership of output-*zero* corresponding with a value of 4.

Value 1.5 is 50 % member of imput-*zero* and 50 % imput-*small*. This means it is 50 % associated with the output-*zero* and –*small* corresponding with values of $50\,\% \times (4+8)=6$.

For all of the imput values modeled output values can be found in this way. The table on page 378, right column shows the results. We perform a logarithmic regression on the fuzzy-modeled outcome data similar to that for the un-modeled output values. The fuzzy-modeld output data provided a much better fit than did the un-modeled output values (lower curve) with an r-square value of 0.852 (F-value = 40.34) as compared to 0.555 (F-value 8.74) for the un-modeled output data.

Conclusion

Fuzzy logic can handle questions to which the answers may be "yes" at one time and "no" at the other, or may be partially true and untrue. Dose response data deal with questions like "does a patient respond to a particular drug dose or not", or "does a drug cause the same effects at the same time in the same subject or not". Such questions are typically of a fuzzy nature, and might, therefore, benefit from an analysis based on fuzzy logic.

Note

More background theoretical and mathematical information of analyses using fuzzy logic is given in Machine learning in medicine part one, Chap. 19, pp 241–253, Springer Heidelberg Germany, 2012, from the same authors.

Chapter 61
Automatic Data Mining for the Best Treatment of a Disease (90 Patients)

General Purpose

SPSS modeler is a work bench for automatic data mining (current chapter) and data modeling (Chaps. 64 and 65). So far it is virtually unused in medicine, and mainly applied by econo-/sociometrists. We will assess whether it can also be used for multiple outcome analysis of clinical data.

Specific Scientific Question

Patients with sepsis have been given one of three treatments. Various outcome variables are used to assess which one of the treatments performs best.

Example

In data mining the question "is a treatment a predictor of clinical improvement" is assessed by the question "is the outcome, clinical improvement, a predictor of the chance of having had a treatment". This approach may seem incorrect, but is also used with discriminant analysis, and works fine, because it does not suffer from strong correlations between outcome variables (Machine Learning in Medicine Part One, Chap. 17, Discriminant analysis of supervised data, pp 215–224, Springer

This chapter was previously published in "Machine learning in medicine-cookbook 2" as Chap. 15, 2014.

T.J. Cleophas, A.H. Zwinderman, *Machine Learning in Medicine - a Complete Overview*, DOI 10.1007/978-3-319-15195-3_61

Heidelberg Germany, 2013). In this example, 90 patients with sepsis are treated with three different treatments. Various outcome values are used as predictors of the output treatment.

asat	alat	ureum	creat	crp	leucos	treat	low bp	death
5,00	29,00	2,40	79,00	18,00	16,00	1,00	1	0
10,00	30,00	2,10	94,00	15,00	15,00	1,00	1	0
8,00	31,00	2,30	79,00	16,00	14,00	1,00	1	0
6,00	16,00	2,70	80,00	17,00	19,00	1,00	1	0
6,00	16,00	2,20	84,00	18,00	20,00	1,00	1	0
5,00	13,00	2,10	78,00	17,00	21,00	1,00	1	0
10,00	16,00	3,10	85,00	20,00	18,00	1,00	1	0
8,00	28,00	8,00	68,00	15,00	18,00	1,00	1	0
7,00	27,00	7,80	74,00	16,00	17,00	1,00	1	0
6,00	26,00	8,40	69,00	18,00	16,00	1,00	1	0
12,00	22,00	2,70	75,00	14,00	19,00	1,00	1	0
21,00	21,00	3,00	70,00	15,00	20,00	1,00	1	0
10,00	20,00	23,00	74,00	15,00	18,00	1,00	1	0
19,00	19,00	2,10	75,00	16,00	16,00	1,00	1	0
8,00	32,00	2,00	85,00	18,00	19,00	1,00	2	0
20,00	11,00	2,90	63,00	18,00	18,00	1,00	1	0
7,00	30,00	6,80	72,00	17,00	18,00	1,00	1	0
1973,00	846,00	73,80	563,00	18,00	38,00	3,00	2	0
1863,00	757,00	41,70	574,00	15,00	34,00	3,00	2	1
1973,00	646,00	38,90	861,00	16,00	38,00	3,00	2	1

asat = aspartate aminotransferase
alat = alanine aminotransferase
creat = creatinine
crp = c-reactive protein
treat = treatments 1–3
low bp = low blood pressure (1 no, 2 slight, 3 severe)
death = death (0 no, 1 yes)

Only the first 20 patients are above, the entire data file is in extra.springer.com and is entitled "spssmodeler.sav". SPSS modeler version 14.2 is used for the analysis. Start by opening SPSS modeler.

Step 1 Open SPSS Modeler

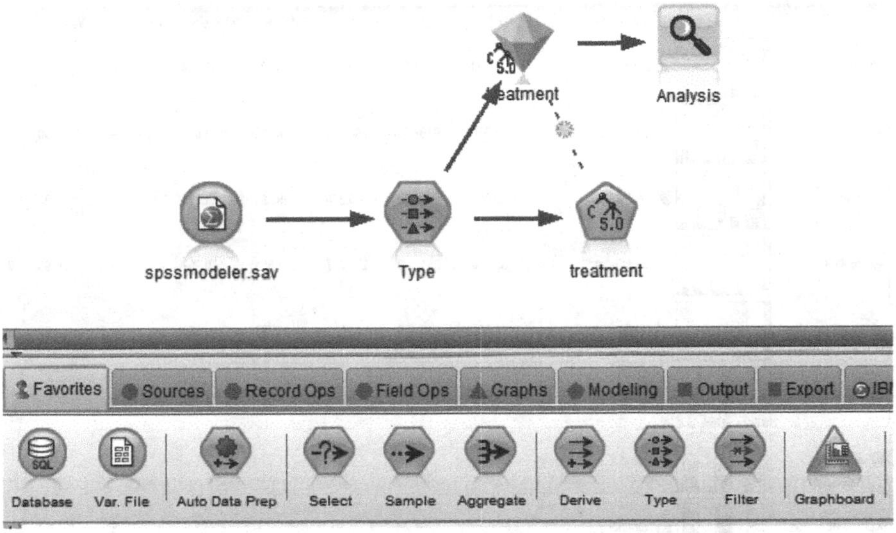

In the palettes at the bottom of the screen full of nodes, look and find the **Statistics File node**, and drag it to the canvas. Double-click on it….Import file: browse and enter the file "spssmodeler.sav"….click OK….in the palette find **Distribution node** and drag to canvas….right-click on the Statistics File node….a Connect symbol comes up….click on the Distribution node….an arrow is displayed….double-click on the Distribution Node….after a second or two the underneath graph with information from the Distribution node is observed.

Step 2 The Distribution Node

Value	Proportion	%	Count
1.00		38.89	35
2.00		40.0	36
3.00		21.11	19

It gives the frequency distribution of the three treatments in the 90 patient data file. All of the treatments are substantially present.

Next remove the Distribution node by clicking on it and press delete on the key board of your computer. Continue by dragging the Data audit node to the canvas…. perform the connecting manoeuvres as above….double-click it again.

Step 3 The Data Audit Node

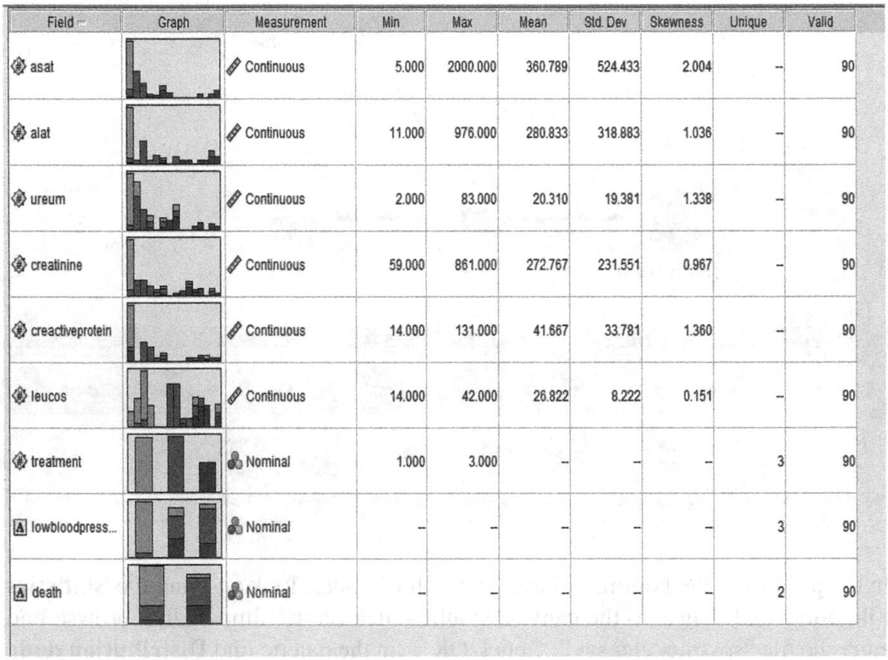

Field	Graph	Measurement	Min	Max	Mean	Std. Dev	Skewness	Unique	Valid
asat		Continuous	5.000	2000.000	360.789	524.433	2.004	–	90
alat		Continuous	11.000	976.000	280.833	318.883	1.036	–	90
ureum		Continuous	2.000	83.000	20.310	19.381	1.338	–	90
creatinine		Continuous	59.000	861.000	272.767	231.551	0.967	–	90
creactiveprotein		Continuous	14.000	131.000	41.667	33.781	1.360	–	90
leucos		Continuous	14.000	42.000	26.822	8.222	0.151	–	90
treatment		Nominal	1.000	3.000	–	–	–	3	90
lowbloodpress...		Nominal	–	–	–	–	–	3	90
death		Nominal	–	–	–	–	–	2	90

The Data audit will be edited. Select "treatment" as target field (field is variable here)....click Run. The information from this node is now given in the form of a Data audit plot, showing that due to the treatment low values are frequently more often observed than the high values. Particularly, the treatments 1 and 2 (light blue and red) are often associated with low values, these are probably the best treatments. Next remove the Data audit node by clicking on it and press delete on the key board of your computer. Continue by dragging the Plot node to the canvas….perform the connecting manoeuvres as above….double-click it again.

Step 4 The Plot Node

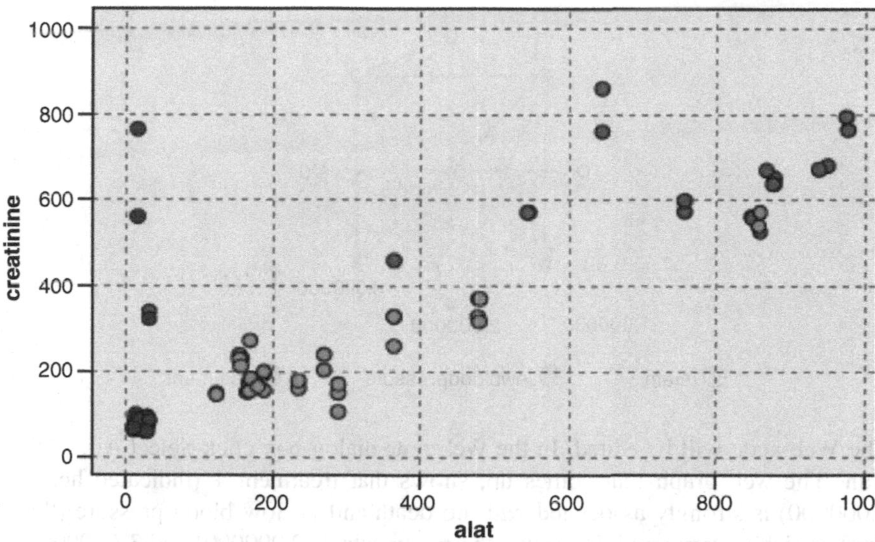

The Plot node will be edited. On the Plot tab select creatinine as y-variable and alat as x-variable, and treatment in the Overlay field at Color….click Run. The information from this node is now given in the form of a scatter plot of patients. This scatter plot of alat versus creatinine values shows that the three treatments are somewhat separately clustered. Treatment 1 (blue) in the left lower part, 2 (green) in the middle, and 3 in the right upper part. Low values means adequate effect of treatment. So treatment 1 (and also some patients with treatment 2) again perform pretty well. Next remove the Plot node by clicking on it and press delete on the key board of your computer. Continue by dragging the Web node to the canvas….perform the connecting manoeuvres as above….double-click it again.

Step 5 The Web Node

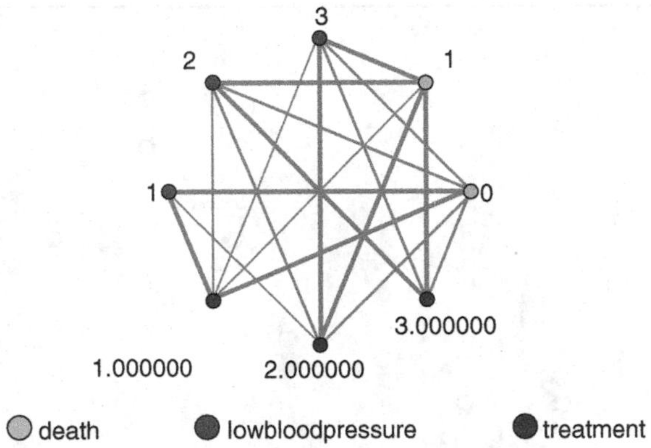

The Web node will be edited. In the Web note dialog box click Select All....click Run. The web graph that comes up, shows that treatment 1 (indicated here as 1.000000) is strongly associated with no death and no low blood pressure (thick line), which is very good. However, the treatments 2 (2.000000) and 3 (3.000000) are strongly associated with death and treatment 2 (2.000000) is also associated with the severest form of low blood pressure. Next remove the Web node by clicking on it and press delete on the key board of your computer. Continue by dragging both the Type and C5.0 nodes to the canvas....perform the connecting manoeuvres respectively as indicated in the first graph of this chapter....double-click it again...a gold nugget is placed as shown above....click the gold nugget.

Step 6 The Type and c5.0 Nodes

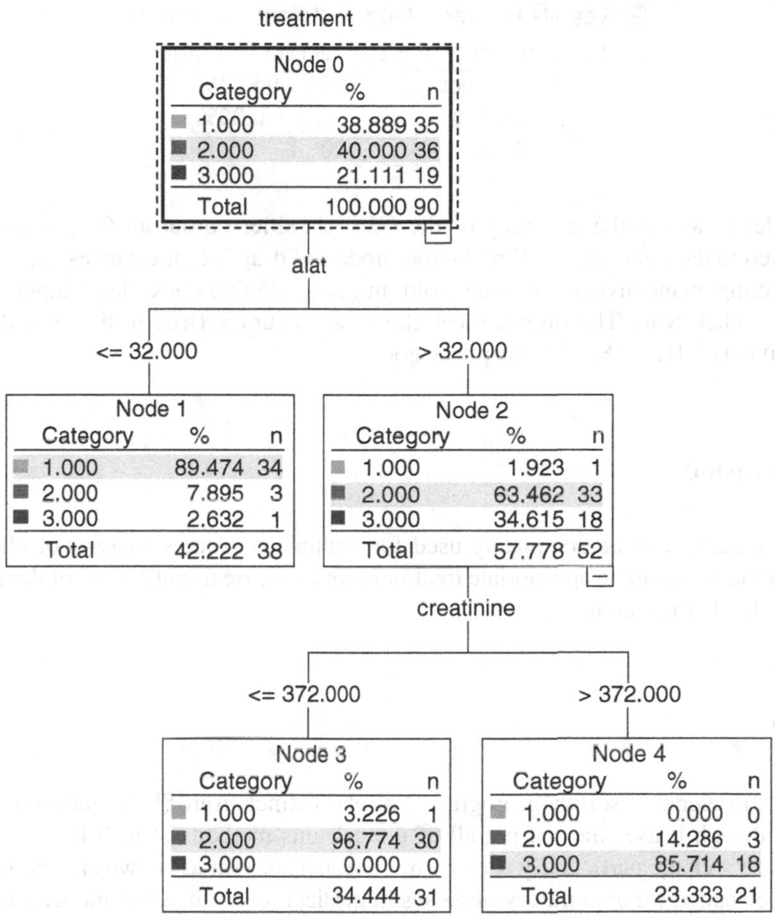

The output sheets give various interactive graphs and tables. One of them is the above C5.0 decision tree. C5.0 decision trees are an improved version of the traditional Quinlan decision trees with less, but more-relevant information.

The C5.0 classifier underscores the previous findings. The variable alat is the best classifier of the treatments with alat <32 over 89 % of the patients having had treatment 1, and with alat>32 over 63 % of the patients having had treatment 2. Furthermore, in the high alat class patients with a creatinine over 372 around 86 % has treatment 3. And so all in all, the treatment 1 would seem the best treatment and treatment 3 the worst one.

Step 7 The Output Node

Results for output field treatment

Comparing $C-treatment with treatment

Correct	82	91,11%
Wrong	8	8,89%
Total	90	

In order to assess the accuracy of the C5.0 classifier output an Output node is attached to the gold nugget. Find Output node and drag it to the canvas….perform connecting manoeuvres with the gold nugget….double-click the Output node again….click Run. The output sheet shows an accuracy (true positives and true negatives) of 91,11 %, which is pretty good.

Conclusion

SPSS modeler can be adequately used for multiple outcomes analysis of clinical data. Finding the most appropriate treatment for a disease might be one of the goals of this kind of research.

Note

SPSS modeler is a software program entirely distinct from SPSS statistical software, though it uses most if not all of the calculus methods of it. It is a standard software package particularly used by market analysts, but as shown can, perfectly, well be applied for exploratory purposes in medical research. SPSS modeler is also applied in the Chaps. 64 and 65.

Chapter 62
Pareto Charts for Identifying the Main Factors of Multifactorial Outcomes (2,000 Admissions to Hospital)

General Purpose

In 1906 the Italian economist Pareto observed that 20 % of the Italian population possessed 80 % of the land, and, looking at other countries, virtually the same seemed to be true. The Pareto principle is currently used to identify the main factors of multifactorial outcomes. Pareto charts is available in SPSS, and this chapter is to assess whether it is useful, not only in marketing science, but also in medicine.

Primary Scientific Question

To assess whether pareto charts can be applied to identify in a study of hospital admissions the main causes of iatrogenic admissions.

This chapter was previously published in "Machine learning in medicine-cookbook 2" as Chap. 16, 2014.

T.J. Cleophas, A.H. Zwinderman, *Machine Learning in Medicine - a Complete Overview*, DOI 10.1007/978-3-319-15195-3_62

Example

Two thousand subsequent admissions to a general hospital in the Netherlands were classified.

Indications for admission	Numbers	%	confidence intervals (95 %)
1. Cardiac condition and hypertension	810	40.5	38.0–42.1
2. Gastrointestinal condition	254	12.7	11.9–14.2
3. Infectious disease	200	10.0	9.2–12.0
4. Pulmonary disease	137	6.9	6.5–7.7
5. Hematological condition	109	5.5	4.0–6.2
6. Malignancy	74	3.7	2.7–4.9
7. Mental disease	54	2.7	1.9–3.8
8. Endocrine condition	49	2.5	1.7–3.5
9. Bleedings with acetyl salicyl/NSAIDS	47	2.4	1.6–3.4
10. Other	41	2.1	1.4–3.1
11. Unintentional overdose	31	1.6	1.0–2.5
12. Bleeding with acenocoumarol/dalteparin	28	1.4	0.8–2.2
13. Fever after chemotherapy	26	1.3	0.7–2.1
14. Electrolyte disturbance	26	1.3	0.7–2.1
15. Dehydration	23	1.2	0.7–2.0
16. Other problems after chemotherapy	20	1.0	0.5–1.8
17. Allergic reaction	17	0.9	0.4–1.7
18. Renal disease	16	0.8	0.3–1.5
19. Pain syndrome	8	0.4	0.1–1.0
20. Hypotension	8	0.4	0.1–1.0
21. Neurological disease	7	0.4	0.1–1.0
22. Vascular disease	6	0.3	0.06–0.7
23. Rheumatoid arthritis/arthrosis/osteoporosis	6	0.3	0.06–0.7
24. Dermatological condition	3	0.2	0.02–0.7
	2,000	100	

NSAIDS non-steroidal anti-inflammatory drugs

The data file is in extras.springer.com and is entitled "paretocharts.sav". Open it.

Command:

Analyze....Quality Control....Pareto Charts....click Simple....mark Value of individual cases....click Define....Values: enter "alladmissions"....mark Variable: enter "diagnosisgroups"....click OK.

The underneath graph shows that over 50 % of the admissions is in the first two diagnosis groups. A general rule as postulated by Pareto says: when analyzing observational studies with multifactorial effects, usually less than 20 % of the factors determines over 80 % of the effect. This postulate seems to be true in this example. The graph shows that the first five diagnosis groups out of 24 % determine around 80 % of the effect (admission). When launching a program to reduce hospital admissions in general, it would make sense to prioritize these five diagnosis groups, and to neglect the other diagnosis groups.

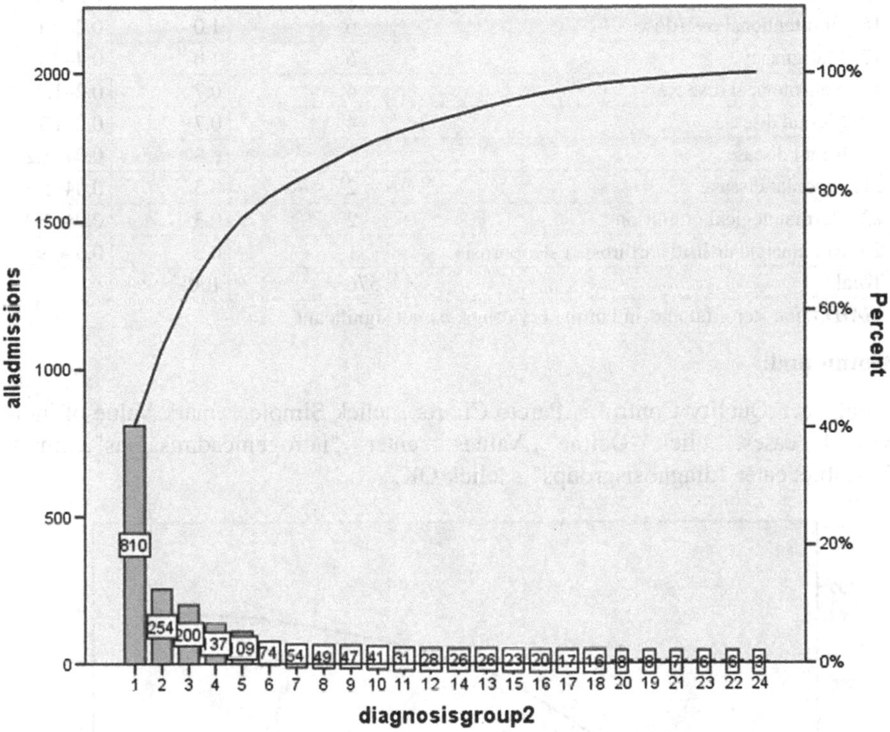

In order to find out how diagnosis groups contributed to the numbers of iatrogenic admissions, a pareto chart was constructed. The data are underneath, and are the variables 4 and 5 in "paretocharts.sav".

	Numbers	%	95 % CIs
1. Cardiac condition and hypertension	202	35.1	31.1–38.9
2. Gastrointestinal condition	89	15.5	12.2–18.1
3. Bleedings with acetyl salicyl/NSAIDS	46	8.0	5.9–10.4
4. Infectious disease	31	5.4	3.6–7.4
5. Bleeding with acenocoumarol/dalteparin	28	4.9	3.1–6.8
6. Fever after chemotherapy	26	4.5	2.9–6.4
7. Hematological condition	24	4.2	2.7–6.1
8. Other problems after chemotherapy	20	3.5	2.1–5.3
9. Endocrine condition	19	3.3	2.0–5.1
10. Dehydration	18	3.1	1.9–4.9
11. Electrolyte disturbance	14	2.4	1.3–3.8
12. Pulmonary disease	9	1.6	0.8–3.0
13. Allergic reaction	8	1.4	0.6–2.8

(continued)

	Numbers	%	95 % CIs
14. Hypotension not due to antihypertensives	8	1.4	0.6–2.8
15. Other	7	1.2	0.5–2.4
16. Unintentional overdose	6	1.0	0.4–2.1
17. Malignancy	6	1.0	0.4–2.1
18. Neurological disease	4	0.7	0.2–1.7
19. Mental disease	4	0.7	0.2–1.7
20. Renal disease	2	0.3	0.04–1.2
21. Vascular disease	2	0.3	0.04–1.2
22. Dermatological condition	2	0.3	0.04–1.2
23. Rheumatoid arthritis/arthrosis/osteoporosis	1	0.2	0.0–0.9
Total	576	100	

NSAIDS non-steroidal anti-inflammatory drugs, *ns* not significant

Command:

Analyze….Quality Control….Pareto Charts….click Simple….mark Value of individual cases….click Define….Values: enter "iatrogenicadmissions"….mark Variable: enter "diagnosisgroups"….click OK.

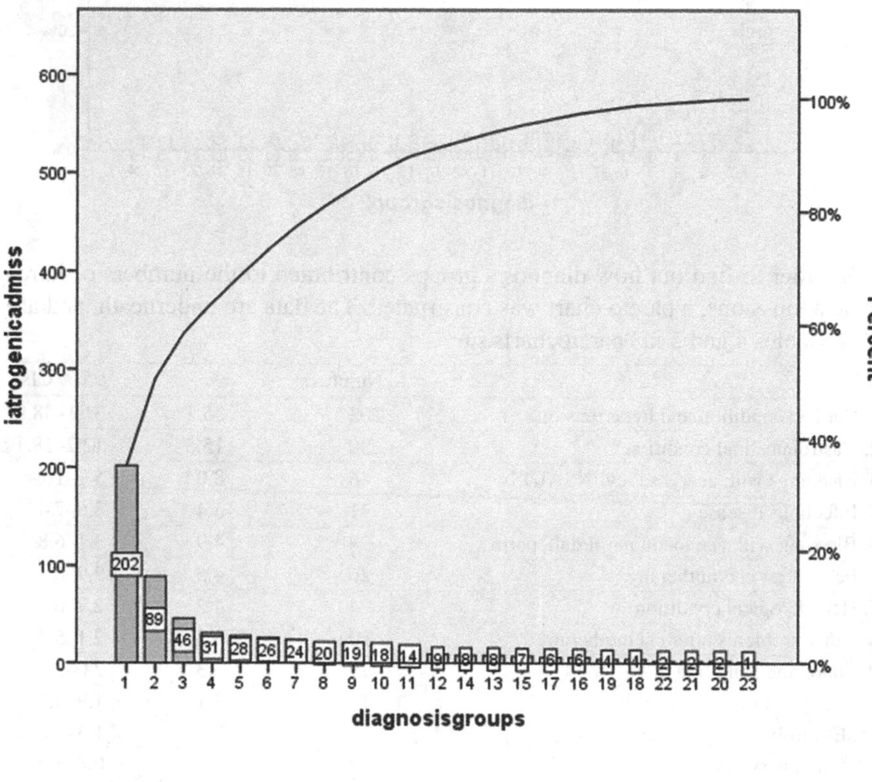

The above pareto chart has a breakpoint at 50 %. Generally, a breakpoint is observed at around 50 % of the effect with around 10 % of the factors before the breakpoint. The breakpoint would be helpful for setting priorities, when addressing the problem of iatrogenic admissions. The diagnosis groups, cardiac condition and gastrointestinal condition, cause over 50 % of all of the iatrogenic admissions.

In order to find which medicines were responsible for the iatrogenic admissions, again a pareto chart was constructed. The variables 1 and 2 of the data file "paretocharts.sav" will be used.

Command:

Analyze....Quality Control....Pareto Charts....click Simple....mark Value of individual cases....click Define....Values: enter "iatrogenicad"....mark Variable: enter "medicinecat"....click OK.

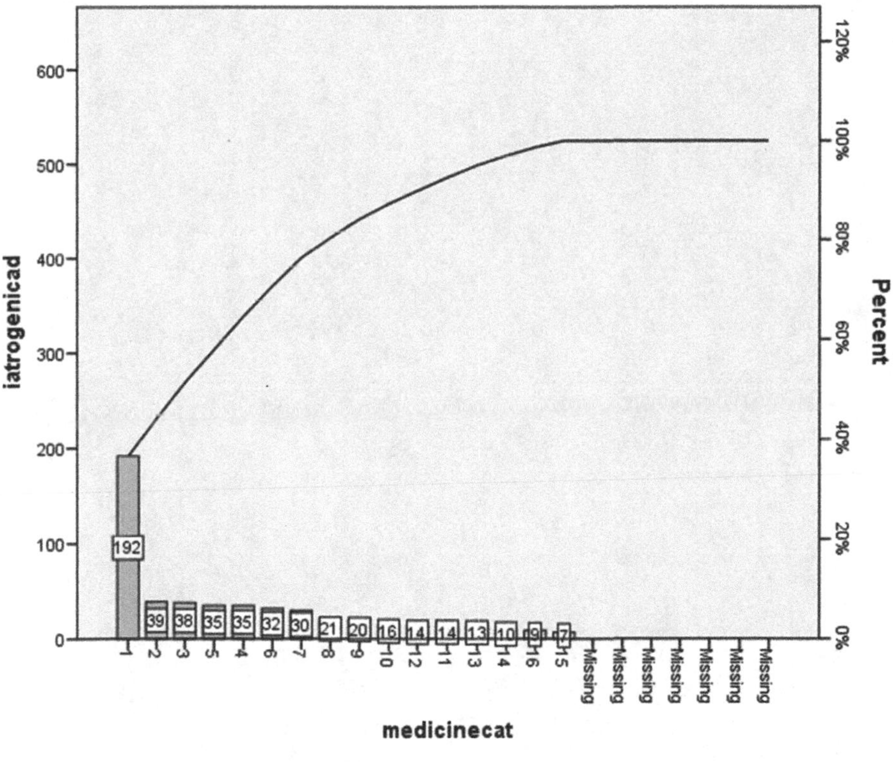

No breakpoint is observed, but the first two medicine categories were responsible for 50 % of the entire number of iatrogenic admissions. We can conclude, that over 50 % of the iatrogenic admissions were in two diagnosis groups, and over 50 % of the medicines responsible were also in two main medicine categories.

Conclusion

Pareto charts are useful for identifying the main factors of multifactorial outcomes, not only in marketing science but also in medicine.

Note

In addition to flow charts, scattergrams, histograms, control charts, cause effects diagrams, and checklists, pareto charts are basic graphical tools of data analysis. All of them require little training in statistics.

Chapter 63
Radial Basis Neural Networks for Multidimensional Gaussian Data (90 Persons)

General Purpose

Radial basis functions may better than multilayer neural network (Chap. 50), predict medical data, because it uses a Gaussian activation function, but it is rarely used. This chapter is to assess its performance in clinical research.

Specific Scientific Question

Body surface area is an indicator for metabolic body mass, and is used for adjusting oxygen, CO_2 transport parameters, blood volumes, urine creatinine clearance, protein/ creatinine ratios and other parameters. Can a radial basis neural network be applied to accurately predict the body surface from gender, age, weight and height?

Example

The body surfaces of 90 persons were calculated using direct photometric measurements. These previously measured outcome data will be used as the socalled learning sample, and the computer will be commanded to teach itself making predictions about the body surface from the predictor variables gender, age, weight and height. The first 20 patients are underneath. The entire data file is in "radialbasisnn".

This chapter was previously published in "Machine learning in medicine-cookbook 2" as Chap. 17, 2013.

T.J. Cleophas, A.H. Zwinderman, *Machine Learning in Medicine - a Complete Overview*, DOI 10.1007/978-3-319-15195-3_63

1,00	13,00	30,50	138,50	10072,90
0,00	5,00	15,00	101,00	6189,00
0,00	0,00	2,50	51,50	1906,20
1,00	11,00	30,00	141,00	10290,60
1,00	15,00	40,50	154,00	13221,60
0,00	11,00	27,00	136,00	9654,50
0,00	5,00	15,00	106,00	6768,20
1,00	5,00	15,00	103,00	6194,10
1,00	3,00	13,50	96,00	5830,20
0,00	13,00	36,00	150,00	11759,00
0,00	3,00	12,00	92,00	5299,40
1,00	0,00	2,50	51,00	2094,50
0,00	7,00	19,00	121,00	7490,80
1,00	13,00	28,00	130,50	9521,70
1,00	0,00	3,00	54,00	2446,20
0,00	0,00	3,00	51,00	1632,50
0,00	7,00	21,00	123,00	7958,80
1,00	11,00	31,00	139,00	10580,80
1,00	7,00	24,50	122,50	8756,10
1,00	11,00	26,00	133,00	9573,00

Var 1 gender
Var 2 age
Var 3 weight (kg)
Var 4 height (m)
Var 5 body surface measured (cm^2)

The Computer Teaches Itself to Make Predictions

The SPSS module Neural Networks is used for training and outcome prediction. It uses XML (exTended Markup Language) files to store the neural network. Start by opening the data file.

Command:

click Transform….click Random Number Generators….click Set Starting Point…. click Fixed Value (2000000)….click OK….click Analyze…. Neural Networks…. Radial Basis Function….Dependent Variables: enter Body surface measured…. Factors: enter gender, age, weight, and height….Partitions: Training 7….Test 3…. Holdout 0….click Output: mark Description….Diagram…. Model summary…. Predicted by observed chart….Case processing summary ….click Save: mark Save predicted value of category for each dependent variable….automatically generate unique names….click Export….mark Export synaptic weights estimates to XML file….click Browse….File Name: enter "exportradialbasisnn" and save in the appropriate folder of your computer….click OK.

The output warns that in the testing sample some cases have been excluded from analysis, because of values not occurring in the training sample. Minimizing the output sheets shows the data file with predicted values. They are pretty much the same as the measured body surface values. We will use linear regression to estimate the association between the two.

Command:

Analyze....Regression....Linear....Dependent: bodysurface ....Independent: RBF_PredictedValue....OK.

The output sheets show that the r-value is 0.931, p<0.0001. The saved XML file will now be used to compute the body surface in six individual patients.

gender	age	weight	height
1,00	9,00	29,00	138,00
1,00	1,00	8,00	76,00
,00	15,00	42,00	165,00
1,00	15,00	40,00	151,00
1,00	1,00	9,00	80,00
1,00	7,00	22,00	123,00

gender
age (years)
weight (kg)
height (m)

Enter the above data in a new SPSS data file.

Command:

Utilities....click Scoring Wizard....click Browse....click Select....Folder: enter the exportradialbasisnn.xml file....click Select....in Scoring Wizard click Next....click Use value substitution....click Next....click Finish.

The underneath data file now gives the body surfaces computed by the neural network with the help of the XML file.

gender	age	weight	height	predicted body surface
1,00	9,00	29,00	138,00	9219,71
1,00	1,00	8,00	76,00	5307,81
,00	15,00	42,00	165,00	13520,13
1,00	15,00	40,00	151,00	13300,79
1,00	1,00	9,00	80,00	5170,13
1,00	7,00	22,00	123,00	8460,05

gender
age (years)
weight (kg)
height (m)
predicted body surface (cm^2)

Conclusion

Radial basis neural networks can be readily trained to provide accurate body surface values of individual patients.

Note

More background, theoretical and mathematical information of neural networks is available in Machine learning in medicine part one, Chaps. 12 and 13, entitled "Artificial intelligence, multilayer perceptron" and "Artificial intelligence, radial basis functions", pp 145–156 and 157–166, Springer Heidelberg Germany 2013, and in the Chap. 50 of the current book.

Chapter 64
Automatic Modeling of Drug Efficacy Prediction (250 Patients)

General Purpose

SPSS modeler is a work bench for automatic data mining (Chap. 61) and modeling (see also the Chap. 65). So far it is virtually unused in medicine, and mainly applied by econo-/sociometrics. Automatic modeling of continuous outcomes computes the ensembled result of a number of best fit models for a particular data set, and provides better sensitivity than the separate models do. This chapter is to demonstrate its performance with drug efficacy prediction.

Specific Scientific Question

The expression of a cluster of genes can be used as a functional unit to predict the efficacy of cytostatic treatment. Can ensembled modeling with three best fit statistical models provide better precision than the separate analysis with single statistical models does.

Example

A 250 patients' data file includes 28 variables consistent of patients' gene expression levels and their drug efficacy scores. Only the first 12 patients are shown underneath. The entire data file is in extras.springer.com, and is entitled "ensembledmodelcontinuous". All of the variables were standardized by scoring

---

This chapter was previously published in "Machine learning in medicine-cookbook 2" as Chap. 18, 2014.

T.J. Cleophas, A.H. Zwinderman, *Machine Learning in Medicine - a Complete Overview*, DOI 10.1007/978-3-319-15195-3_64

them on 11 points linear scales. The following genes were highly expressed: the genes 1–4, 16–19, and 24–27.

G1	G2	G3	G4	G16	G17	G18	G19	G24	G25	G26	G27	O
8,00	8,00	9,00	5,00	7,00	10,00	5,00	6,00	9,00	9,00	6,00	6,00	7,00
9,00	9,00	10,00	9,00	8,00	8,00	7,00	8,00	8,00	9,00	8,00	8,00	7,00
9,00	8,00	8,00	8,00	8,00	9,00	7,00	8,00	9,00	8,00	9,00	9,00	8,00
8,00	9,00	8,00	9,00	6,00	7,00	6,00	4,00	6,00	6,00	5,00	5,00	7,00
10,00	10,00	8,00	10,00	9,00	10,00	10,00	8,00	8,00	9,00	9,00	9,00	8,00
7,00	8,00	8,00	8,00	8,00	7,00	6,00	5,00	7,00	8,00	8,00	7,00	6,00
5,00	5,00	5,00	5,00	5,00	6,00	4,00	5,00	5,00	6,00	6,00	5,00	5,00
9,00	9,00	9,00	9,00	8,00	8,00	8,00	8,00	9,00	8,00	3,00	8,00	8,00
9,00	8,00	9,00	8,00	9,00	8,00	7,00	7,00	7,00	7,00	5,00	8,00	7,00
10,00	10,00	10,00	10,00	10,00	10,00	10,00	10,00	10,00	8,00	8,00	10,00	10,00
2,00	2,00	8,00	5,00	7,00	8,00	8,00	8,00	9,00	3,00	9,00	8,00	7,00
7,00	8,00	8,00	7,00	8,00	6,00	6,00	7,00	8,00	8,00	8,00	7,00	7,00

G gene (gene expression levels), *O* outcome (score)

Step 1 Open SPSS Modeler (14.2)

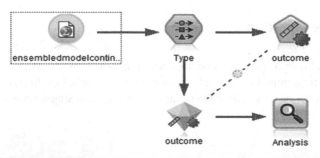

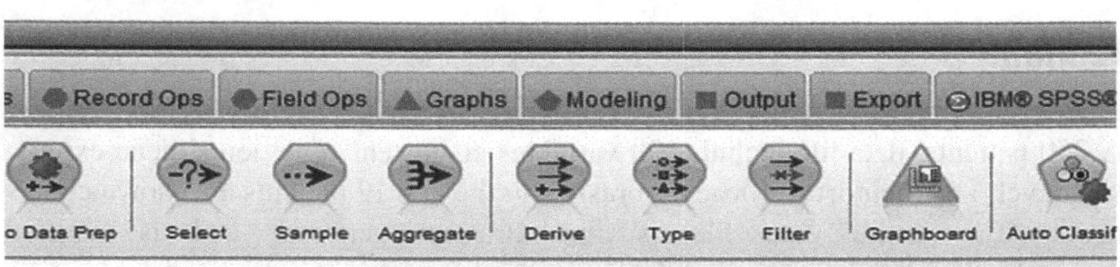

Step 2 The Statistics File Node

The canvas is, initially, blank, and above a screen view is of the final "completed ensemble" model, otherwise called stream of nodes, which we are going to build. First, in the palettes at the bottom of the screen full of nodes, look and find the **Statistics File node**, and drag it to the canvas. Double-click on it....Import file: browse and enter the file "ensembledmodelcontinuous" ....click OK. The graph below shows that the data file is open for analysis.

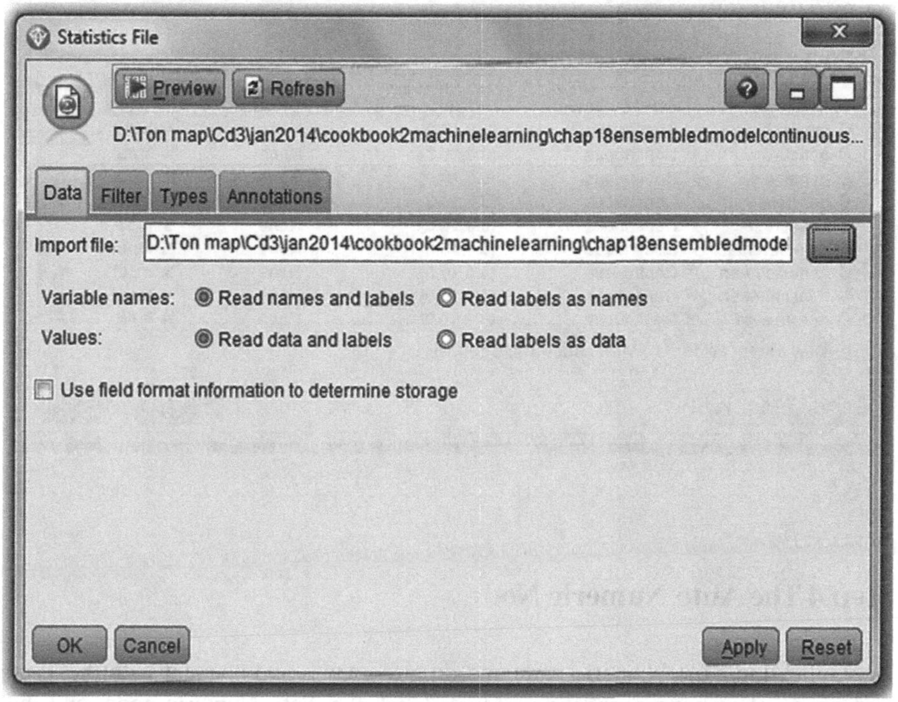

Step 3 The Type Node

In the palette at the bottom of screen find Type node and drag to the canvas....right-click on the Statistics File node....a Connect symbol comes up....click on the Type node....an arrow is displayed....double-click on the Type Node....after a second or two the underneath graph with information from the Type node is observed. Type nodes are used to access the properties of the variables (often called fields here) like type, role, unit etc. in the data file. As shown below, the variables are appropriately set: 14 predictor variables, 1 outcome (= target) variable, all of them continuous.

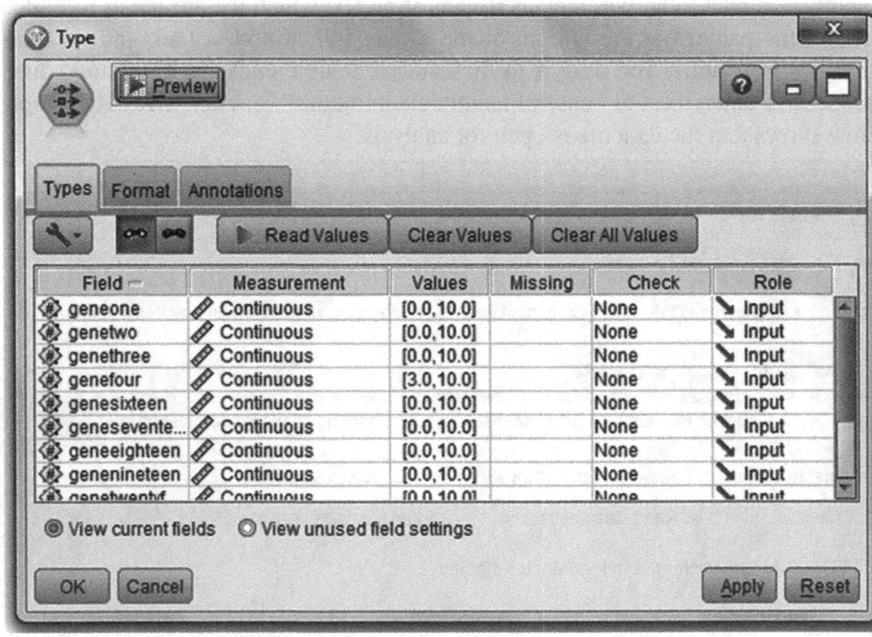

Step 4 The Auto Numeric Node

Now, click the Auto Numeric node and drag to canvas and connect with the Type node using the above connect-procedure. Click the Auto Numeric node, and the underneath graph comes up….now click Model….select Correlation as metric to rank quality of the various analysis methods used…. the additional manoeuvres are as indicated below….in Numbers of models to use: type the number 3.

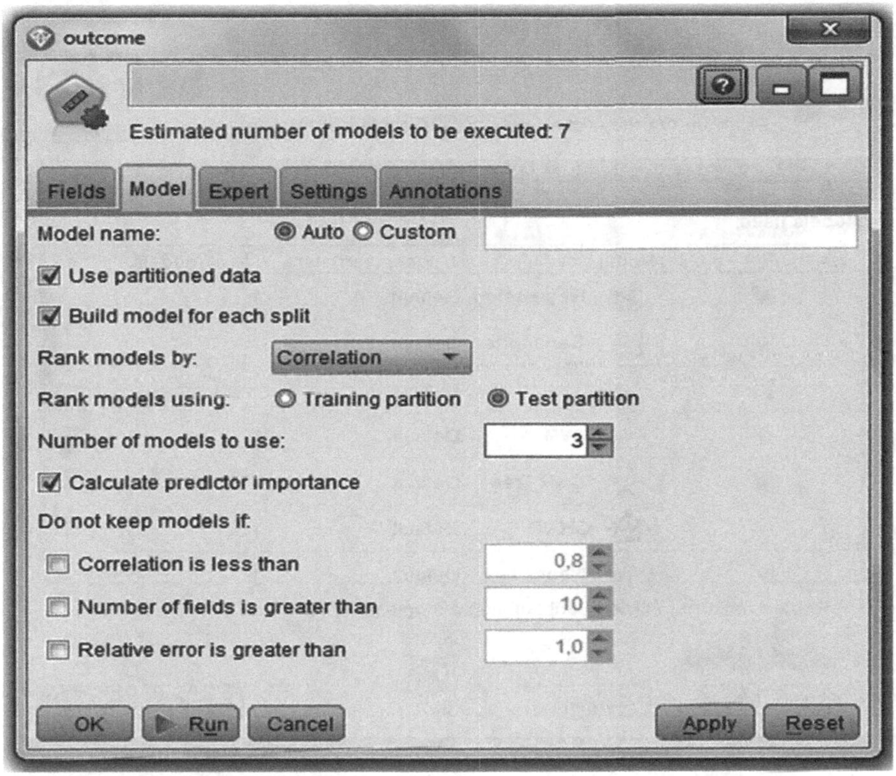

Step 5 The Expert Node

Then click the Expert tab. It is shown below. Out of seven statistical models the three best fit ones are used by SPSS modeler for the ensembled model.

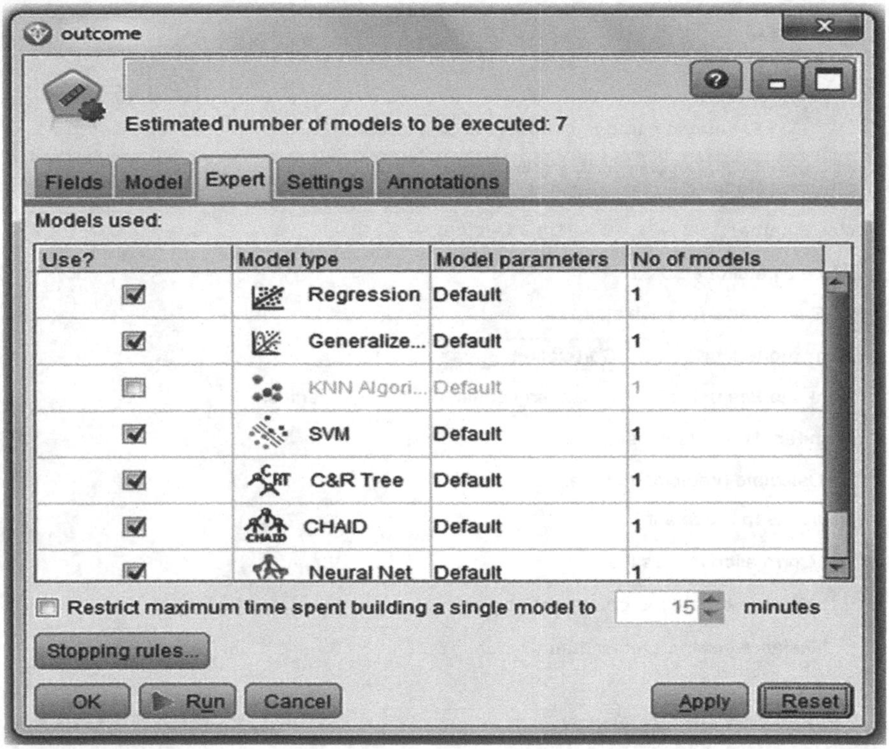

The seven statistical models include:

1. Linear regression (Regression)
2. Generalized linear model (Generalized….)
3. K nearest neighbor clustering (KNN Algorithm)
4. Support vector machine (SVM)
5. Classification and regression tree (C&R Tree)
6. Chi square automatic interaction detection (CHAID Tree)
7. Neural network (Neural Net)

More background information of the above methods are available at

1. SPSS for Starters Part One, Chap. 5, Linear regression, pp 15–18, Springer Heidelberg Germany 2010
2. The Chaps. 20 and 21 of current book.
3. Chapter 1 of current work.
4. Machine Learning in Medicine Part Two, Chap. 15, Support vector machines, pp 155–161, Springer Heidelberg Germany, 2013.
5. Chapter 53 of current book.
6. Machine Learning in Medicine Part Three, Chap. 14, Decision trees, pp 137–150, Springer Heidelberg Germany 2013.

7. Machine Learning in Medicine Part One, Chap. 12, Artificial intelligence, multilayer perceptron modeling, pp 145–154, Springer Heidelberg Germany 2013.

All of the seven above references are from the same authors as the current work.

Step 6 The Settings Tab

In the above graph click the Settings tab….click the Run button….now a gold nugget is placed on the canvas….click the gold nugget….the model created is shown below.

Use?	Graph	Model	Build Time (mins)	Correlation	No. Fields Used	Relative Error
☑		CHAID 1	<1	0,854	8	0,271
☑		SVM 1	<1	0,836	12	0,304
☑		Regressi...	<1	0,821	12	0,326

The correlation coefficients of the three best models are close to 0.8, and, thus, pretty good. We will now perform the ensembled procedure.

Step 7 The Analysis Node

Find in the palettes below the screen the Analysis node and drag it to the canvas. With the above connect procedure connect it with the gold nugget….click the Analysis node.

Comparing $XR-outcome with outcome

Minimum Error	-2,878
Maximum Error	3,863
Mean Error	-0,014
Mean Absolute Error	0,77
Standard Deviation	1,016
Linear Correlation	0,859
Occurrences	250

The above table is shown and gives the statistics of the ensembled model created. The ensembled outcome is the average score of the scores from the three best fit statistical models. Adjustment for multiple testing and for variance stabilization with Fisher transformation is automatically carried out. The ensembled outcome (named the $XR-outcome) is compared with the outcomes of the three best fit statistical models, namely, CHAID (chi square automatic interaction detector), SVM (support vector machine), and Regression (linear regression). The ensembled correlation coefficient is larger (0.859) than the correlation coefficients from the three best fit models (0.854, 0.836, 0.821), and so ensembled procedures make sense, because they can provide increased precision in the analysis. The ensembled model can now be stored as an SPSS Modeler Stream file for future use in the appropriate folder of your computer. For the readers' convenience it is in extras.springer.com, and it is entitled "ensembledmodelcontinuous".

Conclusion

In the example given in this chapter, the ensembled correlation coefficient is larger (0.859) than the correlation coefficients from the three best fit models (0.854, 0.836, 0.821), and, so, ensembled procedures do make sense, because they can provide increased precision in the analysis.

Note

SPSS modeler is a software program entirely distinct from SPSS statistical software, though it uses most if not all of the calculus methods of it. It is a standard software package particularly used by market analysts, but, as shown, can, perfectly, well be applied for exploratory purposes in medical research. It is also applied in the Chaps. 61 and 65.

Chapter 65
Automatic Modeling for Clinical Event Prediction (200 Patients)

General Purpose

SPSS modeler is a work bench for automatic data mining (Chap. 61) and modeling (see also the Chap. 64). So far it is virtually unused in medicine, and mainly applied by econo-/sociometrists. Automatic modeling of binary outcomes computes the ensembled result of a number of best fit models for a particular data set, and provides better sensitivity than the separate models do. This chapter is to demonstrate its performance with clinical event prediction.

Specific Scientific Question

Multiple laboratory values can predict events like health, death, morbidities etc. Can ensembled modeling with four best fit statistical models provide better precision than the separate analysis with single statistical models does.

Example

A 200 patients' data file includes 11 variables consistent of patients' laboratory values and their subsequent outcome (death or alive). Only the first 12 patients are shown underneath. The entire data file is in extras.springer.com, and is entitled "ensembledmodelbinary".

This chapter was previously published in "Machine learning in medicine-cookbook 2" as Chap. 19, 2014.

T.J. Cleophas, A.H. Zwinderman, *Machine Learning in Medicine - a Complete Overview*, DOI 10.1007/978-3-319-15195-3_65

Death	ggt	asat	alat	bili	ureum	creat	c-clear	esr	crp	leucos
,00	20,00	23,00	34,00	2,00	3,40	89,00	−111,00	2,00	2,00	5,00
,00	14,00	21,00	33,00	3,00	2,00	67,00	−112,00	7,00	3,00	6,00
,00	30,00	35,00	32,00	4,00	5,60	58,00	−116,00	8,00	4,00	4,00
,00	35,00	34,00	40,00	4,00	6,00	76,00	−110,00	6,00	5,00	7,00
,00	23,00	33,00	22,00	4,00	6,10	95,00	−120,00	9,00	6,00	6,00
,00	26,00	31,00	24,00	3,00	5,40	78,00	−132,00	8,00	4,00	8,00
,00	15,00	29,00	26,00	2,00	5,30	47,00	−120,00	12,00	5,00	5,00
,00	13,00	26,00	24,00	1,00	6,30	65,00	−132,00	13,00	6,00	6,00
,00	26,00	27,00	27,00	4,00	6,00	97,00	−112,00	14,00	6,00	7,00
,00	34,00	25,00	13,00	3,00	4,00	67,00	−125,00	15,00	7,00	6,00
,00	32,00	26,00	24,00	3,00	3,60	58,00	−110,00	13,00	8,00	6,00
,00	21,00	13,00	15,00	3,00	3,60	69,00	−102,00	12,00	2,00	4,00

death = death yes no (0 = no)
ggt = gamma glutamyl transferase (u/l)
asat = aspartate aminotransferase (u/l)
alat = alanine aminotransferase (u/l)
bili = bilirubine (micromol/l)
ureum = ureum (mmol/l)
creat = creatinine (mmicromol/l)
c-clear = creatinine clearance (ml/min)
esr = erythrocyte sedimentation rate (mm)
crp = c-reactive protein (mg/l)
leucos = leucocyte count ($.10^9$/l)

Step 1 Open SPSS Modeler (14.2)

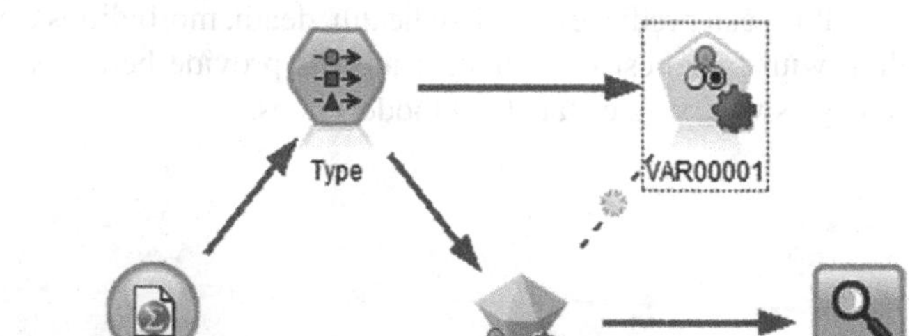

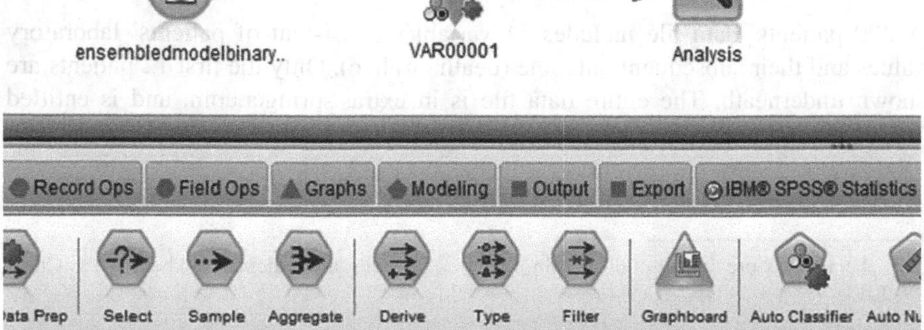

Step 2 The Statistics File Node

The canvas is, initially, blank, and above is given a screen view of the completed ensembled model, otherwise called stream of nodes, which we are going to build. First, in the palettes at the bottom of the screen full of nodes, look and find the **Statistics File node**, and drag it to the canvas, pressing the mouse left side. Double-click on this node….Import file: browse and enter the file "ensembledmodelbinary" ….click OK. The graph below shows, that the data file is open for analysis.

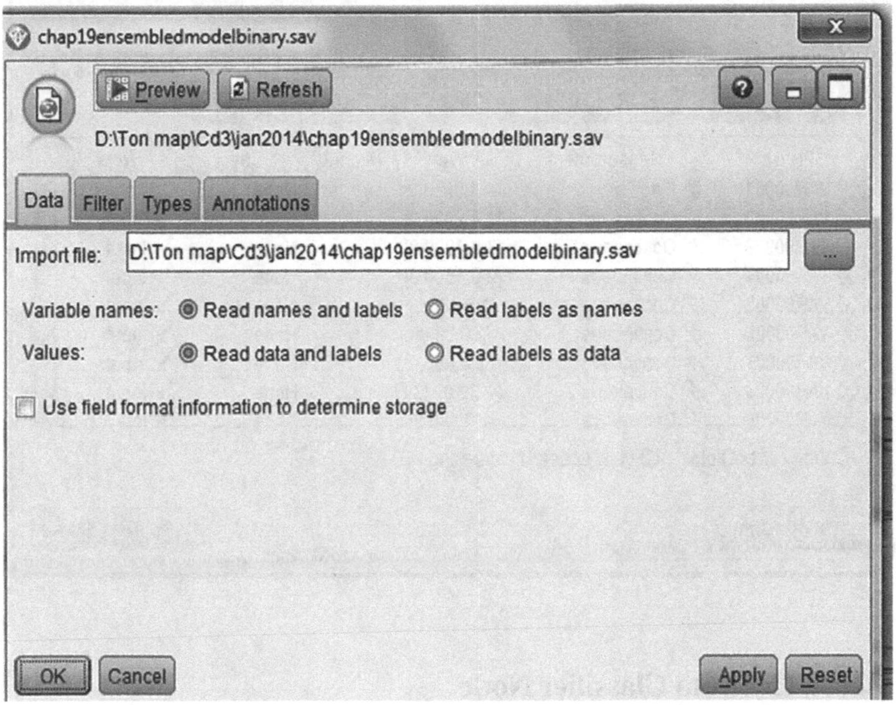

Step 3 The Type Node

In the palette at the bottom of screen find Type node and drag to the canvas….right-click on the Statistics File node….a Connect symbol comes up….click on the Type node….an arrow is displayed….double-click on the Type Node….after a second or two the underneath graph with information from the Type node is observed. Type nodes are used to access the properties of the variables (often called fields here) like type, role, unit etc. in the data file. As shown below, 10 predictor variables (all of them continuous) are appropriately set. However, VAR 00001 (death) is the outcome (= target) variable, and is binary. Click in the row of variable VAR00001 on the measurement column and replace "Continuous" with "Flag". Click Apply and OK. The underneath figure is removed and the canvas is displayed again.

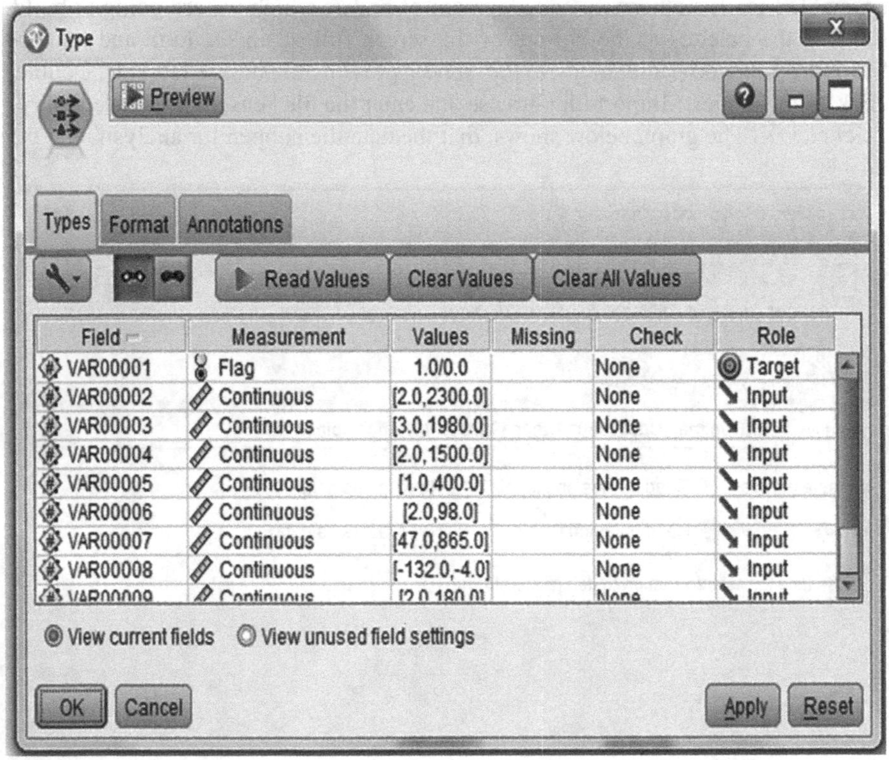

Step 4 The Auto Classifier Node

Now, click the Auto Classifier node and drag to the canvas, and connect with the Type node using the above connect-procedure. Click the Auto Classifier node, and the underneath graph comes up….now click Model….select Lift as Rank model of the various analysis models used…. the additional manoeuvres are as indicated below….in Numbers of models to use: type the number 4.

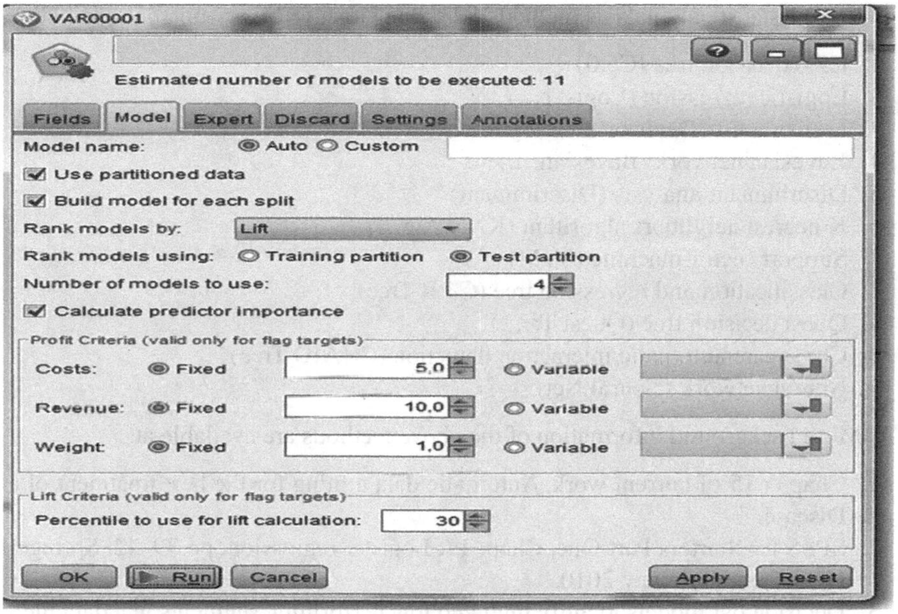

Step 5 The Expert Tab

Then click the Expert tab. It is shown below. Out of 11 statistical models the four best fit ones are selected by SPSS modeler for constructing an ensembled model.

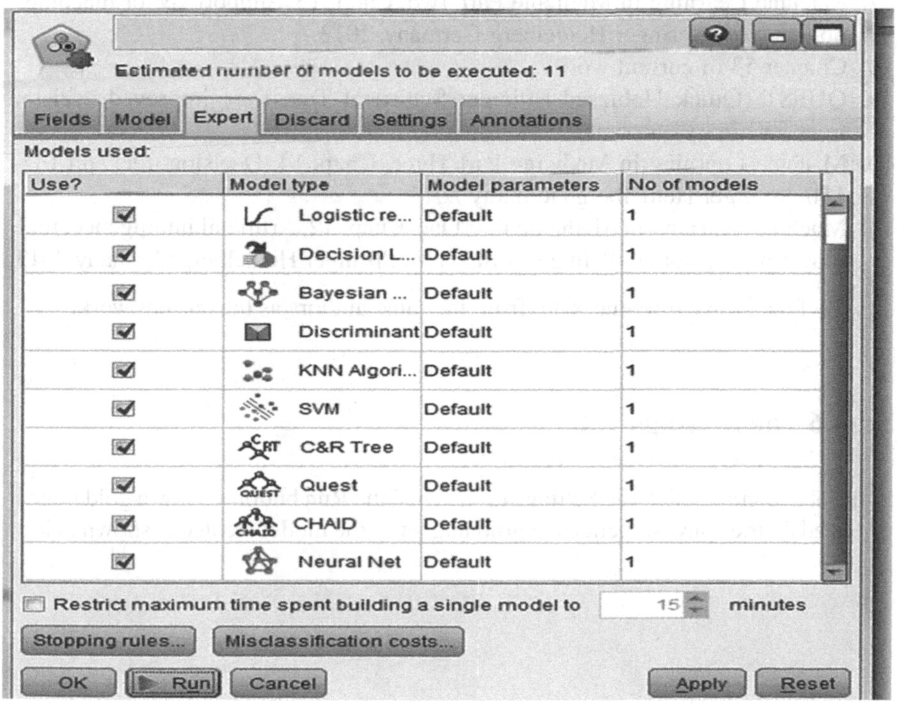

The 11 statistical analysis methods for a flag target (= binary outcome) include:

1. C5.0 decision tree (C5.0)
2. Logistic regression (Logist r…)
3. Decision list (Decision….)
4. Bayesian network (Bayesian….)
5. Discriminant analysis (Discriminant)
6. K nearest neighbors algorithm (KNN Alg…)
7. Support vector machine (SVM)
8. Classification and regression tree (C&R Tree)
9. Quest decision tree (Quest Tr….)
10. Chi square automatic interaction detection (CHAID Tree)
11. Neural network (Neural Net)

More background information of the above methods are available at.

1. Chapter 15 of current work, Automatic data mining for the best treatment of a Disease.
2. SPSS for Starters Part One, Chap. 11, Logistic regression, pp 39–42, Springer Heidelberg Germany 2010.
3. Decision list models identify high and low performing segments in a data file,
4. Machine Learning in Medicine Part Two, Chap. 16, Bayesian networks, pp 163–170, Springer Heidelberg Germany, 2013.
5. Machine Learning in Medicine Part One, Chap. 17, Discriminant analysis for supervised data, pp 215–224, Springer Heidelberg Germany 2013.
6. Chapter 4 of current work, Nearest neighbors for classifying new medicines.
7. Machine Learning in Medicine Part Two, Chap. 15, Support vector machines, pp 155–161, Springer Heidelberg Germany, 2013.
8. Chapter 53 of current work.
9. QUEST (Quick Unbiased Efficient Statistical Trees) are improved decision trees for binary outcomes.
10. Machine Learning in Medicine Part Three, Chap. 14, Decision trees, pp 137–150, Springer Heidelberg Germany 2013.
11. Machine Learning in Medicine Part One, Chap. 12, Artificial intelligence, multilayer perceptron modeling, pp 145–154, Springer Heidelberg Germany 2013.

All of the above references are from the same authors as the current work.

Step 6 The Settings Tab

In the above graph click the Settings tab….click the Run button….now a gold nugget is placed on the canvas….click the gold nugget….the model created is shown below.

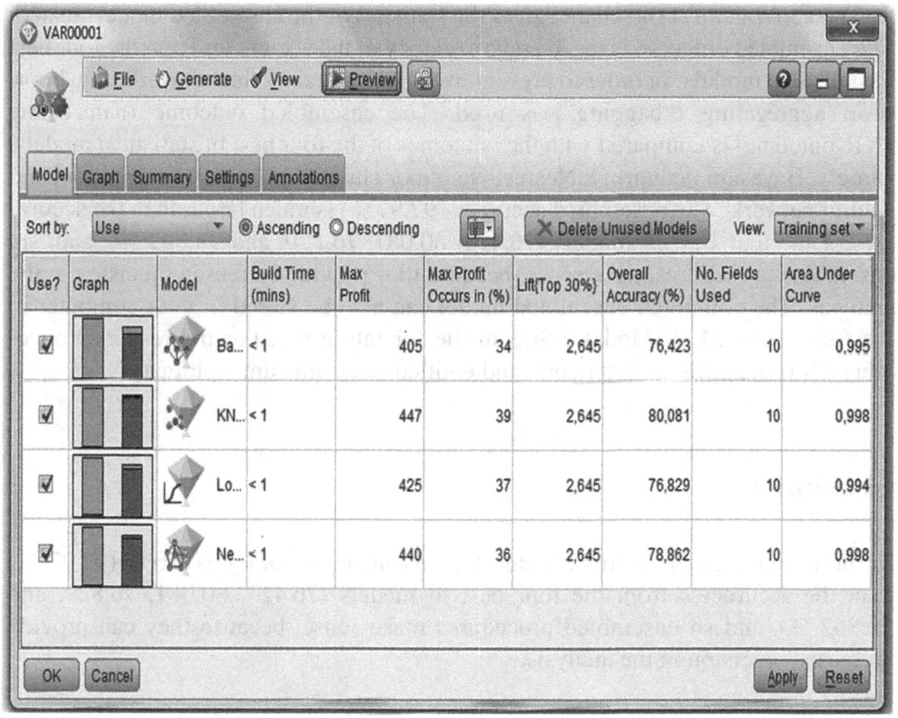

The overall accuracies (%) of the four best fit models are close to 0.8, and are, thus, pretty good. We will now perform the ensembled procedure.

Step 7 The Analysis Node

Find in the palettes at the bottom of the screen the Analysis node and drag it to the canvas. With above connect procedure connect it with the gold nugget….click the Analysis node.

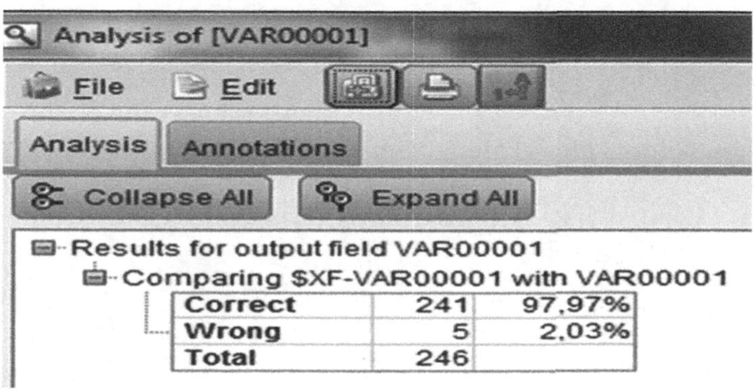

The above table is shown and gives the statistics of the ensembled model created. The ensembled outcome is the average accuracy of the accuracies from the four best fit statistical models. In order to prevent overstated certainty due to overfitting, bootstrap aggregating ("bagging") is used. The ensembled outcome (named the $XR-outcome) is compared with the outcomes of the four best fit statistical models, namely, Bayesian network, k Nearest Neighbor clustering, Logistic regression, and Neural network. The ensembled accuracy (97.97 %) is much larger than the accuracies of the four best fit models (76.423, 80,081, 76,829, and 78,862 %), and, so, ensembled procedures make sense, because they provide increased precision in the analysis. The computed ensembled model can now be stored in your computer in the form of an SPSS Modeler Stream file for future use. For the readers' convenience it is in extras.springer.com, and entitled "ensembledmodelbinary".

Conclusion

In the example given in this chapter, the ensembled accuracy is larger (97,97 %) than the accuracies from the four best fit models (76.423, 80,081, 76,829, and 78,862 %), and so ensembled procedures make sense, because they can provide increased precision in the analysis.

Note

SPSS modeler is a software program entirely distinct from SPSS statistical software, though it uses most if not all of the calculus methods of it. It is a standard software package particularly used by market analysts, but, as shown, can perfectly well be applied for exploratory purposes in medical research. It is also applied in the Chaps. 61 and 64.

Chapter 66
Automatic Newton Modeling in Clinical Pharmacology (15 Alfentanil Dosages, 15 Quinidine Time-Concentration Relationships)

General Purpose

Traditional regression analysis selects a mathematical function, and, then, uses the data to find the best fit parameters. For example, the parameters a and b for a linear regression function with the equation $y = a + bx$ have to be calculated according to

$$b = \text{regression coefficient} = \frac{\sum (x-\bar{x})(y-\bar{y})}{\sum (x-\bar{x})^2}$$

$$a = \text{intercept} = \bar{y} - b\bar{x}$$

With a quadratic function, $y = a + b_1x + b_2x^2$ (and other functions) the calculations are similar, but more complex. Newton's method works differently. Instead of selecting a mathematical function and using the data for finding the best fit parameter-values, it uses arbitrary parameter-values for a, b_1, b_2, and, then, iteratively measures the distance between the data and the modeled curve until the shortest distance is obtained. Calculations are much more easy than those of traditional regression analysis, making the method, particularly, interesting for comparing multiple functions to one data set. Newton's method is mainly used for computer solutions of engineering problems, but is little used in clinical research. This chapter is to assess whether it is also suitable for the latter purpose.

This chapter was previously published in "Machine learning in medicine-cookbook 2" as Chap. 20, 2014.

T.J. Cleophas, A.H. Zwinderman, *Machine Learning in Medicine - a Complete Overview*, DOI 10.1007/978-3-319-15195-3_66

Specific Scientific Question

Can Newton's methods provide appropriate mathematical functions for dose-effectiveness and time-concentration studies?

Examples

Dose-Effectiveness Study

Alfentanil dose x-axis mg/m^2	effectiveness y-axis [1- pain scale]
0,10	0,1701
0,20	0,2009
0,30	0,2709
0,40	0,2648
0,50	0,3013
0,60	0,4278
0,70	0,3466
0,80	0,2663
0,90	0,3201
1,00	0,4140
1,10	0,3677
1,20	0,3476
1,30	0,3656
1,40	0,3879
1,50	0,3649

The above table gives the data of a dose-effectiveness study. Newton's algorithm is performed. We will apply the online Nonlinear Regression Calculator of Xuru's website. This website is made available by Xuru, the world largest business network based in Auckland CA, USA. We simply copy or paste the data of the above table into the spreadsheet given be the website, then click "allow comma as decimal separator" and click "calculate". Alternatively the SPSS file available at extras.springer.com entitled "newtonmethod" can be opened if SPSS is installed in your computer and the copy and paste commands are similarly given.

Since Newton's method can be applied to (almost) any function, most computer programs fit a given dataset to over 100 functions including Gaussians, sigmoids, ratios, sinusoids etc. For the data given 18 significantly ($P<0.05$) fitting non-linear functions were found, the first six of them are shown underneath.

	Non-linear function	residual sum of squares	P value
1.	$y=0.42x/(x+0.17)$	0.023	0.003
2.	$y=-1/(38.4x+1)^{0.12}+1$	0.024	0.003
3.	$y=0.08 \ln x+0.36$	0.025	0.004
4.	$y=0.40e^{-0.11/x}$	0.025	0.004
5.	$y=0.36x^{0.26}$	0.027	0.004
6.	$y=-0.024/x+0.37$	0.029	0.005

The first one gives the best fit. Its measure of certainty, given as residual sum of squares, is 0.023. It is the function of a hyperbola:

$$y = 0.42x / (x + 0.17).$$

This is convenient, because, dose-effectiveness curves are, often, successfully assessed with hyperbolas mimicking the Michaelis-Menten equation. The parameters of the equation can be readily interpreted as $\text{effectiveness}_{\text{maximum}}=0.42$, and dissociation constant$=0.17$. It is usually very laborious to obtain these parameters from traditional regression modeling of the quantal effect histograms and cumulative histograms requiring data samples of at least 100 or so to be meaningful. The underneath figure shows an Excel graph of the fitted non-linear function for the data, using Newton's method (the best fit curve is here a hyperbola). A cubic spline goes smoothly through every point, and does this by ensuring that the first and second derivatives of the segments match those that are adjacent.

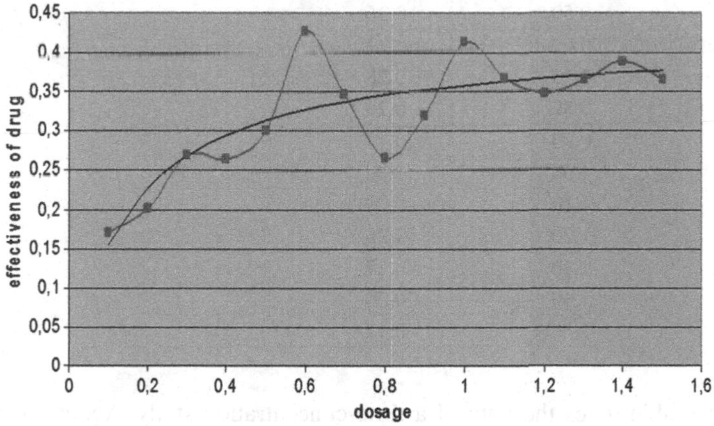

The Newton's equation better fits the data than traditional modeling with linear, logistic, quadratic, and polynomial modeling does as shown underneath.

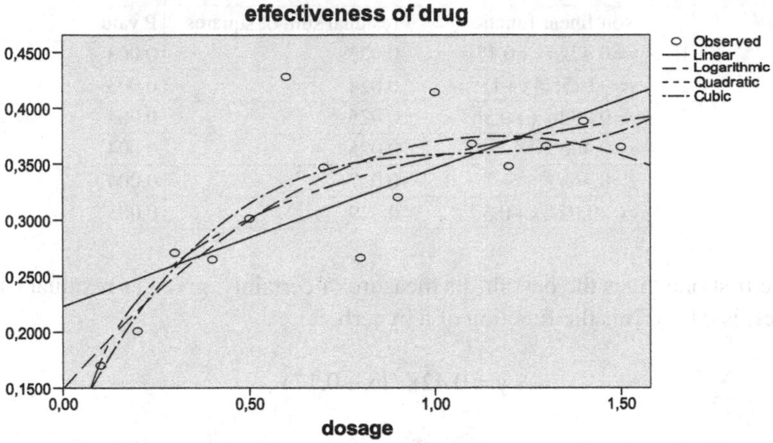

Time-Concentration Study

Time x-axis hours	quinidine concentration μg/ml
0,10	0,41
0,20	0,38
0,30	0,36
0,40	0,34
0,50	0,36
0,60	0,23
0,70	0,28
0,80	0,26
0,90	0,17
1,00	0,30
1,10	0,30
1,20	0,26
1,30	0,27
1,40	0,20
1,50	0,17

The above table gives the data of a time-concentration study. Again a non-linear regression using Newton's algorithm is performed. We use the online Nonlinear Regression Calculator of Xuru's website. We copy or paste the data of the above table into the spreadsheet, then click "allow comma as decimal separator" and click "calculate". Alternatively the SPSS file available at extras.springer.com entitled "newtonmethod" can be opened if SPSS is installed in your computer and the copy and paste commands are similarly given. For the data given 10 statistically significantly ($P<0.05$) fitting non-linear functions were found and shown. For further assessment of the data an exponential function, which is among the first five shown by the software, is chosen, because relevant pharmacokinetic parameters can be conveniently calculated from it:

$$y = 0.41e^{-0.48x}.$$

This function's measure of uncertainty (residual sums of squares) value is 0.027, (with a p-value of 0.003). The following pharmacokinetic parameters are derived:

$$0.41 = C_0 = (\text{administration dosage drug}) / (\text{distribution volume})$$
$$-0.48 = \text{elimination constant}.$$

Below an Excel graph of the exponential function fitted to the data is given. Also, a cubic spline curve going smoothly through every point and to be considered as a perfect fit curve is again given. It can be observed from the figure that the exponential function curve matches the cubic spline curve well.

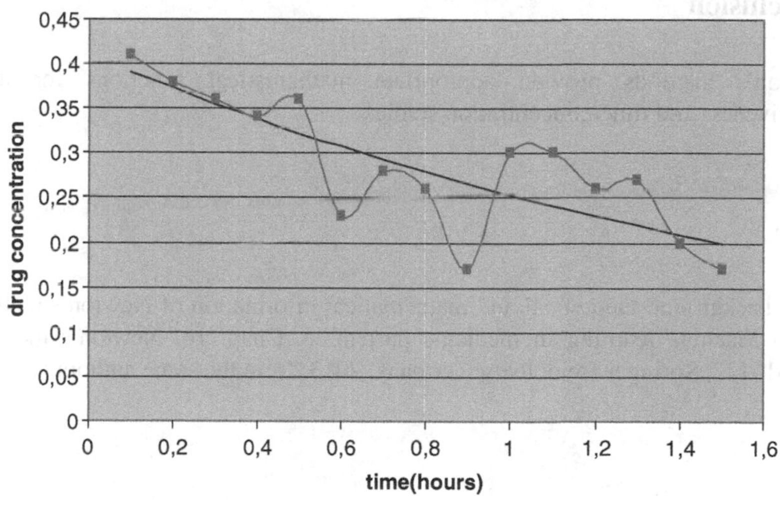

The Newton's equation fits the data approximately equally well as do traditional best fit models with linear, logistic, quadratic, and polynomial modeling shown underneath. However, traditional models do not allow for the computation of pharmacokinetic parameters.

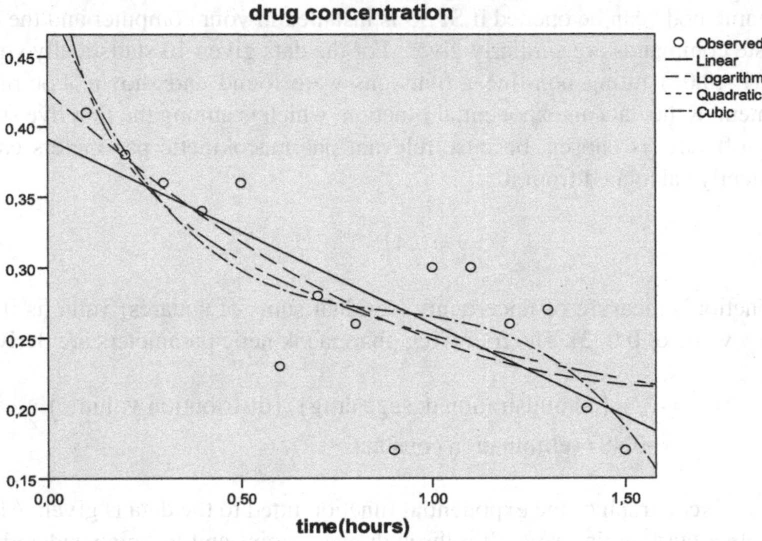

Conclusion

Newton's methods provide appropriate mathematical functions for dose-effectiveness and time-concentration studies.

Note

More background theoretical and mathematical information of Newton's methods are in Machine learning in medicine part three, Chap. 16, Newton's methods, pp 161–172, Springer Heidelberg Germany, 2013, from the same authors.

Chapter 67
Spectral Plots for High Sensitivity Assessment of Periodicity (6 Years' Monthly C Reactive Protein Levels)

General Purpose

In clinical research times series often show many peaks and irregular spaces.

Spectral plots is based on traditional Fourier analyses, and may be more sensitive than traditional autocorrelation analysis in this situation.

Specific Scientific Question

To assess whether, in monthly C reactive Protein (CRP) levels with inconclusive scattergrams and autocorrelation analysis, spectral plot methodology is able to demonstrate periodicity even so.

Example

A data file of 6 years' mean monthly CRP levels from a target population was assessed for seasonality. The first 2 years' values are given underneath. The entire data file is in "spectralanalysis" as available on the internet at extras.springer.com.

First day of month	CRP level (mg/l)
1993/07/01	1.29
1993/08/01	1.43
1993/09/01	1.54

(continued)

This chapter was previously published in "Machine learning in medicine-cookbook 3" as Chap. 9, 2014.

T.J. Cleophas, A.H. Zwinderman, *Machine Learning in Medicine - a Complete Overview*, DOI 10.1007/978-3-319-15195-3_67

First day of month	CRP level (mg/l)
1993/10/01	1.68
1993/11/01	1.54
1993/12/01	2.78
1994/01/01	1.27
1994/02/01	1.26
1994/03/01	1.26
1994/04/01	1.54
1994/05/01	1.13
1994/06/01	1.60
1994/07/01	1.47
1994/08/01	1.78
1994/09/01	2.69
1994/10/01	1.91
1994/11/01	1.74
1994/12/01	3.11

Start by opening the data file in SPSS.

Command:

Click Graphs….click Legacy Dialogs….click Scatter/Dot…. Click Simple Scatter…..click Define….y-axis: enter "mean crp mg/l"….x-axis: enter date…. click OK.

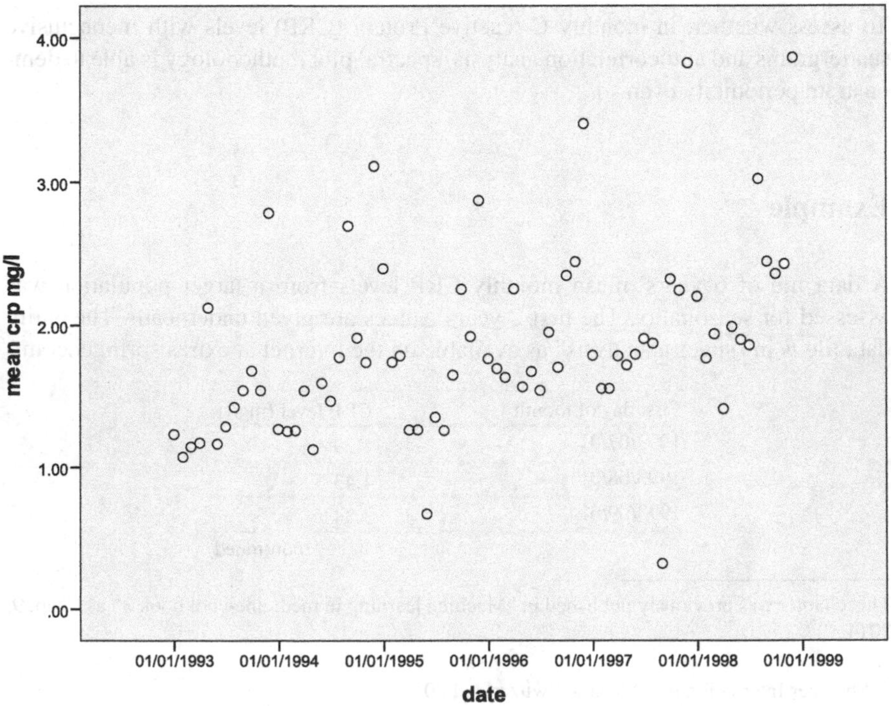

In the output the above figure is displayed. Many peaks and irregularities are observed, and the presence of periodicity is not unequivocal.

Subsequently, autocorrelation coefficients are computed.

Command:

click Analyze....click Forecast....click Autocorrelations....Variables: enter "mean crp mg/l"....click OK.

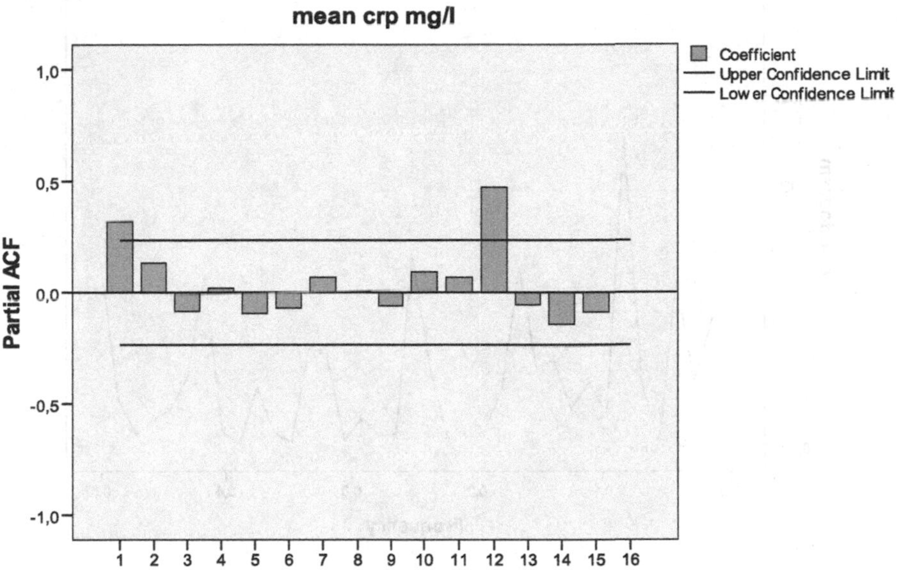

In the output the above autocorrelation coefficients are given. It suggests the presence of periodicity. However, this conclusion is based on a single value, i.e., the 12th month value, and, for concluding unequivocal periodicity not only autocorrelation coefficients significantly larger than 0 but also significantly smaller than 0 should have been observed.

Spectral plots may be helpful for support.

Command:

Analyze....Forecasting....Spectral Analysis....select CRP and enter into Variable(s)....select Spectral density in Plot....click Paste....change in syntax text: TSET PRINT-DEFAULT into TSET PRINT-DETAILED.... click Run....click All.

In the output sheets underneath the *periodogram* is observed (upper part) with mean CRP values on the y-axis and frequencies on the x-axis. Of the peaks CRP-values observed the first one has a frequency of slightly less than 0.1. We assumed that CRP had an annual periodicity. Twelve months are in a year, months is the unit applied. As period is the inverted value of frequency a period of 12 months would equal a frequency of 1/12=0.0833. An annual periodicity would produce a peak CRP-value with a frequency of 1/12=0.0833. Indeed, the table underneath shows that at a frequency of 0.0833 the highest CRP value is observed. However, many more peaks are observed, and how to interpret them. For that purpose we use *spectral density analysis* (lower figure underneath).

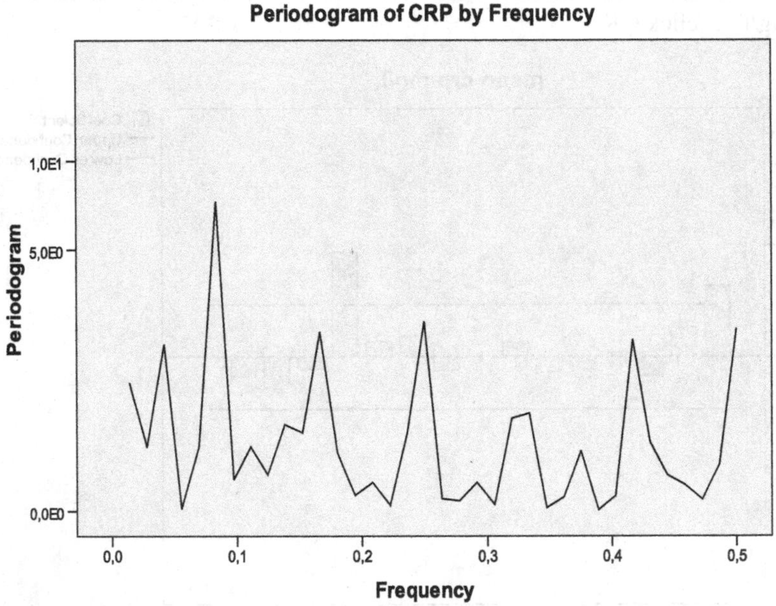

Univariate statistics						
Series name:mean crp mg/l						
	Frequency	Period	Sine transform	Cosine transform	Periodogram	Spectral density estimate
1	,00000		,000	1,852	,000	8,767
2	,01389		–,197	,020	1,416	12,285
3	,02778		–,123	,012	,552	9,223
4	,04167		–,231	,078	2,144	10,429
5	,05556		,019	,010	,016	23,564
6	,06944		–,040	–,117	,552	22,985
7	,08333		–,365	,267	7,355	19,519
8	,09722		–,057	–,060	,243	20,068
9	,11111		–,101	–,072	,556	20,505
10	,12500		–,004	–,089	,286	5,815
11	,13889		,065	–,135	,811	10,653
12	,15278		–,024	,139	,715	10,559

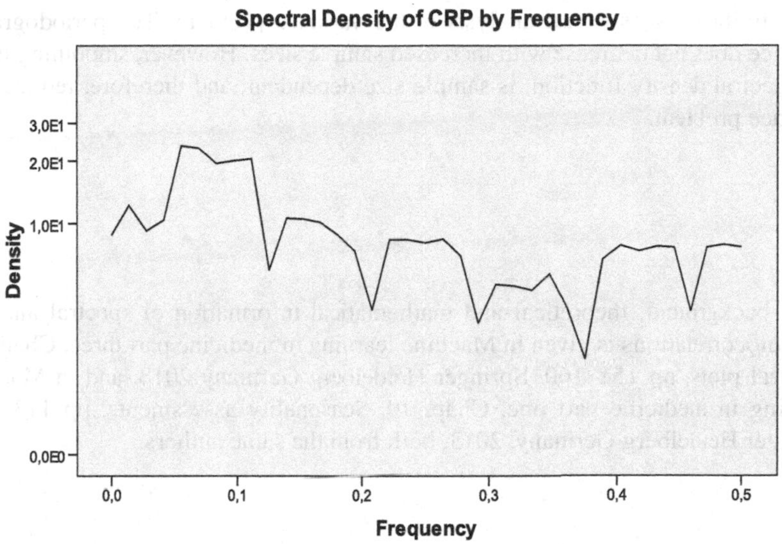

The spectral density curve is a filtered, otherwise called smoothed, version of the usual periodogram with irregularities beyond a given threshold (noise) filtered out. The above spectral density curve shows five distinct peaks with a rather regular pattern. The lowest frequency simply displays the yearly peak at a frequency of 0.0833. The other peaks at higher frequencies are the result of the Fourier model consistent of sine and cosine functions, and do not indicate additional periodicities. Even so much so that they demonstrate the absence of further periodicities.

Conclusion

Seasonal patterns are assumed in many fields of medicine. Usually, the mean differences between the data of different seasons or months are used. E.g., the number of hospital admissions in the month of January may be roughly twice that of July. However, biological processes are full of variations and the possibility of chance findings can not be fully ruled out. Autocorrelations can be adequately used for the purpose. It is a technique that cuts time curves into pieces. These pieces are, subsequently, compared with the original data-curve using linear regression analysis. Autocorrelation coefficients significantly larger and smaller than 0 must be observed in order to conclude periodicity. If not, spectral analysis is often helpful.

It displays a peak outcome at the frequency of the expected periodicity (months, years, weeks etc.). The current chapter shows that spectral analysis can be adequately used with very irregular patterns and inconclusive autocorrelation analysis, and is able to demonstrate unequivocal periodicities where visual methods like scatter-grams and traditional methods like autocorrelations are inconclusive.

A limitation of spectral analysis is the variance problem. The periodogram's variance does not decrease with increased sample sizes. However, smoothing using the spectral density function, is sample size dependent, and therefore, reduces the variance problem.

Note

More background, theoretical and mathematical information of spectral analysis and autocorrelations is given in Machine learning in medicine part three, Chap. 15, Spectral plots, pp 151–160, Springer Heidelberg Germany 2013, and in Machine learning in medicine part one, Chap. 10, Seasonality assessments, pp 113–126, Springer Heidelberg Germany, 2013, both from the same authors.

Chapter 68
Runs Test for Identifying Best Regression Models (21 Estimates of Quantity and Quality of Patient Care)

General Purpose

R-square values are often used to test the appropriateness of diagnostic models.

However, in practice, pretty large r-square values (squared correlation coefficients) may be observed even if data do not fit the model very well. This chapter assesses whether the runs test is a better alternative to the traditional r-square test for addressing the differences between the data and the best fit regression models.

Primary Scientific Question

A real data example was given comparing quantity of care with quality of care scores.

Example

Doctors were assessed for the relationship between their quantity and quality of care. The quantity of care was estimated with the numbers of daily interventions like endoscopies and small operations per doctor, the quality of care with quality of care scores. The data file is given below, and is also available in "runstest" on the internet at extras.springer.com.

This chapter was previously published in "Machine learning in medicine-cookbook 3" as Chap. 10, 2014.

T.J. Cleophas, A.H. Zwinderman, *Machine Learning in Medicine - a Complete Overview*, DOI 10.1007/978-3-319-15195-3_68

Quantity of care	Quality of care
19,00	2,00
20,00	3,00
23,00	4,00
24,00	5,00
26,00	6,00
27,00	7,00
28,00	8,00
29,00	9,00
29,00	10,00
29,00	11,00
28,00	12,00
27,00	13,00
27,00	14,00
26,00	15,00
25,00	16,00
24,00	17,00
23,00	18,00
22,00	19,00
22,00	20,00
21,00	21,00
21,00	22,00

Quantity of care = numbers of daily interventions per doctor; Quality of care = quality of care scores

The relationship seemed not to be linear, and curvilinear regression in SPSS was used to find the best fit curve to describe the data and eventually use them as prediction model. First, we will make a graph of the data.

Command:

Analyze....Graphs....Chart builder....click: Scatter/Dot....Click quality of care and drag to the Y-Axis....Click Intervention per doctor and drag to the X-Axis.... OK.

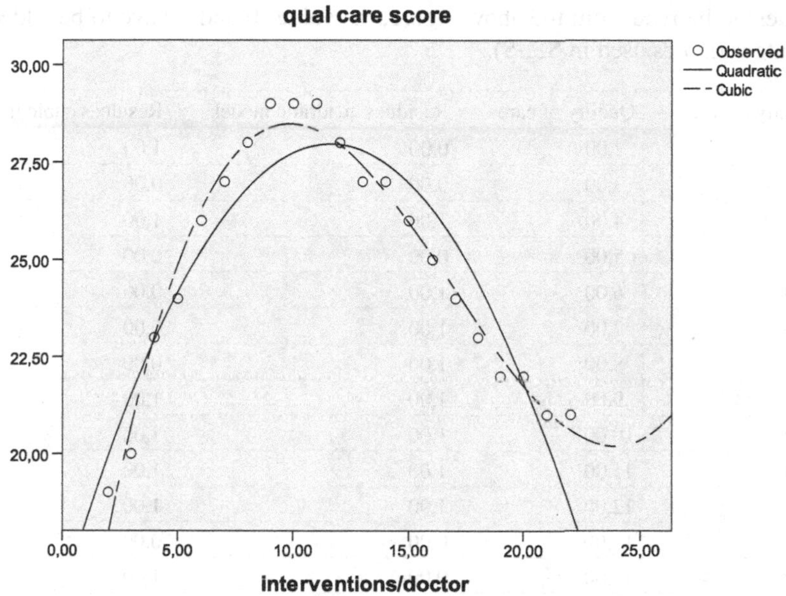

The above figure shows the scattergram of the data. A non-linear relationship is indeed suggested, and the curvilinear regression option in SPSS was helpful to find the best fit model.

Command:

Analyze....Regression....Curve Estimation....mark: Quadratic, Cubic....mark: Display ANOVA Table....OK.

The quadratic (best fit second order, parabolic, relationship) and cubic (best fit third order, hyperbolic, relationship) were the best options, with very good r-squares and p-values < 0.0001 as shown in the table given by the software.

Model summary and parameter estimates

Dependent variable:qual care score

	Model summary					Parameter estimates			
Equation	R square	F	df1	df2	Sig.	Constant	b1	b2	b3
Quadratic	,866	58,321	2	18	,000	16,259	2,017	–,087	
Cubic	,977	236,005	3	17	,000	10,679	4,195	–,301	,006

The independent variable is interventions/doctor

The runs test requires the residues from respectively the best fit quadratic and the cubic models of the data (instead of – and + distances from the modeled curves (the residues) to be read from the above figure, the values 0 and 1 have to be added as separate variables used in SPSS).

Quantity of care	Quality of care	Residues quadratic model	Residues cubic model
19,00	2,00	0,00	1,00
20,00	3,00	0,00	0,00
23,00	4,00	1,00	1,00
24,00	5,00	0,00	0,00
26,00	6,00	1,00	0,00
27,00	7,00	1,00	0,00
28,00	8,00	1,00	0,00
29,00	9,00	1,00	1,00
29,00	10,00	1,00	1,00
29,00	11,00	1,00	1,00
28,00	12,00	1,00	1,00
27,00	13,00	0,00	0,00
27,00	14,00	0,00	1,00
26,00	15,00	0,00	1,00
25,00	16,00	0,00	0,00
24,00	17,00	0,00	0,00
23,00	18,00	0,00	0,00
22,00	19,00	0,00	0,00
22,00	20,00	1,00	1,00
21,00	21,00	1,00	0,00
21,00	22,00	1,00	1,00

Command:

Analyze....Nonparametric tests....Runs Test....move the runsquadratic model residues variable to Test Variable List....click Options....click Descriptives....click Continue....click Cut Point....mark Median....click OK.

The output table shows that in the runs test the quadratic model differs from the actual data with p=0.02. It means that the quadratic model is systematically different from the data.

Runs test	
	Runsquadraticmodel
Test value[a]	1,00
Cases < test value	10
Cases >= test value	11
Total cases	21
Number of runs	6
Z	−2,234

(continued)

Runs test	
	Runsquadraticmodel
Asymp. sig. (2-tailed)	,026
Exact sig. (2-tailed)	,022
Point probability	,009

[a]Median

When the similar procedure is followed for the best fit cubic model, the result is very insignificant with a p-value of 1.00. The cubic model was, thus, a much better predicting model for the data than the quadratic model.

Runs test 2	
	Runscubicmodel
Test value[a]	,4762
Cases<test value	11
Cases>= test value	10
Total cases	21
Number of runs	11
Z	,000
Asymp. sig. (2-tailed)	1,000
Exact sig. (2-tailed)	1,000
Point probability	,165

[a]Mean

Conclusion

The runs test is appropriate both for testing whether fitted theoretical curves are systematically different or not from a given data set. The fit of regression models is traditionally assessed with r-square tests. However, the runs test is more appropriate for the purpose, because large r-square value do not exclude poor systematic data fit, and because the runs test assesses the entire pattern in the data, rather than mean distances between data and model.

Note

More background, theoretical and mathematical information of the runs test is given in Machine learning in medicine part three, Chap. 13, Runs test, pp 127–135, Springer Heidelberg Germany 2013, from the same authors.

Chapter 69
Evolutionary Operations for Process Improvement (8 Operation Room Air Condition Settings)

General Purpose

Evolutionary operations (evops) try and find improved processes by exploring the effect of small changes in an experimental setting. It stems from evolutionary algorithms (see Machine learning in medicine part three, Chap. 2, Evolutionary operations, pp 11–18, Springer Heidelberg Germany, 2013, from the same authors), which uses rules based on biological evolution mechanisms where each next generation is slightly different and generally somewhat improved as compared to its ancestors. It is widely used not only in genetic research, but also in chemical and technical processes. So much so that the internet nowadays offers free evop calculators suitable not only for the optimization of the above processes, but also for the optimization of your pet's food, your car costs, and many other daily life standard issues. This chapter is to assess how evops can be helpful to optimize the air quality of operation rooms.

Specific Scientific Question

The air quality of operation rooms is important for infection prevention. Particularly, the factors (1) humidity (30–60 %), (2) filter capacity (70–90 %), and (3) air volume change (20–30 % per hour) are supposed to be important determinants. Can an evolutionary operation be used for process improvement.

This chapter was previously published in "Machine learning in medicine-cookbook 3" as Chap. 11, 2014.

T.J. Cleophas, A.H. Zwinderman, *Machine Learning in Medicine - a Complete Overview*, DOI 10.1007/978-3-319-15195-3_69

Example

Eight operation room air condition settings were investigated, and the results are underneath.

Operation Setting	humidity (30 % = 1, 60 % = 4)	filter capacity (70 % = 1, 90 % = 3)	air volume change (20 % = 1, 30 % = 3)	infections number of
1	1	1	1	99
2	2	1	1	90
3	1	2	1	75
4	2	2	1	73
5	1	1	2	99
6	2	1	2	99
7	1	2	2	61
8	2	2	2	52

We will use multiple linear regression in SPSS with the number of infections as outcome and the three factors as predictors to identify the significant predictors.

First, the data file available as "evops" in extras.springer.com is opened in SPSS.

Command:

Analyze….Regression….Linear….Dependent: enter "Var00004"…. Independent(s): enter "Var00001-00003"….click OK.

The underneath table in the output shows that all of the determinants are statistically significant at $p < 0.10$. A higher humidity, filtering level, and air volume change better prevents infections.

Coefficients[a]

Model		Unstandardized coefficients		Standardized coefficients		
		B	Std. error	Beta	t	Sig.
1	(Constant)	103,250	18,243		5,660	,005
	Humidity1	−12,250	3,649	−,408	−3,357	,028
	Filter capacity1	−21,250	3,649	−,707	−5,824	,004
	Air volume change1	15,750	3,649	,524	4,317	,012

[a]Dependent Variable: infections1

In the next eight operation settings higher determinant levels were assessed.

Operation Setting	humidity (30 % = 1, 60 % = 4)	filter capacity (70 % = 1, 90 % = 3)	air volume change (20 % = 1, 30 % = 3)	infections number of
1	3	2	2	51
2	4	2	2	45

(continued)

Operation Setting	humidity (30 %=1, 60 %=4)	filter capacity (70 %=1, 90 %=3)	air volume change (20 %=1, 30 %=3)	infections number of
3	3	3	2	33
4	4	3	2	26
5	3	2	3	73
6	4	2	3	60
7	3	3	3	54
8	4	3	3	31

We will use again multiple linear regression in SPSS with the number of infections as outcome and the three factors as predictors to identify the significant predictors.

Command:

Analyze....Regression....Linear....Dependent: enter "Var00008".... Independent(s): enter "Var00005-00007"....click OK.

Coefficients[a]

Model		Unstandardized coefficients		Standardized coefficients		
		B	Std. error	Beta	t	Sig.
1	(Constant)	145,500	15,512		9,380	,001
	Humidity2	−5,000	5,863	−,145	−,853	,442
	Filter capacity2	−31,500	5,863	−,910	−5,373	,006
	Air volume change2	−6,500	5,863	−,188	−1,109	,330

[a]Dependent Variable: infections2

The underneath table in the output shows that only Var 00006 (the filter capacity) is still statistically significant. Filter capacity 3 performs better than 2, while humidity levels and air volume changes were not significantly different. We could go one step further to find out how higher levels would perform, but for now we will conclude that humidity level 2–4, filter capacity level 3, and air flow change level 2–4 are efficacious level combinations. Higher levels of humidity and air flow change is not meaningful. An additional benefit of a higher level of filter capacity cannot be excluded, but requires additional testing.

Conclusion

Evolutionary operations can be used to improve the process of air quality maintenance in operation rooms. This methodology can similarly be applied for finding the best settings for numerous clinical, and laboratory settings. We have to add that interaction between the predictors was not taken into account in the current example. For a meaningful assessment of 2- and 3-factor interactions larger samples would be required, however. Moreover, we have clinical arguments that no important interactions are to be expected.

Note

More background, theoretical and mathematical information of evops is given in Machine learning in medicine part three, Chap. 2, Evolutionary operations, pp 11–18, Springer Heidelberg Germany, 2013, from the same authors.

Chapter 70
Bayesian Networks for Cause Effect Modeling (600 Patients)

General Purpose

Bayesian networks are probabilistic graphical models using nodes and arrows, respectively representing variables, and probabilistic dependencies between two variables. Computations in a Bayesian network are performed using weighted likelihood methodology and marginalization, meaning that irrelevant variables are integrated or summed out. Additional theoretical information is given in Machine Learning in medicine part two, Chap. 16, Bayesian networks, pp 163–170, Springer Heidelberg Germany, 2013 (from the same authors). This chapter is to assess if Bayesian networks is able to determine direct and indirect predictors of binary outcomes like morbidity/mortality outcomes.

Primary Scientific Question

Longevity is multifactorial, and logistic regression is adequate to assess the chance of longevity in patients with various predictor scores like physical, psychological, and family scores. However, some factors may have both direct and indirect effects. Can a best fit Bayesian network demonstrate not only direct but also indirect effects of factors on the outcome?

This chapter was previously published in "Machine learning in medicine-cookbook 3" as Chap. 12, 2014.

T.J. Cleophas, A.H. Zwinderman, *Machine Learning in Medicine - a Complete Overview*, DOI 10.1007/978-3-319-15195-3_70

Example

In 600 patients, 70 years of age, a score sampling of factors predicting longevity was performed. The outcome was death after 10 years of follow-up. The first 12 patients are underneath, the entire data file is in "longevity", and is available at extras.springer.com. We will first perform a logistic regression of these data using SPSS statistical software. Start by opening SPSS. Enter the above data file.

Variables					
1	2	3	4	5	6
death	econ	psychol	physic	family	educ
0	70	117	76	77	120
0	70	68	76	56	114
0	70	74	71	57	109
0	90	114	82	79	125
0	90	117	100	68	123
0	70	74	100	57	121
1	70	77	103	62	145
0	70	62	71	56	100
0	90	86	88	65	114
0	90	77	88	61	111
0	110	56	65	59	130
0	70	68	50	60	118

death (0 = no)
econ = economy score
psychol = psychological score
physic = physical score
family = familial risk score of longevity
educ = educational score

Binary Logistic Regression in SPSS

Command:

Analyze....Regression....Binary Logistic....Dependent: enter "death"....Covariates: enter "econ, psychol, physical, family, educ"....OK.

The underneath output table shows the results. With $p < 0.10$ as cut-off for statistical significance, all of the covariates, except economical score, were significant predictors of longevity (death), although both negative and positive b-values were observed.

Variables in the equation							
		B	S.E.	Wald	df	Sig.	Exp(B)
Step 1[a]	ecom	,003	,006	,306	1	,580	1,003
	psychol	–,056	,009	43,047	1	,000	,946
	physical	–,019	,007	8,589	1	,003	,981
	family	,045	,017	7,297	1	,007	1,046
	educ	,017	,009	3,593	1	,058	1,018
	Constant	–,563	,922	,373	1	,541	,569

[a]Variable(s) entered on step 1: ecom, psychol, physical, family, educ

For these data we hypothesized that all of these scores would independently affect longevity. However, indirect effects were not taken into account, like the effect of psychological on physical scores, and the effect of family on educational scores etc. In order to assess both direct and indirect effects, a Bayesian network DAG (directed acyclic graph) was fitted to the data. The Konstanz information miner (Knime) was used for the analysis. In order to enter the SPSS data file in Knime, an excel version of the data file is required. For that purpose open the file in SPSS and follow the commands.

Command in SPSS:

click File....click Save as....in "Save as" type: enter Comma Delimited (*.csv).... click Save.

For convenience the excel file has been added to extras.springer.com, and is, just like the SPSS file, entitled "longevity".

Konstanz Information Miner (Knime)

In Google enter the term "knime". Click Download and follow instructions. After completing the pretty easy download procedure, open the knime workbench by clicking the knime welcome screen. The center of the screen displays the workflow editor like the canvas in SPSS modeler. It is empty, and can be used to build a stream of nodes, called workflow in knime. The node repository is in the left lower angle of the screen, and the nodes can be dragged to the workflow editor simply by left-clicking. The nodes are computer tools for data analysis like visualization and statistical processes. Node description is in the right upper angle of the screen. Before the nodes can be used, they have to be connected with the file reader and with one another by arrows drawn again simply by left clicking the small triangles attached to the nodes. Right clicking on the file reader enables to configure from your computer a requested data file....click Browse....and download from the appropriate folder a csv type Excel file. You are almost set for analysis now, but in order to perform a Bayesian analysis Weka software 3.6 for windows (statistical software from the University of Waikato (New Zealand)) is required. Simply type the term Weka software, and find the site. The software can be freely downloaded from the internet, following a few simple instructions, and it can, subsequently, be readily opened in Knime. Once it has been opened, it is stored in your Knime node repository, and you will be able to routinely use it.

Knime Workflow

A knime workflow for the analysis of the above data example is built, and the final result is shown in the underneath figure, by dragging and connecting as explained above.

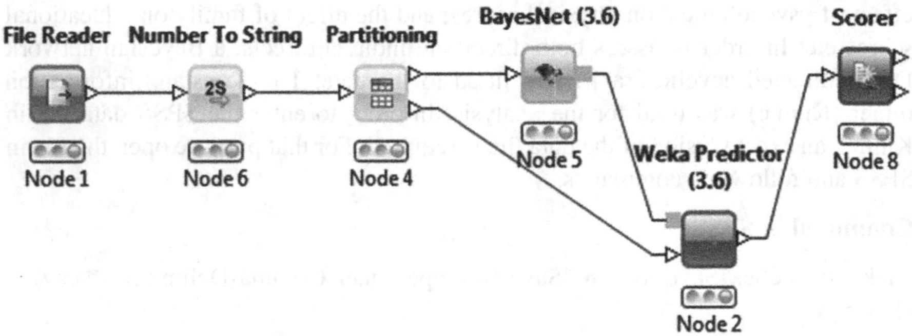

In the node repository click and type File Reader and drag to workflow editor in the node repository click again File reader....click the ESCbutton of your computer....in the node repository click again and type Number to String....the node is displayed....drag it to the workflow editor....perform the same kind of actions for all of the nodes as shown in the above figure....connect, by left clicking, all of the nodes with arrows as indicated above....click File Reader....click Browse....and type the requested data file ("longevity.csv")....click OK....the data file is given....right click all of the nodes and then right click Configurate and execute all of the nodes by right clicking the nodes and then the texts "Configurate" and "Execute"....the red lights will successively turn orange and then green....right click the Weka Predictor node.... right click the Weka Node View....right click Graph.

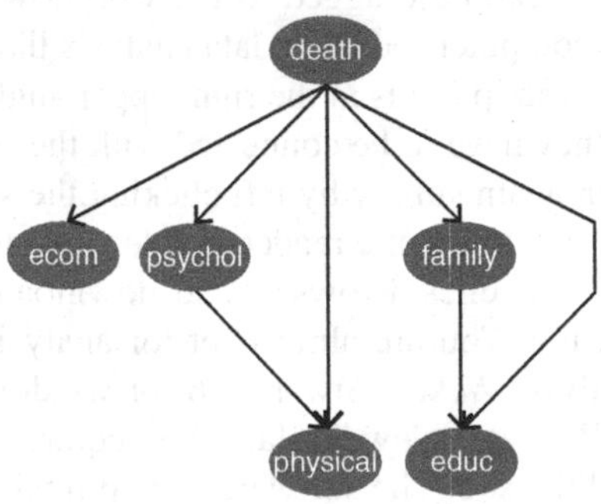

The above graph, a socalled directed acyclic graph (DAG) shows the Bayesian network obtained from the analysis. This best fitting DAG was, obviously, more complex than expected from the logistic model. Longevity was directly determined by all of the five predictors, but additional indirect effects were between physical and psychological scores, and between educational and family scores. In order to assess the validity of the Bayesian model, a confusion matrix and accuracy statistics were computed.

Right click the Scorer node....right click Confusion matrix

Confusion matrix

Table "spec_name" - Rows: 2 | Spec - Columns: 2 | Properties | Flow Variables

Row ID	0	1
0	295	70
1	91	44

The observed and predicted values are summarized. Subsequently, right click Accuracy statistics.

Accuracy statistics

Row ID	TruePo...	FalsePo...	TrueNe...	FalseN...	Recall	Precision	Sensitivity	Specifity
0	295	91	44	70	0.808	0.764	0.808	0.326
1	44	70	295	91	0.326	0.386	0.326	0.808
Overall	?	?	?	?	?	?	?	?

The sensitivity of the Bayesian model to predict longevity was pretty good, 80.8 %. However, the specificity was pretty bad. "No deaths" were rightly predicted in 80.8 % of the patients, "deaths", however, were rightly predicted in only 32.6 % of the patients.

Conclusion

Bayesian networks are probabilistic graphical models for assessing cause effect relationships. This chapter is to assess if Bayesian networks is able to determine direct and indirect predictors of binary outcomes like morbidity/mortality outcomes. As an example a longevity study is used. Longevity is multifactorial, and logistic regression is adequate to assess the chance of longevity in patients with various predictor scores like physical, psychological, and family scores. However, factors may have both direct and indirect effects. A best fit Bayesian network demonstrated not only direct but also indirect effects of the factors on the outcome.

Note

More background, theoretical and mathematical information of Bayesian networks is in Machine learning in medicine part two, Chap. 16, Bayesian networks, pp 163–170, Springer Heidelberg Germany, 2013, from the same authors.

Chapter 71
Support Vector Machines for Imperfect Nonlinear Data (200 Patients with Sepsis)

General Purpose

The basic aim of support vector machines is to construct the best fit separation line (or with three dimensional data separation plane), separating cases and controls as good as possible. Discriminant analysis, classification trees, and neural networks (see Machine Learning in medicine part one, Chap. 17, Discriminant analysis for supervised data, pp 215–224, Chap. 13, Artificial intelligence, Chaps. 12 and 13, pp 145–165, 2013, and Machine Learning in medicine part three, Chap. 14, Decision trees, pp 137–150, 2013, Springer Heidelberg Germany, by the same authors as the current chapter) are alternative methods for the purpose, but support vector machines are generally more stable and sensitive, although heuristic studies to indicate when they perform better are missing. Support vector machines are also often used in automatic modeling that computes the ensembled results of several best fit models (see the Chaps. 64 and 65).

This chapter uses the Konstanz information miner (Knime), a free data mining software package developed at the University of Konstanz, and also used in the chaps. 7 and 8.

Primary Scientific Question

Is support vector machines adequate to classify cases and controls in a cohort of admitted because of sepsis?

This chapter was previously published in "Machine learning in medicine-cookbook 3" as Chap. 13, 2014.

T.J. Cleophas, A.H. Zwinderman, *Machine Learning in Medicine - a Complete Overview*, DOI 10.1007/978-3-319-15195-3_71

Example

Two hundred patients were admitted because of sepsis. The laboratory values and the outcome death or alive were registered. We wish to use support vector machines to predict from the laboratory values the outcome, death or alive, including information on the error rate. The data of the first 12 patients are underneath. The entire data file is in extras.springer.com. Konstanz information miner (Knime) does not use SPSS files, and, so, the file has to be transformed into a csv excel file (click Save As....in "Save as" type: replace SPSS Statistics(*sav) with SPSS Statistics(*csv)). For convenience the csv file is in extras.springer.com and is entitled "svm".

Death 1=yes	Ggt	asat	alat	bili	ureum	creat	c-clear	esr	crp	leucos
var1	var2	var3	var4	var5	var6	var7	var8	var9	Var10	var11
0	20	23	34	2	3,4	89	−111	2	2	5
0	14	21	33	3	2	67	−112	7	3	6
0	30	35	32	4	5,6	58	−116	8	4	4
0	35	34	40	4	6	76	−110	6	5	7
0	23	33	22	4	6,1	95	−120	9	6	6
0	26	31	24	3	5,4	78	−132	8	4	8
0	15	29	26	2	5,3	47	−120	12	5	5
0	13	26	24	1	6,3	65	−132	13	6	6
0	26	27	27	4	6	97	−112	14	6	7
0	34	25	13	3	4	67	−125	15	7	6
0	32	26	24	3	3,6	58	−110	13	8	6
0	21	13	15	3	3,6	69	−102	12	2	4

Var 1 death 1=yes
Var 2 gammagt (Var=variable) (U/l)
Var 3 asat (U/l)
Var 4 alat (U/l)
Var 5 bili (mumol/l)
Var 6 ureum (mmol/l)
Var 7 creatinine (mumol/l)
Var 8 creatinine clearance (ml/min)
Var 9 esr (erythrocyte sedimentation rate) (mm)
Var 10 c-reactive protein (mg/l)
Var 11 leucos ($\times 10^9$/l)

Knime Data Miner

In Google enter the term "knime". Click Download and follow instructions. After completing the pretty easy download procedure, open the knime workbench by clicking the knime welcome screen. The center of the screen displays the workflow editor like the canvas in SPSS modeler. It is empty, and can be used to build a stream of nodes, called workflow in knime. The node repository is in the left lower angle of the screen, and the nodes can be dragged to the workflow editor simply by left-clicking. The nodes are computer tools for data analysis like visualization and statistical processes. Node description is in the right upper angle of the screen. Before the nodes can be used they have to be connected with the file reader and with one another by arrows drawn again simply by left clicking the small triangles attached to the nodes. Right clicking on the file reader enables to configure from your computer a requested data file.

Knime Workflow

A knime workflow for the analysis of thc above data example will be built, and the final result is shown in the underneath figure

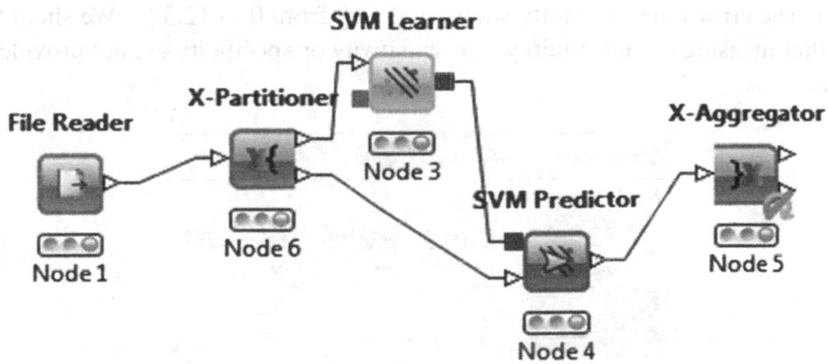

File Reader Node

In the node repository find the node File Reader. Drag the node to the workflow editor by left clicking....click Browse....and download from extras.springer.com the csv type Excel file entitled "svm". You are set for analysis now. By left clicking the node the file is displayed. The File Reader has chosen Var 0006 (ureum) as S variable (dependent). However, we wish to replace it with Var 0001 (death yes = 1).... click the column header of Var 0006....mark "Don't include column in output".... click OK....in the column header of Var 0001 leave unmarked "Don't include column in output" click OK.

The outcome variable is now rightly the Var 0001 and is indicated with S, the Var 0006 has obtained the term "SKIP" between brackets.

The Nodes X-Partitioner, svm Learner, svm Predictor, X-Aggregator

Find the above nodes in the node repository and drag them to the workflow editor and connect them with one another according to the above figure. Configurate and execute all them by right clicking the nodes and the texts "Configurate" and "Execute". The red lights under the nodes get, subsequently, yellow and, then, green. The miner has accomplished its task.

Error Rates

Right click the X-Aggregator node once more, and then right click Error rates. The underneath table is shown. The svm model is used to make predictions about death or not from the other variables of your file. Nine random samples of 25 patients are shown. The error rates are pretty small, and vary from 0 to 12.5 %. We should add that other measures of uncertainty like sensitivity or specificity are not provided by knime.

Error rates - 0:5 - X-Aggregator

File

Table "default" - Rows: 10 | Spec - Columns: 3 | Properties | Flow Variables

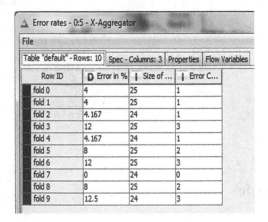

Row ID	D Error in %	I Size of ...	I Error C...
fold 0	4	25	1
fold 1	4	25	1
fold 2	4.167	24	1
fold 3	12	25	3
fold 4	4.167	24	1
fold 5	8	25	2
fold 6	12	25	3
fold 7	0	24	0
fold 8	8	25	2
fold 9	12.5	24	3

Prediction Table

Right click the x-aggregator node once more, and then right click Prediction Table. The underneath table is shown. The svm model is used to make predictions about death or not from the other variables of your file.

The left column gives the outcome values (death yes = 1), the right one gives the predicted values. It can be observed that the two results very well match one another.

Prediction table - 0:5 - X-Aggregator

File

Table "default" - Rows: 246 | Spec - Columns: 11 | Properties | Flow Variables

Row ID	S i>¿VAR...	I VAR00...	I VAR00...	I VAR00...	I VAR00...	I VAR00...	I VAR00...	I VAR00...	I VAR00...	I VAR00...	S Predicti...
Row4	0	23	33	22	4	95	-120	9	6	6	0
Row6	0	15	29	26	2	47	-120	12	5	5	0
Row9	0	34	25	13	3	67	-125	15	7	6	0
Row14	0	19	16	9	4	80	-113	8	4	7	0
Row18	0	24	24	27	4	84	-120	15	6	6	0
Row36	0	19	236	15	2	78	-113	7	6	6	0
Row42	0	27	17	27	4	98	-101	14	4	3	0
Row47	0	15	17	15	2	89	-112	13	9	6	0
Row62	0	16	14	19	4	67	-102	14	7	2	0
Row64	0	14	14	27	2	76	-109	18	5	5	0
Row66	0	16	27	29	3	77	-102	14	4	6	0
Row67	0	24	25	24	2	69	-110	16	5	7	0
Row68	0	21	29	25	4	78	-112	15	7	4	0
Row73	0	21	15	13	2	92	-120	17	7	4	0
Row114	1	900	759	856	287	532	-8	109	103	23	1
Row144	1	376	459	389	135	267	-29	97	33	20	1
Row151	1	169	154	267	75	244	-50	42	21	15	1
Row155	1	175	250	276	95	231	-41	36	28	15	1
Row170	1	276	230	156	79	235	-54	34	23	15	1
Row181	1	75	84	145	39	137	-66	28	18	14	1

Conclusion

The basic aim of support vector machines is to construct the best fit separation line (or with three dimensional data separation plane), separating cases and controls as good as possible. This chapter uses the Konstanz information miner, a free data mining software package developed at the University of Konstanz, and also used in the chaps. 1 and 2. The example shows that support vector machines is adequate to predict the presence of a disease or not in a cohort of patients at risk of a disease.

Note

More background, theoretical and mathematical information of support vector machines is given in Machine in medicine part two, Chap. 14, Support vector machines, pp 155–162, Springer Heidelberg Germany, from the same authors.

Chapter 72
Multiple Response Sets for Visualizing Clinical Data Trends (811 Patient Visits)

General Purpose

Multiple response methodology answers multiple qualitative questions about a single group of patients, and uses for the purpose summary tables. The method visualizes trends and similarities in the data, but no statistical test is given.

Specific Scientific Question

Can multiple response sets better than traditional frequency tables demonstrate results that could be selected for formal trend tests.

Example

An 811 person health questionnaire addressed the reasons for visiting general practitioners (gps) in 1 month. Nine qualitative questions addressed various aspects of health as primary reasons for visits. SPSS statistical software was used to analyze the data.

This chapter was previously published in "Machine learning in medicine-cookbook 3" as Chap. 14, 2014.

T.J. Cleophas, A.H. Zwinderman, *Machine Learning in Medicine - a Complete Overview*, DOI 10.1007/978-3-319-15195-3_72

ill	alcohol	weight	tired	cold	family	mental	physical	social	no
0	0	1	1	0	0	0	0	1	0
1	1	1	1	1	1	1	1	1	0
0	0	0	0	0	0	0	0	0	1
1	0	0	1	0	0	0	0	0	0
1	0	0	0	1	1	1	1	0	0
0	0	0	0	0	1	1	1	0	0
0	0	0	0	0	0	0	0	0	1
1	1	0	1	1	1	1	1	1	0
0	0	0	0	0	0	1	0	0	0
1	1	0	1	0	1	1	1	1	0
0	0	0	0	0	0	0	0	0	1
0	0	0	0	0	1	1	1	0	0
1	1	0	1	1	1	0	1	1	0
1	0	0	0	1	0	1	0	0	0
1	0	0	1	0	0	0	1	1	0

ill = ill feeling
alcohol = alcohol abuse
weight = weight problems
tired + tiredness
cold = common cold
family = family problem
mental = mental problem
physical = physical problem
social = social problem
no = no answer

The first 15 patient data are given. The entire data file is entitled "multipleresponse", and can be downloaded from extras.springer.com. SPSS statistical software is used for analysis. We will start by the descriptive statistics.

Command:

Descriptive Statistics….Frequencies….Variables: enter the variables between "illfeeling" to "no answer"….click Statistics….click Sum….click Continue….click OK.

The output is in the underneath 10 tables. It is pretty hard to observe trends across the tables. Also redundant information as given is not helpful for overall conclusion about the relationships between the different questions.

Illfeeling

		Frequency	Percent	Valid percent	Cumulative percent
Valid	No	420	43,3	51,8	51,8
	Yes	391	40,3	48,2	100,0
	Total	811	83,6	100,0	
Missing	System	159	16,4		
Total		970	100,0		

Alcohol					
		Frequency	Percent	Valid percent	Cumulative percent
Valid	No	569	58,7	70,2	70,2
	Yes	242	24,9	29,8	100,0
	Total	811	83,6	100,0	
Missing	System	159	16,4		
Total		970	100,0		

Weight problem					
		Frequency	Percent	Valid percent	Cumulative percent
Valid	No	597	61,5	73,6	73,6
	Yes	214	22,1	26,4	100,0
	Total	811	83,6	100,0	
Missing	System	159	16,4		
Total		970	100,0		

Tiredness					
		Frequency	Percent	Valid percent	Cumulative percent
Valid	No	511	52,7	63,0	63,0
	Yes	300	30,9	37,0	100,0
	Total	811	83,6	100,0	
Missing	System	159	16,4		
Total		970	100,0		

Cold					
		Frequency	Percent	Valid percent	Cumulative percent
Valid	No	422	43,5	52,0	52,0
	Yes	389	40,1	48,0	100,0
	Total	811	83,6	100,0	
Missing	System	159	16,4		
Total		970	100,0		

Family problem					
		Frequency	Percent	Valid percent	Cumulative percent
Valid	No	416	42,9	51,3	51,3
	Yes	395	40,7	48,7	100,0
	Total	811	83,6	100,0	
Missing	System	159	16,4		
Total		970	100,0		

Mental problem					
		Frequency	Percent	Valid percent	Cumulative percent
Valid	No	410	42,3	50,6	50,6
	Yes	401	41,3	49,4	100,0
	Total	811	83,6	100,0	
Missing	System	159	16,4		
Total		970	100,0		

Physical problem					
		Frequency	Percent	Valid percent	Cumulative percent
Valid	No	402	41,4	49,6	49,6
	Yes	409	42,2	50,4	100,0
	Total	811	83,6	100,0	
Missing	System	159	16,4		
Total		970	100,0		

Social problem					
		Frequency	Percent	Valid percent	Cumulative percent
Valid	No	518	53,4	63,9	63,9
	Yes	293	30,2	36,1	100,0
	Total	811	83,6	100,0	
Missing	System	159	16,4		
Total		970	100,0		

No answer					
		Frequency	Percent	Valid percent	Cumulative percent
Valid	,00	722	74,4	89,0	89,0
	1,00	89	9,2	11,0	100,0
	Total	811	83,6	100,0	
Missing	System	159	16,4		
Total		970	100,0		

In order to find out more about trends in de data a multiple response analysis will be performed next.

Command:

Analyze….Multiple Response….Define Variable Sets….move "ill feeling, alcohol, tiredness, cold, family problem, mental problem, physical problem, social problem" from Set Definition to Variables in Set….Counted Values enter 1….Name enter "health"….Label enter "health"….Multiple Response Set: click Add….click Close….click Analyze….Multiple Response….click Frequencies….move $health from Multiple Response Sets to Table(s)….click OK.

The underneath Case Summary table show that of all visitants 25.6 % did not answer any question, here called the missing cases.

Case summary						
	Cases					
	Valid		Missing		Total	
	N	Percent	N	Percent	N	Percent
$health[a]	722	74,4 %	248	25,6 %	970	100,0 %

[a]Dichotomy group tabulated at value 1

$health frequencies		Responses		
		N	Percent	Percent of cases
Health[a]	Illfeeling	391	12,9 %	54,2 %
	Alcohol	242	8,0 %	33,5 %
	Weight problem	214	7,1 %	29,6 %
	Tiredness	300	9,9 %	41,6 %
	Cold	389	12,8 %	53,9 %
	Family problem	395	13,0 %	54,7 %
	Mental problem	401	13,2 %	55,5 %
	Physical problem	409	13,5 %	56,6 %
	Social problem	293	9,7 %	40,6 %
Total		3,034	100,0 %	420,2 %

[a]Dichotomy group tabulated at value 1

The letter N gives the numbers of yes-answers per question, "Percent of Cases" gives the yes-answers per question in those who answered at least once (missing data not taken into account), and Percent gives the percentages of these yes-answers per question

The above output shows the number of patients who answered yes to at least one question. Of all visitants 25.6 % did not answer any question, here called the missing cases. In the second table the letter N gives the numbers of yes-answers per question, "Percent of Cases" gives the yes-answers per question in those who answered at least once (missing data not taken into account), and "Percent" gives the percentages of these yes-answers per question. The gp consultation burden of mental and physical problems was about twice the size of that of alcohol and weight problems. Tiredness and social problems were in-between. In order to assess these data against all visitants, the missing cases have to be analyzed first.

Command:

Transform....Compute Variable....Target Variable: type "none"....Numeric Expression: enter "1-max(illfeeling, …….., social problem)" ....click Type and Label....LabelL enter "no answer"....click Continue....click OK....Analyze .... Multiple Response ....Define Variable sets....click Define Multiple Response Sets....click $health....move "no answer" to Variables in Set....click Change.... click Close.

The data file now contains the novel "no answer" variable and a novel multiple response variable including the missing cases but the latter is not shown. It is now also possible to produce crosstabs with the different questions as rows and other variables like personal characteristics as columns. In this way the interaction with the personal characteristics can be assessed.

Command:

Analyze....Multiple Response....Multiple Response Crosstabs....Rows: enter $health....Columns: enter ed (= level of education)....click Define Range.... Minimum: enter 1....Maximum: enter 5....Continue....Click Options....Cell Percentages: click Columns.... click Continue....click OK.

$heatth*ed crosstabulatlon

			Level of education					
			No high school	No high school	College	University	Completed university	Total
Health[a]	Ill feeling	Count	45	101	87	115	43	391
		% within ed	27,6 %	43,3 %	50,9 %	60,2 %	81,1 %	
	Alcohol	Count	18	55	52	83	34	242
		% within ed	11,0 %	23,6 %	30,4 %	43,5 %	64,2 %	
	Weight problem	Count	13	51	43	82	25	214
		% within ed	8,0 %	21,9 %	25,1 %	42,9 %	47,2 %	
	Tiredness	Count	10	55	71	122	42	300
		% within ed	6,1 %	23,6 %	41,5 %	63,9 %	79,2 %	
	Cold	Count	71	116	85	96	21	389
		% within ed	43,6 %	49,8 %	49,7 %	50,3 %	39,6 %	
	Family problem	Count	75	118	84	93	25	395
		% within ed	46,0 %	50,6 %	49,1 %	48,7 %	47,2 %	
	Mental problem	Count	78	112	91	94	26	401
		% within ed	47,9 %	48,1 %	53,2 %	49,2 %	49,1 %	
	Physical problem	Count	78	123	87	95	26	409
		% within ed	47,9 %	52,8 %	50,9 %	49,7 %	49,1 %	
	Social problem	Count	11	67	68	111	36	293
		% within ed	6,7 %	28,8 %	39,8 %	58,1 %	67,9 %	
	No answer	Count	39	29	13	6	2	89
		% within ed	23,9 %	12,4 %	7,6 %	3,1 %	3,8 %	
Total		Count	163	233	171	191	53	811

Percentages and totals are based on respondents
[a]Dichotomy group tabulated at value 1

The output table gives the results. Various trends are observed. E.g., there is a decreasing trend of patients not answering any question with increased levels of education. Also there is an increasing trend of ill feeling, alcohol problems, weight problems, tiredness and social problems with increased levels of education. If we wish to test whether the increasing trend of tiredness with increased level of education is statistically significant, a formal trend test can be performed.

Command:

Analyze....Descriptive Statistics....Crosstabs....Rows: enter tiredness....Columns: enter level of education....click Statistics....mark Chi-square....click Continue.... click OK.

Underneath a formal trend test is given. It tests whether an increasing trend of tiredness is associated with increased levels of education.

Chi-square tests

	Value	df	Asymp. sig. (2-sided)
Pearson Chi-square	185,824[a]	4	,000
Likelihood ratio	202,764	4	,000
Linear-by-linear association	184,979	1	,000
N of valid cases	811		

[a]0 cells (,0 %) have expected countless than 5. The minimum expected count is 19,61

In the output chi-square tests are given. The linear-by-linear association data show a chi-square value of 184.979 and 1 degree of freedom. This means that a statistically very significant linear trend with $p<0.0001$ is in these data.

Also interactions and trends of any other health problems with all of the other variables including gender, age, marriage, income, period of constant address or employment can be similarly analyzed.

Conclusion

The answers to a set of multiple questions about a single underlying disease / condition can be assessed as multiple dimensions of a complex variable. Multiple response methodology is adequate for the purpose. The most important advantage of the multiple response methodology versus traditional frequency table analysis is that it is possible to observe relevant trends and similarities directly from data tables. A disadvantage is that only summaries but no statistical tests are given, but observed trends can, of course, be, additionally, tested statistically with formal trend tests.

Note

More background, theoretical and mathematical information of multiple response sets are in Machine Learning in medicine part three, Chap. 11, pp 105–115, Multiple response sets, Springer Heidelberg Germany, 2013, from the same authors.

Chapter 73
Protein and DNA Sequence Mining

General Purpose

Sequence similarity searching is a method that can be applied by almost anybody for finding similarities between his/her query sequences of amino acids and DNA and the sequences known to be associated with different clinical effects. The latter have been included in database systems like the BLAST (Basic Local Alignment Search Tool) database system from the US National Center of Biotechnology Information (NCBI), and the MOTIF data base system, a joint website from different European and American institutions, and they are available through the internet for the benefit of individual researchers trying and finding a match for novel sequences from their own research. This chapter is to demonstrate that sequence similarity searching is a method that can be applied by almost anybody for finding similarities between his/her sequences and the sequences known to be associated with different clinical effects.

Specific Scientific Question

Amino acid	Three-letter abbreviation	One-letter symbol
Alanine	Ala	A
Arginine	Arg	R
Asparagine	Asn	N
Aspartic acid	Asp	D
Asparagine or aspartic acid	Asx	B

(continued)

This chapter was previously published in "Machine learning in medicine-cookbook 3" as Chap. 15, 2014.

T.J. Cleophas, A.H. Zwinderman, *Machine Learning in Medicine - a Complete Overview*, DOI 10.1007/978-3-319-15195-3_73

Amino acid	Three-letter abbreviation	One-letter symbol
Cysteine	Cys	C
Glutamine	Gln	Q
Glutamic acid	Glu	E
Glutamine or glutamic acid	Glx	Z
Glycine	Gly	G
Histidine	His	H
Isoleucine	Ile	I
Leucine	Leu	L
Lysine	Lys	K
Methionine	Met	M
Phenylalanine	Phe	F
Proline	Pro	P
Serine	Ser	S
Threonine	Thr	T
Tryptophan	Trp	W
Tyrosine	Tyr	Y
Valine	Val	V

In this chapter amino acid sequences are analyzed, but nucleic acids sequences can similarly be assessed. The above table gives the one letter abbreviations of amino acids. The specific scientific question is: can sequence similarity search be applied for finding similarities between the sequences found in your own research and the sequences known to be associated with different clinical effects.

Data Base Systems on the Internet

The BLAST (http://blast.ncbi.nlm.nih.gov/Blast.cgi) program reports several terms:

1. Max score = best bit score between query sequence and database sequence (the bit score = the standardized score, i.e. the score that is independent of any unit).
2. Total score = best bit score if some amino acid pairs in the data have been used more often than just once.
3. Query coverage = percentage of amino acids used in the analysis.
4. E-value = expected number of large similarity alignment scores.

If the E-value is very small for the score observed, then a chance finding can be rejected. The sequences are then really related. An E-value = p-value adjusted for multiple testing = the chance that the association found is a chance finding. It indicates that the match between a novel and already known sequence is closer than could happen by chance, and that the novel and known sequence are thus homologous (philogenetically from the same ancestor, whatever that means).

Example 1

We isolated the following amino acid sequence: serine, isoleucine, lysine, leucine, tryptophan, proline, proline. The one letter abbreviation code for this sequence is SIKLWPP. The BLAST Search site is explored, while giving the following commands.

Open BLAST Search site at appropriate address (Reference 1).
Choose Protein BLAST
Click Enter Sequences and enter the amino acid sequence SIKLWPP
Click BLAST

The output tables use the term blast hit which means here a database sequence selected by the provider's software to be largely similar to the unknown sequence, and the term query, which means here an unknown sequence that the investigator has entered for sequence testing against known sequences from the database. The output tables report

1. No putative conserved domains have been detected.
2. In the Distribution of 100 Blast Hits on the Query sequence all of the Blast Hits have a very low alignment score (<40).
3. In spite of the low scores their precise alignment values are given next, e.g. the best one has

   a max score of 21.8,
   total score of 21.8,
   query coverage of 100 %, and
   adjusted p-value of 1956 (not significant).

As a contrast search the MOTIF Search site is explored. We command.

Open MOTIF Search site at appropriate address (MOTIF Search. http://www.genome.jp/tools/motif).
Choose: Searching Protein Sequence Motifs
Click: Enter your query sequence and enter the amino acid sequence SIKLWPP
Select motif libraries: click various databases given
Then click Search.

The output table reports: 1 motif found in PROSITE database (found motif PKC_PHOSPHO_SITE; description: protein kinase C phosphorylation site). Obviously, it is worthwhile to search other databases if one does not provide any hits.

Example 2

We wish to examine a 12 amino acid sequence that we isolated at our laboratory, use again BLAST. We command.

Open BLAST Search site at appropriate address (Reference 1).
Choose Protein BLAST
Click Enter Sequences and enter the amino acid sequence ILVFMCWLVFQC
Click BLAST

The output tables report

1. No putative conserved domains have been detected.
2. In the Distribution of 100 Blast Hits on the Query sequence all of the Blast Hits have a very low alignment score (<40).
3. In spite of the low scores their precise alignment values are given next. Three of them have a significant alignment score at $p<0.05$ with

   max scores of 31.2,
   total scores 31.2,
   query cover of around 60 %, and
   E-values (adjusted p-values) of 4.1, 4.1, and 4.5.

Parts of the novel sequence have been aligned to known sequences of proteins from a streptococcus and a nocardia bacteria and from caenorhabditis, a small soil-dwelling nematode. These findings may not seem clinically very relevant, and may be due to type I errors, with low levels of statistical significance, or material contamination.

Example 3

A somewhat larger amino acid sequence (25 letters) is examined using BLAST. We command.

Open BLAST Search site at appropriate address (Reference 1).
Choose Protein BLAST
Click Enter Sequences and enter the amino acid sequence SIKLWPPSQTTRLLLVERMANNLST
Click BLAST

The output tables report the following.

1. Putative domains have been detected. Specific hits regard the WPP superfamily. The WPP domain is a 90 amino acid protein that serves as a transporter protein for other protein in the plant cell from the cell plasma to the nucleus.
2. In the Distribution of 100 Blast Hits on the Query sequence all of the Blast Hits have a very high alignment score (80–200 for the first 5 hits, over 50 for the remainder, all of them statistically very significant).

3. Precise alignment values are given next. The first 5 hits have the highest scores: with

   max scores of 83.8,
   total scores of 83.8,
   Cover queries of 100 %,
   p-values of 4 e^{-17}, which is much smaller than 0.05 (5 %).

   All of them relate to the WPP superfamily sequence.
   The next 95 hits produced Max scores and Total scores from 68.9 to 62.1, query coverages from 100 to 96 %. and adjusted p-values from 5 e^{-12} to 1 e^{-9}, which is again much smaller than 0.05 (5 %).
4. We can subsequently browse through the 95 hits to see if anything of interest for our purposes can be found. All of the alignments as found regarded plant proteins like those of grasses, maize, nightshade and other plants, no alignments with human or veterinary proteins were established.

Example 4

A 27 amino acid sequence from a laboratory culture of pseudomonas is examined using BLAST. We command.

Open BLAST Search site at appropriate address (Reference 1).
Choose Protein BLAST
Click Enter Sequences and enter the amino acid sequence MTDLNIPHTHAHLVDAFQALGIRAQAL
Click BLAST

The output tables report

1. No putative domains have been detected.
2. The 100 blast hit table shows, however, a very high alignment score for gentamicin acetyl transferase enzyme, recently recognized as being responsible for resistance of pseudomonas to gentamicin. The ailments values were

   max score
   total score of 85.5,
   query coverage of 100 %,
   adjusted p-value of 1 e^{-17}, and so statistically very significant.

3. In the Distribution of the 99 remaining Blast Hits only 5 other significant alignment were detected with

   max score and total scores from 38.5 to 32.9,
   query coverages 55–92 %,
   adjusted p-values between 0.08 and 4.5 (all of them 5 %).

The significant alignments regarded bacterial proteins including the gram negative bacterias, rhizobium, xanthomonas, and morganella, and a mite protein. This may not clinically be very relevant, but our novel sequence was derived from a pseudomonas culture, and we know now that this particular culture contains pathogens very resistant to gentamicin.

Conclusion

Sequence similarity searching is a method that can be applied by almost anybody for finding similarities between his/her query sequences and the sequences known to be associated with different clinical effects.

With sequence similarity searching the use of p-values to distinguish between high and low similarity is relevant. Unlike the BLAST interactive website, the MOTIF interactive website does not give them, which hampers inferences from the alignments to be made.

Note

More background, theoretical and mathematical information of protein and DNA sequence mining is given in Machine learning in medicine part two, Chap. 17, pp 171–185, Protein and DNA sequence mining, Springer Heidelberg Germany 2013, from the same authors.

Chapter 74
Iteration Methods for Crossvalidations (150 Patients with Pneumonia)

General Purpose

In the Chap. 8 of this book validation of a decision tree model is performed splitting a data file into a training and a testing sample. This method performed pretty well with a sensitivity of 90–100 % and an overall accuracy of 94 %. However, measures of error of predictive models like the above one are based on residual methods, assuming a priori defined data distributions, particularly normal distributions. Machine learning data file may not meet such assumptions, and distribution free methods of validation, like crossvalidations may be more safe.

Primary Scientific Question

How does crossvalidation of the data from Chap. 8 perform as compared to the residual method used in the scorer node of the Konstanz information miner (Knime)?

Example

The data file from Chap. 8 is used once more. Four inflammatory markers (CRP (C-reactive protein), ESR (erythrocyte sedimentation rate), leucocyte count (leucos), and fibrinogen) were measured In 150 patients. Based on x-ray chest clinical severity was classified as A (mild infection), B (medium severity), C (severe

---

This chapter was previously published in "Machine learning in medicine-cookbook 3" as Chap. 16, 2014.

T.J. Cleophas, A.H. Zwinderman, *Machine Learning in Medicine - a Complete Overview*, DOI 10.1007/978-3-319-15195-3_74

infection). A major scientific question was to assess what markers were the best predictors of the severity of infection.

CRP	leucos	fibrinogen	ESR	x-ray severity
120,00	5,00	11,00	60,00	A
100,00	5,00	11,00	56,00	A
94,00	4,00	11,00	60,00	A
92,00	5,00	11,00	58,00	A
100,00	5,00	11,00	52,00	A
108,00	6,00	17,00	48,00	A
92,00	5,00	14,00	48,00	A
100,00	5,00	11,00	54,00	A
88,00	5,00	11,00	54,00	A
98,00	5,00	8,00	60,00	A
108,00	5,00	11,00	68,00	A
96,00	5,00	11,00	62,00	A
96,00	5,00	8,00	46,00	A
86,00	4,00	8,00	60,00	A
116,00	4,00	11,00	50,00	A
114,00	5,00	17,00	52,00	A

CRP = C-reactive protein (mg/l)
leucos = leucyte count (*10^9/l)
fibrinogen = fibrinogen level (mg/l)
ESR = erythrocyte sedimentation rate (mm)
x-ray severity = x-chest severity pneumonia score (A – C = mild to severe)

The first 16 patients are in the above table, the entire data file is in "decisiontree" and can be obtained from "extras.springer.com" on the internet.

Downloading the Knime Data Miner

In Google enter the term "knime". Click Download and follow instructions. After completing the pretty easy download procedure, open the knime workbench by clicking the knime welcome screen. The center of the screen displays the workflow editor like the canvas in SPSS modeler. It is empty, and can be used to build a stream of nodes, called workflow in knime. The node repository is in the left lower angle of the screen, and the nodes can be dragged to the workflow editor simply by left-clicking. Start by dragging the file reader node to the workflow. The nodes are computer tools for data analysis like visualization and statistical processes. Node description is in the right upper angle of the screen. Before the nodes can be used, they have to be connected with the file reader node and with one another by arrows drawn again simply by left clicking the small triangles attached to the nodes. Right clicking on the file reader node enables to configure from your computer a requested data file....click Browse....and download from the appropriate folder a csv type Excel file. You are set for analysis now.

Note: the above data file cannot be read by the file reader node as it is an SPSS file, and must first be saved as an csv type Excel file. For that purpose command in SPSS: click File....click Save as....in "Save as" type: enter Comma Delimited (*. csv)....click Save. For your convenience it is available in extras.springer.com, and is also entitled "decisiontree".

Knime Workflow

A knime workflow for the analysis of the above data example is built, and the final result is shown in the underneath figure

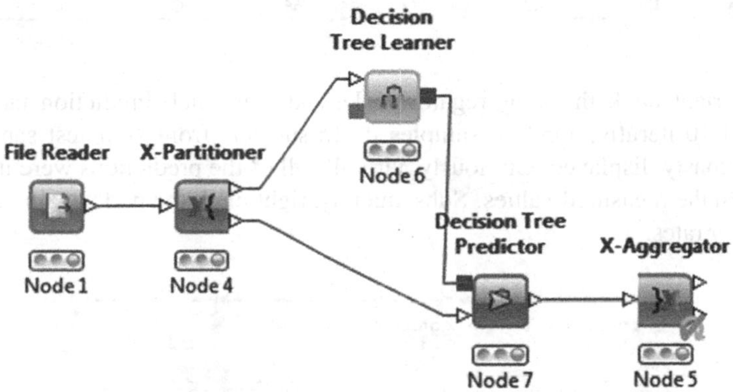

In the node repository click X-Partitioner, Decision Tree Learner, Decision Tree Predictor and X-Aggregator and drag them to the workflow editor. If you have difficulty finding the nodes (the repository contains hundreds of nodes), you may type their names in the small window at the top of the node repository box, and its icon and name will immediately appear. Connect, by left clicking, all of the nodes with arrows as indicated above....Configurate and execute all of the nodes by right clicking the nodes and then the texts "Configurate" and "Execute"....the red lights will successively turn orange and then green....right click the Decision Tree Predictor again....right click the text "View: Decision Tree View". The decision tree comes up, and it is, obviously, identical to the one of Chap. 2.

Crossvalidation

If you, subsequently, right click the Decision Tree Predictor, and then click Classified Data, a table turns up of 15 randomly selected subjects from your test sample. The predicted values are identical to the measured ones. And, so, for this selection the Decision Tree Predictor node performed well.

Row ID	ï»¿CRP	leucos	fibrinogen	ESR	xrayse...	Predicti...
Row5	108	6	17	48	A	A
Row20	108	6	11	60	A	A
Row28	104	4	11	58	A	A
Row39	102	5	11	56	A	A
Row94	112	14	44	76	B	B
Row103	126	19	59	68	C	C
Row111	128	18	62	70	C	C
Row112	136	18	68	72	C	C
Row113	114	17	65	60	C	C
Row120	138	19	74	99	C	C
Row126	124	16	59	84	C	C
Row137	128	18	59	44	C	C
Row138	120	16	59	98	C	C
Row144	134	19	80	100	C	C
Row145	134	17	74	64	C	C

Next, right click the x-aggregator node, and then click Prediction table. The results of 10 iterative random samples of 15 subjects from your test sample are simultaneously displayed. Obviously, virtually all of the predictions were in agreement with the measured values. Subsequently, right click the node again, and then click Error rates.

Error rates - 0:5 - X-Aggregator

File

Table "default" - Rows: 10 | Spec - Columns: 3 | Properties | Flow Variables

Row ID	Error in %	Size of ...	Error C...
fold 0	6.667	15	1
fold 1	6.667	15	1
fold 2	6.667	15	1
fold 3	20	15	3
fold 4	0	15	0
fold 5	0	15	0
fold 6	6.667	15	1
fold 7	6.667	15	1
fold 8	0	15	0
fold 9	0	15	0

The above table comes up. It shows the error rates of the above 10 iterative random samples. The result is pretty good. Virtually, all of them have 0 or 1 erroneous value.

The crossvalidation can also be performed with a novel validation set. For that purpose you need a novel file reader node, and the novel validation set has to be configured and executed. Furthermore, you need to copy and paste the above

Aggregator node, and you need to connect the output port of the above Decision Tree Predictor node to the input port of Aggregator node.

Conclusion

In Chap. 8 of this volume validation of a decision tree model was performed splitting a data file into a training and testing sample. This method performed pretty well with an overall accuracy of 94 %. However, the measure of error is based on the normal distribution assumption, and data may not meet this assumption. Crossvalidation is a distribution free method, and may here be a more safe, and less biased approach to validation.

It performed very well, with errors mostly 0 and 1 out of 15 cases. We should add that Knime does not provide sensitivity and specificity measures here.

Note

More background, theoretical and mathematical information of validations and crossvalidations is given in:

Statistics applied to clinical studies 5th edition, Springer Heidelberg Germany.

Chap. 46, Validating qualitative diagnostic tests, pp 509–517, 2012,
Chap. 47 Uncertainty of qualitative diagnostic tests, pp 519–525, 2012,
Chap. 50 Validating quantitative diagnostic tests, pp 545–552, 2012,
Chap. 51 Summary of validation procedures for diagnostic tests, pp 555–568, 2012.

Machine learning in medicine part one, Springer Heidelberg Germany.

Chap. 1 Introduction to machine learning, p 5, 2012,
Chap. 3 Optimal scaling: discretization, p 28, 2012,
Chap. 4 Optimal scaling, regularization including ridge, lasso, and elastic net regression, p 41, 2012.

All of the above publications are from the same authors as the current work.

Chapter 75
Testing Parallel-Groups with Different Sample Sizes and Variances (5 Parallel-Group Studies)

General Purpose

Unpaired t-tests are traditionally used for testing the significance of difference between parallel-groups according to

$$t \ \text{value} = \left(\text{mean}_1 - \text{mean}_2\right) / \sqrt{\left(\text{SD}_1 / \text{N}_1 + \text{SD}_2 / \text{N}_2\right)}$$

where mean, SD, N are respectively the mean, the standard deviation and the sample size of the parallel groups.

Many calculators on the internet (e.g., the P value calculator-GraphPad) can tell you whether the t-value is significantly smaller than 0.05, and, thus, whether there is a statistically significant difference between the parallel groups.

E.g., open Google and type p-value calculator for t-test....click Enter....click P value calculator -GraphPad....select P from t....t: enter computed t-value....DF: compute $N_1 + N_2$ -2 and enter the result....click Compute P.

This procedure assumes that the two parallel groups have equal variances. However in practice this is virtually never entirely true. This chapter is to assess tests accounting the effect of different variances on the estimated p-values.

Primary Scientific Question

Two methods for adjustment of different variances and different sample sizes are available, the pooled t-test which assumes that the differences in variances are just residual, and that the two variances are equal, and the Welch's test which assumes

---

This chapter was previously published in "Machine learning in medicine-cookbook 3" as Chap. 17, 2014.

T.J. Cleophas, A.H. Zwinderman, *Machine Learning in Medicine - a Complete Overview*, DOI 10.1007/978-3-319-15195-3_75

that they are due to a real effect, like a difference in treatment effect with comcomitant difference in spread of the data. How are the results of the two adjustment procedures.

Examples

In the underneath table the t- test statistics and p-values of 5 parallel-group studies with differences in the means, standard deviations (SDs) and sample sizes (Ns) are given. In the examples 2, 3, 4, and 5 respectively the Ns, SDs, means, and SDs have been changed as compared to example 1.

				unadjusted		adjusted (pooled)		Welch's adjust	
	means	SDs	Ns	t value	p value	t value	p value	t value	p value
1.	**50/40**	**5/3**	**100/200**	**1.715/0.087**		**1.811/0.071**		**1.715/0.088**	
2.			10/20	1.715/0.092		1.814/0.080		1.715/0.100	
3.		10/3		0.958/0.339		1.214/0.226		0.958/0.340	
4.	60/40			3.430/0.007		3.662/0.000		3.430/0.001	
5.		6/2		1.581/0.115		1.963/0.051		1.581/0.117	

Open Google and type GraphPad Software QuickCalcs t test calculator....mark: Enter mean, SEM, N....mark: Unpaired test....label: type Group 1....mean: type 50....SEM: type 5....N: type 100....label: type Group 2.... mean: type 40....SEM: type 3....N: type 200....click Calculate now.

In the output an adjusted t-value of 1.811 is given and a p-value of 0.071, slightly better than the unadjusted p-value of 0.087. Next a Welch's t-test will be performed using the same procedure as above, but with Welch's Unpaired t-test marked instead of just Unpaired t-test. The output sheet shows that the p-value is now worse than the unadjusted p-value instead of better.

In the examples 2–5 slightly different means, SDs, and Ns were used but, otherwise, the data were the same. After computations it can be observed that in all of the examples the adjusted test using pooled variances produced the best p-values. This sometimes lead to a statistically significant effect while the other two test are non-significant, for example with data 5 (p-value = 0.05). The Welch's adjustment produced the worst p-value, while the unadjusted produced the best statistics.

Conclusion

Two methods for adjustment of different variances and different sample sizes are available, the pooled t-test which assumes that the differences in variances are just residual, and the Welch's test which assumes that they are real differences. From five examples it can be observed that the t-tests using pooled variances consistently produced the best p-values sometimes leading to a statistically significant result in otherwise statistically insignificant data. In contrast, the Welch's adjustment consistently produced the worst result. The pooled t-test is probably the best option if we have clinical arguments for residual differences in variances, while the Welch's test would be a scientifically better option, if it can be argued that differences in variance were due to real clinical effects. Moreover, the Welch's test would be more in agreement with the general feature of advanced statistical analyses: tests taking special effects in the data into account are associated with larger p-values (more uncertainties).

Note

More background, theoretical and mathematical information of improved t-tests are in Statistics applied to clinical studies, Chap. 2, The analysis of efficacy data, pp 15–40, Springer Heidelberg Germany 5th edition, 2012, from the same authors.

Chapter 76
Association Rules Between Exposure and Outcome (50 and 60 Patients)

General Purpose

Traditional analysis of exposure outcome relationships is only sensitive with strong relationships. This chapter is to assess whether association rules, based on conditional probabilities, may be more sensitive in case of weak relationships.

Primary Scientific Question

Is association rule analysis better sensitive than regression analysis and paired chi-square tests are for demonstrating significant exposure effects.

Example

The proportions observed in a sample are equal to chances or probabilities. If you observe a 40 % proportion of healthy patients, then the chance or probability (P) of being healthy in this group is 40 %. With two variables, e.g., healthy and happy, the symbol ∩ is often used to indicate "and" (both are present). Underneath a hypothesized example of 5 patients, with 3 of them having overweight and 2 of them coronary artery disease (CAD), is given.

This chapter was previously published in "Machine learning in medicine-cookbook 3" as Chap. 18, 2014.

T.J. Cleophas, A.H. Zwinderman, *Machine Learning in Medicine - a Complete Overview*, DOI 10.1007/978-3-319-15195-3_76

Patient	overweight (predictor)	coronary artery disease
	X	Y
1	1	0
2	0	1
3	0	0
4	1	1
5	1	0

Support rule

$$\text{Support} = \text{PX} \cap \text{Y} = 1/5 = 0.2$$

Confidence rule

$$\text{Confidence} = \text{PX} \cap \text{Y}/\text{PY} = [1/5]/\ [2/5] = 0.5$$

Lift rule (or lift-up rule)

$$\text{Lift} = \text{PX} \cap \text{Y}/[\text{PX} \times \text{PY}] = [1/5]/\ [2/5 \times 2/5] = 1.25$$

Conviction rule

$$\text{Conviction} = [1-\text{PY}]/[1-\text{PX} \cap \text{Y}/\text{PY}] = [1-2/5]/[1\quad 0.5] = 1.20$$

I. The support gives the proportion of patients with both overweight and CAD in the entire population. A support of 0.0 would mean that overweight and CAD are mutually elusive, a support of x.y would mean that the two factors are independent of one another.
II. The confidence gives the fraction of patients with both CAD and overweight in those with CAD. This fraction is obviously larger than that in the entire population, because it rose from 0.2 to 0.5.
III. The lift compares the observed proportion of patients with both overweight and CAD with the expected proportion if CAD and overweight would have occurred independently of one another. Obviously, the observed value is larger than expected, 1.25 versus 1.00, suggesting that overweight does contribute to the risk of CAD.
IV. Finally, the conviction compares the patients with no-CAD in the entire population with those with both no-CAD and the presence of overweight. The ratio is larger than 1.00, namely 1.20. Obviously, the benefit of no-CAD is better for the entire population than it is for the subgroup with overweight.

In order to assess whether the computed values, like 0.2 and 1.25, are significantly different from 0.0 to 1.0 confidence intervals have to be calculated. We will use the McCallum-Layton calculator for proportions, freely available from the Internet (Confidence interval calculator for proportions. www.mccallum-layton.co.uk/).

The calculations will somewhat overestimate the true confidence intervals, because the true confidence intervals are here mostly composed of two or more proportions, and this is not taken into account. Therefore, doubling the p-values may be more adequate (Bonferroni adjustment), but with very small p-values we need not worry.

Example One

A data set of 50 patients with coronary artery disease or not (1 = yes) and overweight as predictor (1 = yes) is given underneath

Patient	Overweight	Coronary artery disease
1	1,00	0,00
2	0,00	1,00
3	0,00	0,00
4	1,00	1,00
5	0,00	0,00
6	1,00	0,00
7	0,00	1,00
8	0,00	0,00
9	1,00	1,00
10	0,00	0,00
11	1,00	0,00
12	0,00	1,00
13	0,00	0,00
14	1,00	1,00
15	0,00	0,00

The first 15 patients are given. The entire data file are the Variables A and B of the data file entitled "associationrule", and are in extras.springer.com.

20/50 of the patients have overweight (predictor), 20/50 have CAD. A paired binary test (McNemar's test) shows no significant difference between the two columns ($p = 1.0$). Binary logistic regression with the predictor as independent variable is equally insignificant ($b = 0.69$, $p = 0.241$).

Applying association rules we find a support of 0.2 and confidence of 0.5. The lift is 1.25 and the conviction is 1.20. The McCallum calculator gives the confidence intervals, respectively 10–34, 36–64, 110–145, and 107–137 %. All of these 95 % confidence intervals indicate a very significant difference from respectively 0 % (support and confidence) and 100 % (lift and conviction) with p-values <0.001 (Bonferroni adjusted $p<0.002$) Indeed, the predictor overweight had a very significant positive effect on the risk of CAD.

Example Two

A data set of 60 patients with coronary artery disease or not (1 = yes) with overweight and "being manager" as predictors (1 = yes)

Patient	Overweight	Manager	Coronary artery disease
1	1,00	1,00	0,00
2	0,00	0,00	1,00
3	1,00	1,00	0,00
4	0,00	1,00	1,00
5	0,00	0,00	0,00
6	1,00	1,00	1,00
7	1,00	1,00	0,00
8	0,00	0,00	1,00
9	1,00	1,00	0,00
10	0,00	1,00	1,00
11	0,00	0,00	0,00
12	1,00	1,00	1,00
13	1,00	1,00	0,00
14	0,00	0,00	1,00
15	1,00	1,00	0,00

The first 15 patients are given. The entire data file are the variables C, D, and E of the data file entitled "associationrule", and is in extras.springer.com.

Instead of a single x –variable now two of them are included. 30/60 of the patients have overweight, 40/60 are manager, and 30/60 have CAD. A paired binary test (Cochran's test, see note section) shows no significant difference between the three columns ($p=0.082$). Binary logistic regression with the two predictors as independent variables is equally insignificant (b-values are – 21.9 and 21.2, p-values are 0.99 and 0.99).

Applying association rules we find a support of 0.1666 and confidence of 0.333. The lift is 2.0 and the conviction is 1.25. The McCallum calculator gives the confidence intervals. Expressed as percentages they are respectively, 8–29, 22–47, and 159–270 and 108–136 %. All of these 95 % confidence intervals indicate a very significant difference from respectively 0 % (support and confidence) and 100 %

(lift and conviction) with p-values <0.001 (Bonferroni adjusted $p < 0.002$ or < 0.003). Indeed, the predictors overweight and being manager had a statistically very significant effect on the risk of CAD.

Conclusion

Association rule analysis is more sensitive than regression analysis and paired chi-square tests, and is able to demonstrate significant predictor effects, when the other methods are not. It can also include multiple variables and very large datasets and is a welcome methodology for clinical predictor research.

Note

More background, theoretical and mathematical information of association rules are in Machine learning in medicine part two, Chap. 11, pp 105–113, Springer Heidelberg Germany, 2013, from the same authors. Cochran's test is explained in SPSS for starters part one, Chap. 14, pp 51–53, Springer Heidelberg Germany, 2010, from the same authors.

Chapter 77
Confidence Intervals for Proportions and Differences in Proportions (100 and 75 Patients)

General Purpose

Proportions, fractions, percentages, risks, hazards are all synonymous terms to indicate what part of a population had events like death, illness, complications etc. Instead of p-values, confidence intervals are often calculated. If you obtained many samples from the same population, 95 % of them would have their mean results between the 95 % confidence intervals. And, likewise, samples from the same population with their proportions outside the 95 % confidence intervals means that they are significantly different from the population with a probability of 5 % ($p<0.05$). This chapter is to assess how confidence intervals can be computed.

Primary Scientific Question

P-values give the type I error, otherwise called the chance of finding a difference where there is none. Confidence intervals tell you the same, but, in addition, they give the range in which the true outcome value lies, and the direction and strength of it. Are confidence intervals more relevant for exploratory studies than p-values, because of the additional information provided.

This chapter was previously published in "Machine learning in medicine-cookbook 3" as Chap. 19, 2014.

T.J. Cleophas, A.H. Zwinderman, *Machine Learning in Medicine - a Complete Overview*, DOI 10.1007/978-3-319-15195-3_77

Example

If in two parallel groups of respectively 100 and 75 patients the numbers of patients with an event are 75 and 50, according to a z-test or chi-square test (see Statistics Applied to Clinical Studies 5th edition, Chap. 3, The analysis of safety data, pp 41–60, 2012, Springer Heidelberg Germany, from the same authors), then the p-value of difference will be 0.23. This means that we have 23 % chance of a type one error, and that this chance is far too large to be statistically significant ($p>0.05$).

In the two above groups the proportions are respectively 75/100 = 0.750 and 50/75 = 0.667. The standard errors of these proportions can be calculated from the equation

$$\text{standard errors} = \pm\sqrt{\left(p(1-p)/\sqrt{n}\right)}$$

where p = proportion and n = sample size.

$$95\%\ \text{confidence intervals} = \pm 1.96\sqrt{\left(p(1-p)/\sqrt{n}\right)}$$

If you have little affinity with computations, then plenty of calculators on the internet are helpful.

Confidence Intervals of Proportions

We will use the free "Matrix Software". Open Google and type Standard Error (SE) of Sample Proportion Calculator-Binomial Standard Deviation....click Enter....click Matrix Software....in Calculate SE Sample Proportion of Standard deviation type 0.75 for Proportion of successes (p)....type 100 for Number of Observations (n).... click Calculate....

$$\begin{aligned} \text{The binomial SE of the Sample proportion} &= \pm 0.04330127\ldots.\\ \text{The 95\% confidence interval of this proportion} &= \pm 1.96 \times 0.04330127\\ &= \pm 0.08487\\ &= \text{between } 0.66513 \text{ and } 0.83487 \end{aligned}$$

Similarly the 95 % confidence interval of the data from group 2 can be calculated.

Confidence Intervals of Differences in Proportions

In order to calculate the confidence interval of the differences between the above two proportions, we will use the free Vassarstats. Open Google en type http://vassarstats.net/prop2_ind.html....click enter....select The Confidence Interval for the Difference Between Two Independent Proportions....Larger Proportion: k_a (number of observations with event) = : type 75....n_a (total number of observations) = : type 100....click Calculate.

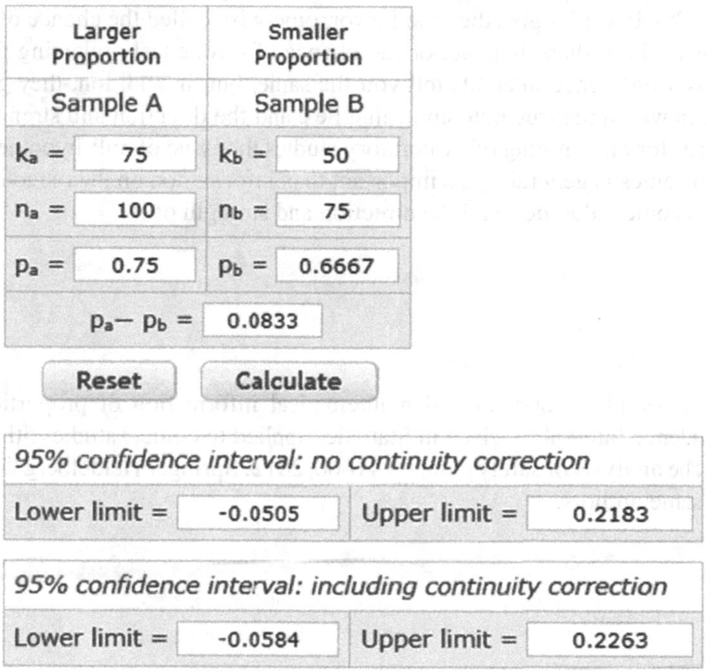

The output is given above. p_a an p_b are the proportions, $p_a - p_b$ the difference. The 95 % confidence interval is between −0.0505 and 0.2183.

Proportions are yes/no data, e.g., a proportion of 75 subjects out of 100 had an event. The normal distribution is used for the calculation of the p-values and confidence intervals. In order to test yes/no data with a normal distribution, a continuity correction can be used to improve the quality of the analysis. In the example given the 75/100 in your sample indicates that the real event rate in your entire population of, e.g., 1,000 may be between 745 and 755/1,000. Because 745/1,000 is, of course, smaller than 750/1,000, it would make sense to use the proportion 745/1,000 for the calculation of the confidence interval instead of 750/1,000. This procedure is called the continuity correction, and as shown above it produces somewhat wider confidence intervals, and, thus, more uncertainty in your data. Unfortunately, higher quality is often associated with larger levels of uncertainty.

Conclusion

Proportions are used to indicate what part of a population had events. Instead of p-values to tell you whether your observed proportion is statistically significantly different from a proportion of 0.0, 95 % confidence intervals are often calculated. If you obtained many samples from the same population, 95 % of them would have their result between the 95 % confidence intervals. And, likewise, samples from the same population having their proportions outside the 95 % confidence intervals means that they are significantly different from the population with a probability of 5 % ($p<0.05$). P-values give the type I error, otherwise called the chance of finding a difference where there is none, or the chance of erroneously rejecting the null-hypothesis. Confidence intervals tell you the same, but, in addition, they give you the range in which the true outcome value lies, and the direction and strength of it. Particularly, for data mining of exploratory studies the issue of null-hypothesis testing with p-values is generally less important than information on the range in which the true outcome value lies, and the direction and strength of it.

Note

More background, theoretical and mathematical information of proportions and their confidence intervals is given in Statistics applied to clinical studies 5th edition, Chap. 3, The analysis of safety data, pp 41–60, 2012, Springer Heidelberg Germany, from the same authors.

Chapter 78
Ratio Statistics for Efficacy Analysis of New Drugs (50 Patients)

General Purpose

Treatment efficacies are often assessed as differences from baseline. However, better treatment efficacies may be observed in patients with high baseline-values than in those with low ones. This was, e.g., the case in the Progress study, a parallel-group study of pravastatin versus placebo (see Statistics applied to clinical studies 5th edition, Chap. 17, Logistic and Cox regression, Markov models, and Laplace transformations, pp 199–218, Springer Heidelberg Germany, 2012, from the same authors). This chapter assesses the performance of ratio statistics for that purpose.

Primary Scientific Question

The differences of treatment efficacy and baseline may be the best fit test statistic, if the treatment efficacies are independent of baseline. However, if not, then ratios of the two may fit the data better.

Example

A 50-patient 5-group parallel-group study was performed with five different cholesterol-lowering compounds. The first 12 patients of the data file is underneath. The entire data file is entitled "ratiostatistics" and is in extra.springer.com.

This chapter was previously published in "Machine learning in medicine-cookbook 2" as Chap. 20, 2014.

T.J. Cleophas, A.H. Zwinderman, *Machine Learning in Medicine - a Complete Overview*, DOI 10.1007/978-3-319-15195-3_78

Variable			
1	2	3	4
Baseline cholesterol (mmol/l)	Treatment cholesterol (mmol/l)	Treatment group no.	Baseline minus treatment cholesterol level (mmol/l)
6.10	5.20	1.00	.90
7.00	7.90	1.00	–.90
8.20	3.90	1.00	4.30
7.60	4.70	1.00	2.90
6.50	5.30	1.00	1.20
8.40	5.40	1.00	3.00
6.90	4.20	1.00	2.70
6.70	6.10	1.00	.60
7.40	3.80	1.00	3.60
5.80	6.30	1.00	–.50
6.20	4.30	2.00	1.90
7.10	6.80	2.00	.30

Start by opening the above data file in SPSS statistical software.

Command:

Graphs….Legacy Dialogs…..Error Bar….mark Summaries of groups of cases…. click Define….Variable: enter "baseline minus treatment"….Category Axis: enter Treatment group….Confidence interval for mean: Level enter 95 %....click OK.

The underneath graph shows that all of the treatments were excellent and significantly lowered cholesterol levels as shown by the 95 % confidence intervals. T-tests are not needed here.

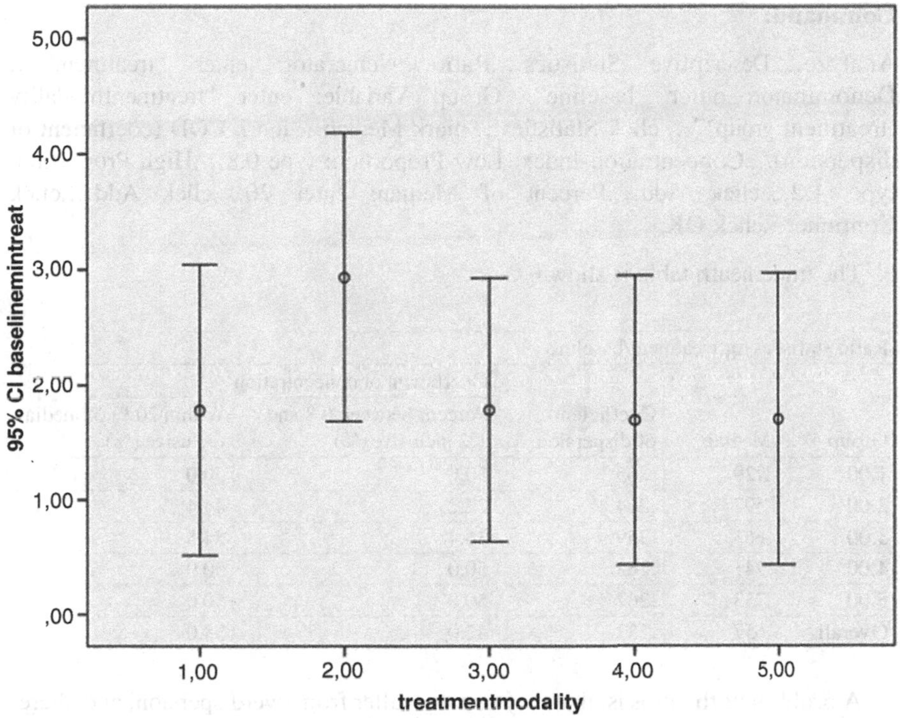

A one-way ANOVA (treatment modality as predictor and "baseline minus treatment" as outcome) will be performed to assess whether any of the treatments significantly outperformed the others.

Command:

Analyze....Compare means....One-Way ANOVA....Dependent List: enter "baseline minus treatment"....Factor: enter Treatment group....click OK.

ANOVA					
Baselinemintreat					
	Sum of squares	df	Mean square	F	Sig.
Between groups	10,603	4	2,651	,886	,480
Within groups	134,681	45	2,993		
Total	145,284	49			

According the above table the differences between the different treatment were statistically insignificant. And, so, according to the above analysis all treatments were excellent and no significance difference between any of the groups were observed. Next, we will try and find out whether ratio statistics can make additional observations.

Command:

Analyze....Descriptive Statistics....Ratio....Numerator: enter "treatment".... Denominator: enter "baseline"....Group Variable: enter "treatmentmodality (treatment group)"....click Statistics....mark Median....mark COD (coefficient of dispersion)....Concentration Index: Low Proportion: type 0.8....High Proportion: type 1.2....click Add....Percent of Median: enter 20....click Add....click Continue....click OK.

The underneath table is shown.

Ratio statistics for treatment/baseline

Group	Median	Coefficient of dispersion	Coefficient of concentration: Percent between 0.8 and 1.2 inclusive (%)	Coefficient of concentration: Within 20 % of median inclusive (%)
1.00	.729	.265	50.0	50.0
2.00	.597	.264	22.2	44.4
3.00	.663	.269	36.4	54.5
4.00	.741	.263	50.0	50.0
5.00	.733	.267	50.0	50.0
Overall	.657	.282	42.0	38.0

A problem with ratios is, that they usually suffer from overdispersion, and, therefore, the spread in the data must be assessed differently from that of normal distributions. First medians are applied, which is not the mean value but the values in the middle of all values. Assessment of spread is then estimated with

(1) the coefficient of dispersion,
(2) the percentual coefficient of concentration (all ratios within 20 % of the median are included),
(3) the interval coefficient of concentration (all ratios between the ratio 0.8*median and 1.2*median are included (*=symbol of multiplication)).

The coefficients (2) and (3) are not the same, if the distribution of the ratios are very skewed.

The above table shows the following.

Treatment 2 (Group 2) performs best with 60 % reduction of cholesterol after treatment, treatment 4 performs worst with only 74 % reduction of cholesterol after treatment. The coefficient (1) is a general measure of variability of the ratios and the coefficient (3) shows the same but is more easy to interpret: around 50 % of the individual ratios are within 20 % distance from the median ratio. The coefficient (2) gives the % of individual ratios between the interval of 0.8 and 1.2 * median ratio. Particularly, groups 2 and 3 have small coefficients indicating little concentration of the individual ratios here. Group 2 may produce the best median ratio, but is also least concentrated, and is thus more uncertain than, e.g., groups 1, 4, 5.

It would make sense to conclude from these observations that treatment group 1 with more certainty is a better treatment choice than treatment group 2.

Conclusion

Treatment efficacies are often assessed as differences from baseline. However, better treatment efficacies may be observed in patients with high baseline-values than in those with low ones. The differences of treatment efficacy and baseline may be the best fit test statistic, if the treatment efficacies are independent of baseline. However, if not, then ratios of the two may fit the data better, and allow for relevant additional conclusions.

Note

More background, theoretical and mathematical information of treatment efficacies that are not independent of baseline is given in Statistics applied to clinical studies 5th edition, Chap. 17, Logistic and Cox regression, Markov models, and Laplace transformations, pp 199–218, Springer Heidelberg Germany, 2012, from the same authors.

Chapter 79
Fifth Order Polynomes of Circadian Rhythms (1 Patient with Hypertension)

General Purpose

Ambulatory blood pressure measurements and other circadian phenomena are traditionally analyzed using mean values of arbitrarily separated daytime hours. The poor reproducibility of these mean values undermines the validity of this diagnostic tool. In 1998 our group demonstrated that polynomial regression lines of the 4th to 7th order generally provided adequate reliability to describe the best fit circadian sinusoidal patterns of ambulatory blood pressure measurements (Van de Luit et al., Eur J Intern Med 1998; 9: 99–103 and 251–256).

We should add that the terms multinomial and polynomial are synonymous. However, in statistics terminology is notoriously confusing, and multinomial analyses are often, though not always, used to indicate logistic regression models with multiple outcome categories. In contrast, polynomial regression analyses are often used to name the extensions of simple linear regression models with multiple order instead of first order relationships between the x and y values (Chap. 16, Curvilinear regression, pp 187–198, in: Statistics applied to clinical studies 5th edition, Springer Heidelberg Germany 2012, from the same authors as the current work). Underneath polynomial regression equations of the first to fifth order are given with y as dependent and x as independent variables.

$y=a+bx$	first order (linear) relationship
$y=a+bx+cx^2$	second order (parabolic) relationship
$y=a+bx+cx^2+dx^3$	third order (hyperbolic) relationship
$y=a+bx+cx^2+dx^3+ex^4$	fourth order (sinusoidal) relationship
$y=a+bx+cx^2+dx^3+ex^4+fx^5$	fifth order relationship

This chapter is to assess whether this method can readily visualize circadian patterns of blood pressure in individual patients with hypertension, and, thus, be helpful for making a precise diagnosis of the type of hypertension, like borderline, diastolic, systolic, white coat, no dipper hypertension.

T.J. Cleophas, A.H. Zwinderman, *Machine Learning in Medicine - a Complete Overview*, DOI 10.1007/978-3-319-15195-3_79

Primary Scientific Question

Can 5th order polynomes readily visualize the ambulatory blood pressure pattern of individual patients?

Example

In an untreated patient with mild hypertension ambulatory blood pressure measurement was performed using a light weight portable equipment (Space Lab Medical Inc, Redmond WA) every 30 min for 24 h. The first 10 measurements are underneath, the entire data file is entitled polynomials and is in extras.springer.com.

Blood pressure mm Hg	Time (30 min intervals)
205,00	1,00
185,00	2,00
191,00	3,00
158,00	4,00
198,00	5,00
135,00	6,00
221,00	7,00
170,00	8,00
197,00	9,00
172,00	10,00
188,00	11,00
173,00	12,00

SPSS statistical software will be used for polynomial modeling of these data. Open the data file in SPSS.

Command:

Analyze....General Linear Model....Univariate....Dependent: enter y (mm Hg).... Covariate(s): enter x (min)....click: Options....mark: Parameter Estimates....click Continue....click Paste....in "/Design=x."replace x with a 5th order polynomial equation tail (* is sign of multiplication)

x x*x x*x*x x*x*x*x x*x*x*x*x

....then click the green triangle in the upper graph row of your screen.

The underneath table is in the output sheets, and gives you the partial regression coefficients (B values) of the 5th order polynomial with blood pressure as outcome and with time as independent variable (–7,135E-6 indicates –0.000007135, which is a pretty small B value). However, in the equation it will have to be multiplied with x^5, and a large term will result even so.

Parameter estimates

Dependent variable: y

Parameter	B	Std. error	t	Sig.	95 % confidence interval Lower bound	Upper bound
Intercept	206,653	17,511	11,801	,000	171,426	241,881
x	–9,112	6,336	–1,438	,157	–21,858	3,634
x*x	,966	,710	1,359	,181	–,463	2,395
x*x*x	–,047	,033	–1,437	,157	–,114	,019
x*x*x*x	,001	,001	1,471	,148	,000	,002
x*x*x*x*x	–7,135E-6	4,948E-6	–1,442	,156	–1,709E-5	2,819E-6

Parameter estimates

Dependent variable:yy

Parameter	B	Std. error	t	Sig.	95 % confidence interval Lower bound	Upper bound
Intercept	170,284	11,120	15,314	,000	147,915	192,654
x	–7,034	4,023	–1,748	,087	–15,127	1,060
x*x	,624	,451	1,384	,173	–,283	1,532
x*x*x	–,027	,021	–1,293	,202	–,069	,015
x*x*x*x	,001	,000	1,274	,209	,000	,001
x*x*x*x*x	–3,951E-6	3,142E 6	–1,257	,215	–1,027E-5	2,370E-6

The entire equations can be written from the above B values:

$$y = 206.653 - 9{,}112x + 0.966x^2 - 0.47x^3 + 0.001x^4 + 0.000007135x^5$$

This equation is entered in the polynomial grapher of David Wees available on the internet at "davidwees.com/polygrapher/", and the underneath graph is drawn. This graph is speculative as none of the x terms is statistically significant. Yet, the actual data have definite patterns with higher values at daytime and lower ones at night. Sometimes even better fit curve are obtained by taking higher order polynomes like 5th order polynomes as previously tested by us (see the above section General Purpose). We should add that in spite of the insignificant p-values in the above tables the two polynomes are not meaningless. The first one suggests some white coat effect, the second one suggests normotension and a normal dipping pattern. With machine learning meaningful visualizations can sometimes be produced of your data, even if statistics are pretty meaningless.

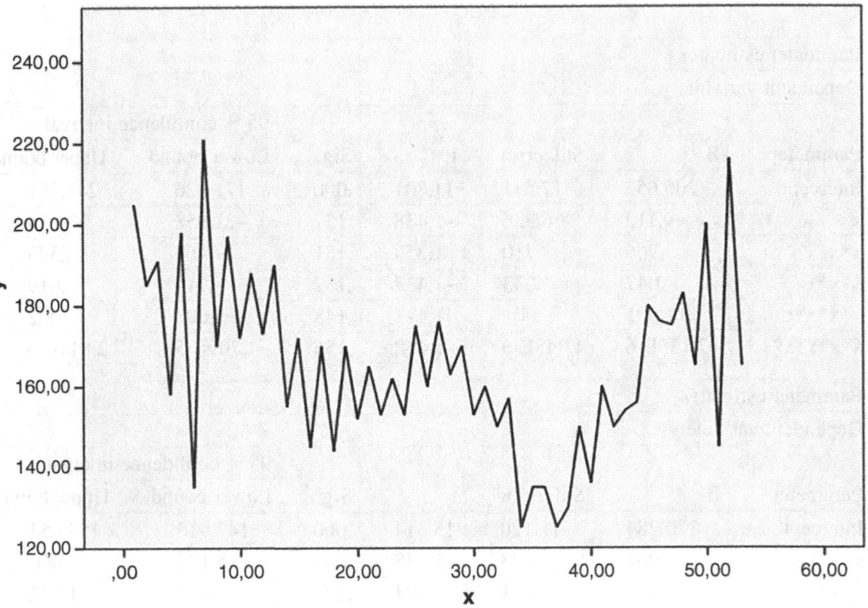

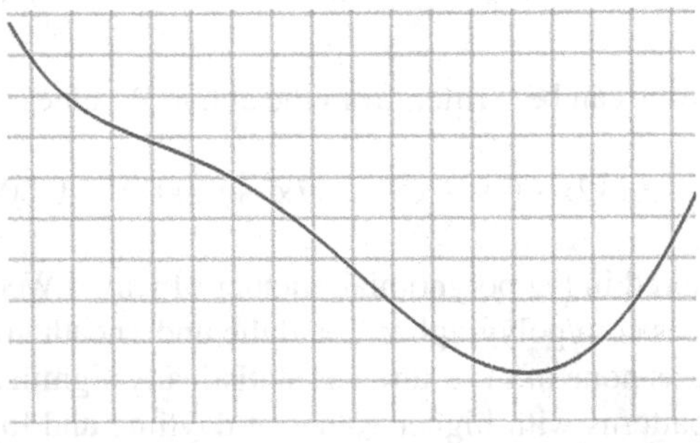

Twenty-four hour ABPM recording (30 min measures) of untreated subject with hypertension and 5th order polynome (suggesting some white coat effect)

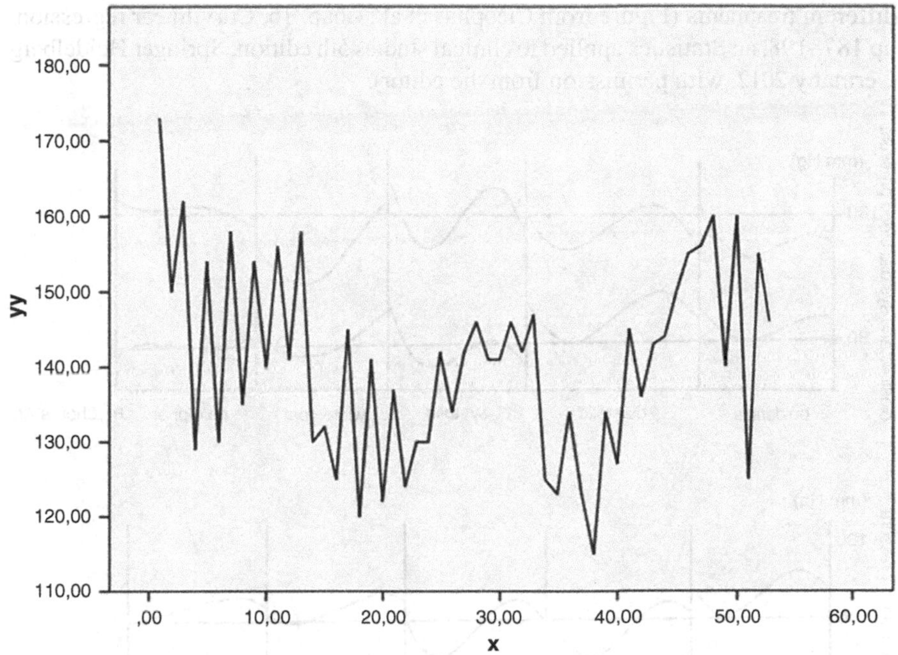

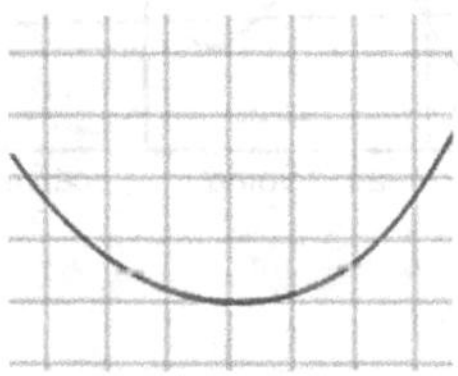

Twenty-four hour ABPM recording (30 min measures) of the above subject treated and 5th order polynome (suggesting normotension and a normal dipping pattern).

Conclusion

Polynomes of ambulatory blood pressure measurements can be applied for visualizing not only hypertension types but also treatment effects, see underneath graphs of circadian patterns in individual patients (upper row) and groups of patients on different treatments (Figure from Cleophas et al., Chap. 16, Curvilinear regression, pp 187–198, in: Statistics applied to clinical studies 5th edition, Springer Heidelberg Germany 2012, with permission from the editor).

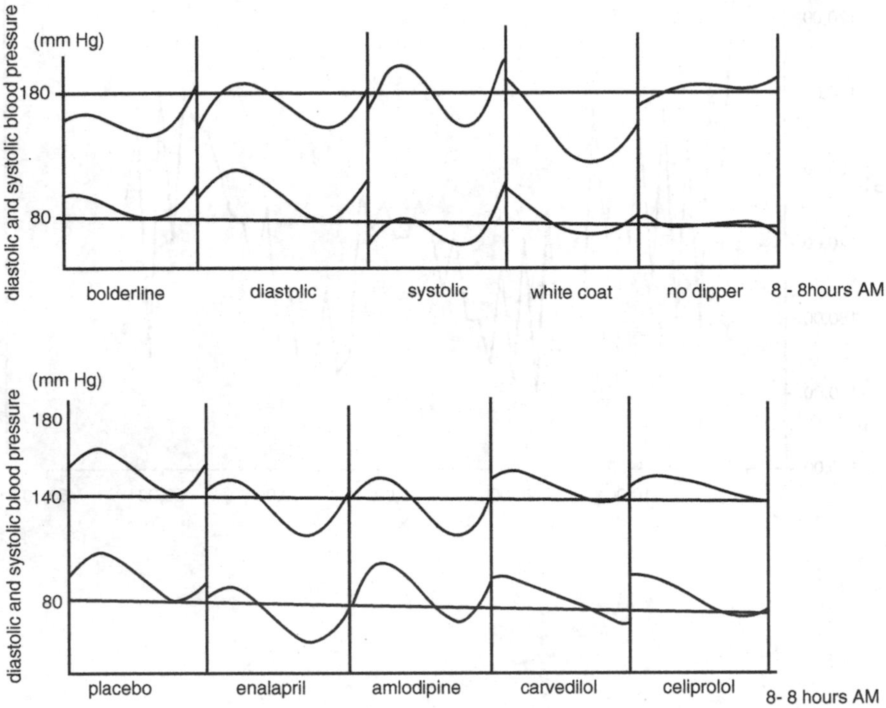

Note

More background, theoretical and mathematical information of polynomes is given in Chap. 16, Curvilinear regression, pp 187–198, in: Statistics applied to clinical studies 5th edition, Springer Heidelberg Germany 2012, from the same authors.

Chapter 80
Gamma Distribution for Estimating the Predictors of Medical Outcome Scores (110 Patients)

General Purpose

The gamma frequency distribution is suitable for statistical testing of nonnegative data with a continuous outcome variable and fits such data often better than does the normal frequency distribution, particularly when magnitudes of benefits or risks is the outcome, like costs. It is often used in marketing research.

By readers not fond of maths the next few lines can be skipped.

The gamma frequency distribution ranges, like the Poisson distribution for rate assessments, from 0 to ∞. It is bell-shaped, like the normal distribution, but not as symmetric, looking a little like the chi-square distribution. Its algebraic approximation is given underneath.

$$y = e \wedge -1/2x^2 \,(\text{standardized normal distribution})$$
$$y = (\lambda x)^r / \gamma * e \wedge -\lambda x \,(\text{gamma distribution})$$

where

λ = scale parameter
r = shape parameter
γ = correction constant.

This chapter is to assess whether gamma distributions are also helpful for the analysis of medical data, particularly those with outcome scores.

T.J. Cleophas, A.H. Zwinderman, *Machine Learning in Medicine - a Complete Overview*, DOI 10.1007/978-3-319-15195-3_80

Primary Scientific Question

Is gamma regression a worthwhile analysis model complementary to traditional linear regression, can it elucidate effects unobserved in the linear models.

Example

In 110 patients the effects of age, psychological and social score on health scores was assessed. The first 10 patients are underneath. The entire data file is entitled "gamma.sav", and is in extras.springer.com.

age	psychologic score	social score	health score
3	5	4	8
1	4	8	7
1	5	13	4
1	4	15	6
1	7	4	10
1	8	8	6
1	9	12	8
1	8	16	2
1	12	4	6
1	13	1	8

age = age class 1–7
psychologicscore = psychological score 1–20
socialscore = social score 1–20
healthscore = health score 1–20

Start by opening the data file in SPSS statistical software. We will first perform linear regressions.

Command:

Analyze....Regression....Linear....Dependent: enter healthscore....Independent(s): enter socialscore....click OK.

The underneath table gives the result. Social score seems to be a very significant predictor of health score.

Coefficients[a]

Model		Unstandardized coefficients		Standardized coefficients		
		B	Std. error	Beta	t	Sig.
1	(Constant)	9.833	.535		18.388	.000
	Social score	–.334	.050	–.541	–6.690	.000

[a]Dependent Variable: health score

Similarly psychological score and age class are tested.

Coefficients[a]

Model		Unstandardized coefficients		Standardized coefficients	t	Sig.
		B	Std. error	Beta		
1	(Constant)	5.152	.607		8.484	.000
	Psychological score	.140	.054	.241	2.575	.011

[a]Dependent Variable: health score

Coefficients[a]

Model		Unstandardized coefficients		Standardized coefficients	t	Sig.
		B	Std. error	Beta		
1	(Constant)	7.162	.588		12.183	.000
	Age class	–.149	.133	–.107	–1.118	.266

[a]Dependent Variable: health score

Linear regression with the 3 predictors as independent variables and health scores as outcome suggests that both psychological and social scores are significant predictors of health but age is not. In order to assess confounding and interaction a multiple linear regression is performed.

Command:

Analyze....Regression....Linear....Dependent: enter healthscore....Independent(s): enter socialscore, psychologicscore, age....click OK.

Coefficients[a]

Model		Unstandardized coefficients		Standardized coefficients	t	Sig.
		B	Std. error	Beta		
1	(Constant)	9.388	.870		10.788	.000
	Social score	–.329	.049	–.533	–6.764	.000
	Psychological score	.111	.046	.190	2.418	.017
	Age class	–.184	.109	–.132	–1.681	.096

[a]Dependent Variable: health score

The above table is shown. Social score is again very significant. Psychological score also, but after Bonferroni adjustment (rejection p-value=0.05/4=0.0125) it would be no more so, because p=0.017 is larger than 0.0125. Age is again not significant. Health score is here a continuous variable of nonnegative values, and perhaps better fit of these data could be obtained by a gamma regression. We will use SPSS statistical software again.

Command:

Analyze....click Generalized Linear Models....click once again Generalized Linear Models....mark Custom....Distribution: select Gamma....Link function: select

Power....Power: type −1....click Response....Dependent Variable: enter healthscore click Predictors....Factors: enter socialscore, psychologicscore, age....Model: enter socialscore, psychologicscore, age....Estimation: Scale Parameter Method: select Pearson chi-square....click EM Means: Displays Means for: enter age, psychologicscore, socialscore....click Save....mark Predict value of linear predictor.... Standardize deviance residual....click OK.

Tests of model effects

	Type III		
Source	Wald Chi-square	df	Sig.
(Intercept)	216.725	1	.000
Ageclass	8.838	6	.183
Psychologicscore	18.542	13	.138
Socialscore	61.207	13	.000

Dependent Variable: health score
Model: (Intercept), ageclass, psychologicscore, socialscore

The above table give the overall result: is similar to that of the multiple linear regression with only social class as significant independent predictor.

Parameter estimates

			95 % Wald confidence interval		Hypothesis test		
Parameter	B	Std. error	Lower	Upper	Wald Chi-square	df	Sig.
(Intercept)	.188	.0796	.032	.344	5.566	1	.018
[ageclass=1]	−.017	.0166	−.050	.015	1.105	1	.293
[ageclass=2]	−.002	.0175	−.036	.032	.010	1	.919
[ageclass=3]	−.015	.0162	−.047	.017	.839	1	.360
[ageclass=4]	.014	.0176	−.020	.049	.658	1	.417
[ageclass=5]	.025	.0190	−.012	.062	1.723	1	.189
[ageclass=6]	.005	.0173	−.029	.039	.087	1	.767
[ageclass=7]	0[a]	.	.	.	.	.	.
[psychologicscore=3]	.057	.0409	−.023	.137	1.930	1	.165
[psychologicscore=4]	.057	.0220	.014	.100	6.754	1	.009
[psychologicscore=5]	.066	.0263	.015	.118	6.352	1	.012
[psychologicscore=7]	.060	.0311	−.001	.121	3.684	1	.055
[psychologicscore=8]	.061	.0213	.019	.102	8.119	1	.004
[psychologicscore=9]	.035	.0301	−.024	.094	1.381	1	.240
[psychologicscore=11]	.057	.0325	−.007	.120	3.059	1	.080
[psychologicscore=12]	.060	.0219	.017	.103	7.492	1	.006
[psychologicscore=13]	.040	.0266	−.012	.092	2.267	1	.132
[psychologicscore=14]	.090	.0986	−.103	.283	.835	1	.361
[psychologicscore=15]	.121	.0639	−.004	.247	3.610	1	.057
[psychologicscore=16]	.041	.0212	−.001	.082	3.698	1	.054
[psychologicscore=17]	.022	.0241	−.025	.069	.841	1	.359

(continued)

Parameter estimates

Parameter	B	Std. error	95 % Wald confidence interval		Hypothesis test		
			Lower	Upper	Wald Chi-square	df	Sig.
[psychologicscore = 18]	0[a]	.	.	.	.	.	.
[socialscore = 4]	−.120	.0761	−.269	.029	2.492	1	.114
[socialscore = 6]	−.028	.0986	−.221	.165	.079	1	.778
[socialscore = 8]	−.100	.0761	−.249	.050	1.712	1	.191
[socialscore = 9]	.002	.1076	−.209	.213	.000	1	.988
[socialscore = 10]	−.123	.0864	−.293	.046	2.042	1	.153
[socialscore = 11]	.015	.0870	−.156	.185	.029	1	.865
[socialscore = 12]	−.064	.0772	−.215	.088	.682	1	.409
[socialscore = 13]	−.065	.0773	−.216	.087	.703	1	.402
[socialscore = 14]	.008	.0875	−.163	.180	.009	1	.925
[socialscore = 15]	−.051	.0793	−.207	.104	.420	1	.517
[socialscore = 16]	.026	.0796	−.130	.182	.107	1	.744
[socialscore = 17]	−.109	.0862	−.277	.060	1.587	1	.208
[socialscore = 18]	−.053	.0986	−.246	.141	.285	1	.593
[socialscore = 19]	0[a]	.	.	.	.	.	.
(Scale)	.088[b]						

Dependent Variable: health score
Model: (Intercept), ageclass, psychologicscore, socialscore
[a]Set to zero because this parameter is redundant
[b]Computed based on the Pearson chi-square

However, as shown in the above large table, gamma regression enables to test various levels of the predictors separately. Age classes were not significant predictors. Of the psychological scores, however, no less than 8 scores produced pretty small p-values, even as small as 0.004 and 0.009. Of the social scores now no one is significant.

In order to better understand what is going on SPSS provides marginal means analysis here.

Estimates

Age class	Mean	Std. error	95 % Wald confidence interval	
			Lower	Upper
1	5.62	.531	4.58	6.66
2	5.17	.461	4.27	6.07
3	5.54	.489	4.59	6.50
4	4.77	.402	3.98	5.56
5	4.54	.391	3.78	5.31
6	4.99	.439	4.13	5.85
7	5.12	.453	4.23	6.01

The mean health scores of the different age classes were, indeed, hardly different.

Estimates

			95 % Wald confidence interval	
Psychological score	Mean	Std. error	Lower	Upper
3	5.03	.997	3.08	6.99
4	5.02	.404	4.23	5.81
5	4.80	.541	3.74	5.86
7	4.96	.695	3.60	6.32
8	4.94	.359	4.23	5.64
9	5.64	.809	4.05	7.22
11	5.03	.752	3.56	6.51
12	4.95	.435	4.10	5.81
13	5.49	.586	4.34	6.64
14	4.31	1.752	.88	7.74
15	3.80	.898	2.04	5.56
16	5.48	.493	4.51	6.44
17	6.10	.681	4.76	7.43
18	7.05	1.075	4.94	9.15

However, increasing psychological scores seem to be associated with increasing levels of health.

Estimates

			95 % Wald confidence interval	
Social score	Mean	Std. error	Lower	Upper
4	8.07	.789	6.52	9.62
6	4.63	1.345	1.99	7.26
8	6.93	.606	5.74	8.11
9	4.07	1.266	1.59	6.55
10	8.29	2.838	2.73	13.86
11	3.87	.634	2.62	5.11
12	5.55	.529	4.51	6.59
13	5.58	.558	4.49	6.68
14	3.96	.711	2.57	5.36
15	5.19	.707	3.81	6.58
16	3.70	.371	2.98	4.43
17	7.39	2.256	2.96	11.81
18	5.23	1.616	2.06	8.40
19	4.10	1.280	1.59	6.61

In contrast, increasing social scores are, obviously, associated with deceasing levels of health, with mean health scores close to 3 in the higher social score patients, and over 8 in the lower social score patients.

Conclusion

Gamma regression is a worthwhile analysis model complementary to linear regression, ands may elucidate effects unobserved in the linear models. Data from sick people may not be normally distributed, but, rather, skewed towards low health scores. Gamma distributions are skewed to the left, and may, therefore, better fit such data than traditional linear regression.

Note

More background, theoretical and mathematical information of linear and nonlinear regression models is given in many chapters of the current book, particularly the chapters in the section entitled (log) linear models.

Index

A
Absolute risk, 251
Absorbing Markov chains, 351
Accuracy, 47, 390
    statistics, 50, 443
    true positives and true negatives, 390
Activation function, 310
Actual % outside specification limits, 106
Adjusted p-values, 462
Advanced analysis of variance, random effects and mixed effects models, 206
Amino acid sequences, 460
Analyses of covariances, 306
Analysis node, 407, 415
Analysis of moment structures (Amos), 295, 301
Analysis of safety data, 65, 70, 75, 85
Analysis of variance (ANOVA), 94, 166
Analysis with two layers, 63
Analyzing predictor categories, 175
Anomaly detection, 33, 170
ANOVA. *See* Analysis of variance (ANOVA)
Apply Models modus, 215
Area under curve (AUC), 251
    of the Gaussian curve, 367
    of the normal distribution, 279
ARIMA. *See* Autoregressive integrated moving average (ARIMA)
Artificial intelligence, 52
    multilayer perceptron, 400
    radial basis functions, 400
Association rules, 475
Auto Classifier node, 412
Autocorrelation analysis, 423
Autocorrelation coefficients, 425
Automatic data mining, 383
Automatic linear regression, 186, 189
Automatic modeling, 445
    of clinical events, 409
    of drug efficacies, 401
Automatic Newton modeling, 417
Automatic non-parametric testing, 175, 179, 182
Automatic regression, 189
Auto Numeric node, 404
Autoregressive integrated moving average (ARIMA), 211
Autoregressive models for longitudinal data, 211
Auxiliary view, 22, 181

B
Balanced iterative reducing and clustering using hierarchies (BIRCH), 31
Bar charts, 36, 53, 67
Basic Local Alignment Search Tool (BLAST) database system, 459
Bayesian network, 295, 301, 414, 439
Bell shape (Gaussian shape), 253
Best fit category
    for making predictions, 25
    and probability of being in it, 171
Best fit separation line, 445
Best unbiased estimate of the variance components, 221
Between-group linkage, 4
Between-subjects factor(s), 272
Bias, 53
    of multiple testing, 321

T.J. Cleophas, A.H. Zwinderman, *Machine Learning in Medicine - a Complete Overview*, DOI 10.1007/978-3-319-15195-3

Binary logistic regression, 118, 248
Binary outcome variable, 179
Binary partitioning, 353
Binning process, 354
Binning Rules in a Syntax file, 26
Binomial SE of the sample proportion, 482
Bins, 26, 41
  variables, 356
Biplot, 323
Bit score = the standardized score (score independent of any unit), 460
Blast hits, 461
Blinding, 241
Bluebit Online Matrix Calculator, 347
Bonferroni-adjusted z-tests, 81
Bonferroni adjustment, 477, 499
Bootstrap aggregating ("bagging"), 416
Bootstrap resampling, 141
Box and whiskers graphs, 180
Box and whiskers plots, 39
Breslow and the Tarone's tests, 74
b-values, 146, 478

C
Canonical analysis, 165
Canonical b-values (regression coefficients), 167
Canonical form, 346
Canonical predictors, 168
Canonical regression, 165, 166
Canonical weights (the multiple b-values of canonical regression), 168
Canvas, 385, 388, 403, 441, 466
Capacity indices, 106
Cases, 7
Categorical analysis of covariates, 179
Categorical and continuous outcome, 47
Categorical data, 182
Categorical variable, 187
Category merging, 189
Causality, 295, 301
Cause effect diagrams, 396
Cause effect relationships, 301
C5.0 classifier, 389
C5.0 decision tree (C5.0), 389, 414
CHAID. *See* Chi square automatic interaction detector (CHAID)
Change points, 211
Checklists, 396
Child Node, 48
Chi-square, 475
Chi square automatic interaction detector (CHAID), 48, 406, 408
Chi-squared automatic interaction model, 328
Chi-square goodness of fit, 253
  for Fit Statistics, 367
Chi-square test, 63, 81, 105, 286
Circadian rhythms, 491
Classification and regression tree (C&R Tree), 406, 414
Classification trees, 445
Classify, 4, 48, 150
Classifying new medicines, 17
Class of drugs, 17
Clinical data where variability is more important than averages, 105, 110, 200
Clinical scores with inconsistent intervals, 223
Clustering Criterion, 32
Cluster membership, 14, 32
Clusters, 6
Cochran and Mantel Haenszel Statistics, 73
Cochran's and Mantel Haenszel tests, 75
Coefficient of dispersion (COD), 488
Cohen's Kappa, 79
Column coordinates, 342
Column proportions, 81
  comparisons of interaction matrices, 85
Comma Delimited (*.csv), 37, 441, 467
Complementary log-log transformations, 54
Complex samples
  methodologies, 313
  statistics, 318
Composite outcome variables, 151
Concentration Index, 488
Concordant cells, 69
Conditional dependencies of nodes, 295, 301
Conditional probabilities, 475
Confidence intervals, 39, 481
  of differences in proportions, 483
  of proportions, 481
  for proportions and differences in proportions, 481
Confidence rule, 476
Configurate and execute commands, 442, 448
Confusion matrix, 443
Conjoint analysis, 359
Conjoint program, 364
Constructing an analysis plan, 359
Contingency coefficient, 63
Contingency table, 61, 67
Continuity correction, 483
Continuous data, 53
Continuous variables, 14
Control charts, 105, 396
Conviction rule, 476
Correlation, 180
  by Kendall's method, 363
  by Pearson, 138

Correlation coefficients, 138
of the three best models, 407
Correlation level, 180
Correlation matrix, 139
Correlations, 94
Correspondence analysis, 321
with multidimensional analyses, 325
Counted rates of events, 261
Covariances, 302
Covariates, 166
Cox regression, 119
with a time-dependent predictor, 371
Crossover studies, 123, 272
Crossover trial, 189
Crosstab, 61, 65, 67, 68, 94, 267
Cross-tables, 321
Crossvalidation, 465
C-statistics, 245
csv file type, 37
csv type Excel file, 38, 49, 441, 466
Cubes, 95
Cubic (best fit third order, hyperbolic) relationship, 431
Cubic spline, 419
Cumulative histograms, 419
Cumulative probabilities (= areas under curve left from the x-value), 258
Curvilinear regression, 430
Cut-off values, 25

D

DAG. *See* Directed acyclic graph (DAG)
Data audit node, 385
Data imputation, 17
Data mining, 35
Data view screen, 33
Davidwees.com/polygrapher, 493
DBSCAN method, 10
Decision analysis, 327
Decision list (Decision..), 414
Decision list models, 414
Decision Tree Learner, 50, 467
Decision Tree Predictor, 50, 467
Decision trees, 28, 47, 327
with binary outcome, 331
with continuous outcome, 331
for decision analysis, 29
model, 469
Decision Tree View, 50
Degenerate solution, 340
Degrees of freedom (df), 166
Demographic data files, 17, 24
Dendrogram, 4
Density-based cluster analysis, 10
Density-based clustering, 7, 9
DeSarbo's and Shepard criteria, 340
Descriptives, 94
Descriptive Statistics, 55, 63, 68, 78, 253, 268, 317, 452, 488
df. *See* Degrees of freedom (df)
Diagonal, 255
Diagonal line, 255
Differences in units, 142
Dimension reduction, 139, 323
Directed acyclic graph (DAG), 295, 301, 441
Discordant cells, 69
Discrete data, 53, 67
Discretize, 145
Discretized variables, 143
Discriminant analysis, 149, 180, 383, 445
for supervised data, 153, 414
Dispersion measures (dispersion accounted for), 340
Dispersion values, 337
Dissociation constant, 419
Distance Measure, 32
Distance network, 181
Distances, 3
Distribution free methods of validation, 465
Distribution node, 385
Dociles, 40
Dose-effectiveness curves, 419
Dose-effectiveness studies, 422
Dotter graph, 7
Doubly multivariate analysis of variance, 271
Drop box, 92
Duplicate observations, 77, 79

E

EAP score table. *See* Expected ability a posteriori (EAP) score table
Elastic net method, 147
Elastic net optimal scaling, 148
Elimination constant, 421
EMS. *See* Expected mean squares (EMS)
Ensembled accuracy, 416
Ensembled correlation coefficient, 408
Ensembled model(ing), 408, 409
of continuous data 387, (DOUBT)
Ensembled outcome, 408, 416
Ensembled procedure, 408
Ensembled results
of best fit models, 445
of a number of best fit models, 401
Entropy method, 353
Eps, 10

Equal intervals, 53
Error rates, 448, 468
Euclidean, 32
E-value = expected number similarity alignment scores, 460
E-value = p-value adjusted for multiple testing, 460
Event-rates, 131–135
Evolutionary operations (evops), 435–437
  calculators, 435
Examine, 94
Excel files, 37
Excel graph, 419
Expected ability a posteriori (EAP) score table, 368
Expected counts, 323
Expected mean squares (EMS), 221
  of error (the residual effect), 222
Expected proportion, 476
Expert Node, 405–407
Expert tab, 413–414
Explanatory variable, 208
Explorative data mining, 3
Exploratory purposes, 390
Exported eXtended Markup Language (XML), 33
Export modeler, 213
Exposure (x-value) variables, 137
eXtended Markup Language (XML), 14, 33, 124, 126, 132, 150, 172, 177, 178, 187, 192, 196, 213, 310, 315, 328, 333, 398
  files, 14, 15, 32, 33, 114, 115, 125
  model, 33
Extras.springer.com, 4, 26, 36, 62, 68, 72, 78, 81, 87, 95, 114, 124, 134, 138, 150, 151, 156, 160, 172, 179, 184, 190, 196, 204, 224, 234, 254, 257, 280, 290, 302, 310, 314, 360, 373, 392, 401, 408, 416, 446, 447, 452, 466, 467, 477

F
Factor analysis, 137–142, 169, 295, 300, 301
False positives, 248
Fifth order polynomes, 491–496
Fifth order polynomial, 492, 493
Fifth order relationship, 491
File reader, 441, 442
File reader node, 38, 447, 466
Filtered periodogram, 427
First order (linear) relationship, 491
Fitting non-linear functions, 418
Fixed and random effects, 203
Fixed intercept log-linear analysis, 184
Fixed intercept models, 187
Flow charts, 396
Forecast, 215, 425
Fourier analyses, 423
Fourth order (sinusoidal) relationship, 491
Frequencies, 94–99
  procedures, 53
  tables, 53, 67
F-tests, 146
Fundamental matrix (F), 347
Fuzzy logic, 377–381
Fuzzy memberships, 379
Fuzzy-model, 381
F-value, 166

G
Gamma, 68, 497–503
Gamma frequency distribution, 497–503
Gamma regression, 498
Gaussian activation function, 397
Gaussian distributions, 175, 179
Gaussian-like patterns, 11
Generalized estimating equations, 126
Generalized linear mixed models, 184, 185, 187, 203–206
Generalized linear models, 123–129, 131–135, 263, 289, 291, 406, 499
General linear models, 94, 166, 220, 272, 314, 492
General loglinear model, 230
GoF. *See* Goodness of fit (GoF)
Gold nugget, 390
Goodman coefficient, 65
Goodness of fit (GoF), 141, 237
Goodness of fit tests, 365
Graphical tools of data analysis, 396
GraphPad Software QuickCalcs t test calculator, 472

H
Health risk cut-offs, 25
Heterogeneity correction factor, 280
Heterogeneity due to chance, 244
Heterogeneity in clinical research, 241–244
Heterogeneity tests, 74
Heterogeneous studies and meta-regression, 244
Heterogeneous target populations, 318
Heteroscedasticity, 158
Heuristic studies, 445

Hidden layers, 310
Hierarchical and k-means clustering, 11
Hierarchical cluster analysis, 4–6
for unsupervised data, 46
Hierarchical clustering, 3–8
Hierarchical cluster modeling, 46
High-Risk-Bin Memberships, 25–29
High risk cut-offs, 27, 353–357
Histogram, 40–41, 197, 254, 258, 419
Holdouts, 360, 363
Homogeneous data, 9–11
Homogenous populations, 7
Homologous (philogenetically from the same ancestors), 461
Homoscedastic, 155
http://blast.ncbi.nlm.nih.gov/Blast.cgi, 460
http://vassarstats.net/prop2_ind.html, 483
Hyperbola, 419
Hyperbolic tangens, 310
Hypotheses, data, stratification, 53

I
Ideal point, 342
Ideal point map, 339
Identity (I) matrix, 347
Improved precision of analysis, 189
Imput and output relationships, 379
Incident rates with varying incident risks, 229–232
Inconsistent spread, 155–158
Index1, 103
Individual proximities, 340
Instrumental variable, 207
Instrument response function (IRF) shape, 367
Integer overflow, 140
Interactions, 37, 159–163
effects, 159–163
matrices, 71, 75, 77, 79, 85
matrix, 65
of nominal variables, 61
between the outcome variables, 150
and trends with multiple response, 457
variable, 160, 161
Interactive histogram, 40
Interactively rotating, 20
Interactive output sheets, 180
Interactive pivot tables, 94
Interactive set of views, 180
Interval censored data analysis, 289–292
Interval censored link function, 289
Interval coefficient of concentration, 488
Interval data, 327
IO option (import/export option nodes), 39
IRF shape. *See* Instrument response function (IRF) shape
Item response modeling, 365–369
Iterate, 6
Iteration methods for crossvalidations, 465–469
Iterations plot, 139
Iterative random samples, 468

J
JAVA Applet, 10

K
Kaplan-Meier curves, 291
Kappa, 78
kappa-value, 79
Kendall's tau-b, 68
Kendall's tau-c, 68
Kinime. *See* Konstanz information miner (Knime)
K-means cluster analysis, 6–7
K-means clustering, 3–8
k-means cluster model, 6
K nearest neighbors (KNN) algorithm, 414
clustering, 406
Kolmogorov Smirnov tests, 253
Konstanz information miner (Knime), 300, 441–443, 446–447, 466–467
data miner, 37–38, 49–50, 446–447, 466 467
software, 35, 45, 441–442
welcome screen, 37, 441, 446, 466
workbench, 37, 441, 446, 466
workflow, 38, 50–51, 442–443
Kruskall-Wallis, 266, 271
Kruskal's stress-I, 340
Kurtosis, 57

L
Lambda, 63, 167
Lambda value, 65
Laplace transformations, 485
Lasso, 145
optimal scaling, 148
regularization model, 146
Latent factors, 137
Layer variable, 73
Learning sample, 397
Legacy Dialogs, 6, 36, 242
Lift Chart, 39–40
Lift rule (lift-up rule), 476

Likelihoods for different powers, 157
Linear-by-linear association, 268, 457
Linear cause-effect relationships, 151
Linear data, 159
Linear equation, 183
Linear, logistic, and Cox regression, 113–121
Linear regression, 142, 144–145, 406
for assessing precision, confounding, interaction, 116, 194
basic approach, 116, 194
Line plot, 41–42
Linguistic membership names, 379
Linguistic rules for the input and output data, 379
Link function: select Power type-1, 499–500
Ljung-Box tests, 214
Logarithmic regression model, 378
Logarithmic transformation, 59
Logical expression, 373
Logistic and Cox regression, Markov models, Laplace transformations, 118, 121
Logistic regression, 116–118, 123, 179
Logit loglinear modeling, 233
Log likelihoods, 353
Loglinear, 229–239
equations, 183
modeling, 229–239, 503
Log odds
of having the disease, 248
otherwise called logit, 279
Log prob (otherwise called probit), 279
Logtime in Target Variable, 59
Log transformed dependent variable, 264
Loss function, 340
Lower confidence limits (LCL), 108, 215
Lower control limit (LCL), 108
LTA-2 (Latent Trait Analysis-2) free software program, 367

M
Machine learning in medicine-cookbook 1, 3, 9, 13, 29, 113, 123, 131, 137, 143, 149, 155, 159, 165, 309, 313, 335, 345, 353, 359
Machine learning in medicine-cookbook 2, 17, 25, 31, 171, 175, 183, 189, 195, 203, 207, 211, 365, 371, 377, 383, 391, 401, 409, 485
Machine learning in medicine-cookbook 3, 35, 47, 219, 223, 229, 233, 241, 245, 423, 429, 435, 439, 445, 451, 459, 465, 471, 475, 481
Machine learning in medicine part one, 46, 47, 52, 102, 104, 142, 148, 163, 169, 180, 206, 295, 301, 312, 353, 369, 375, 381, 383, 400, 407, 414, 428, 445, 469
Machine learning in medicine part three, 29, 158, 206, 222, 276, 277, 279, 287, 319, 334, 351, 357, 364, 406, 414, 422, 428, 433, 445, 457
Machine learning in medicine part two, 8, 11, 15, 33, 34, 174, 210, 217, 245, 251, 325, 344, 406, 414, 439, 444, 449, 464, 479
Magnitude of variance due to residual error (unexplained variance, otherwise called Error), 220
Magnitude of variance due to subgroup effects, 222
MANOVA. *See* Multivariate analysis of variance (MANOVA)
Mantel Haenszel (MH) odds ratio (OR), 74, 75
Marginalization, 439
Marginal means analysis, 501
Markov chains, 351
Markov modeling, 345
Mathematical functions, 417
Matrix algebra, 346
Matrix mean scores, 336
Matrix of scatter plots, 42–43
Matrix software, 482
Max score = best bit score between query and database sequence, 460
McCallum-Layton calculator for proportions, 477
McNemar's test, 477
Mean predicted probabilities, 292
Means and standard deviations, 53
Measuring agreement, 77–79
Median, 57, 180, 488
Menu bar, 90
Meta-analysis, review and update of methodologies, 244
Meta-regression, 244
Michaelis-Menten equation, 419
Microsoft, 187
Microsoft's drawing commands, 6, 338
Missing data, 24
imputation, 24
Mixed data, 203–206
Mixed linear analysis, 103
Mixed linear models, 102
Mixed models, 184
Modeled regression coefficients, 192

Model entropy, 26
Model viewer, 19, 32, 180
Modified hierarchical cluster analysis, 45
Monte Carlo simulation, 195
MOTIF data base system, 459
Multidimensional clustering, 15
Multidimensional data, 87–94
Multidimensional datasets, 95
Multidimensional scaling, 335–344
Multidimensional Unfolding (PREFSCAL), 339, 342
Multilayer neural network, 397
Multilayer perceptron, 310
  modeling, 47
Multinomial and polynomial not synonymous, 491
Multinomial logistic regression, 37
Multinomial, otherwise called polytomous, logistic regression, 174
Multinomial regression
  for outcome categories, 171–174
Multinomial regression, 171–174, 183, 223
Multiple bins for a single case, 29
Multiple dimensions, 87
  with multiple response, 457
Multiple endpoints, 276, 277
Multiple groups chi-square test, 322
Multiple linear regression, 144–145, 176
Multiple paired outcomes and multiple measures of the outcomes, 273
Multiple probit regression, 282–286
Multiple response crosstabs, 456
Multiple response sets, 451–457
Multiple testing, 276, 408
Multiple treatments, 277
Multistage regression, 295, 300
Multivariate analysis of time series, 217
Multivariate analysis of variance (MANOVA), 140, 162, 164, 180, 271

N
Nearest neighbors, 17–24, 414
  methodology, 17, 24
Nested term, 104
Neural network (neural net), 47, 52, 309–312, 397–400, 445
Newton's method, 417
Node box plot, 39
Node dialog, 39
Node repository, 39, 49, 441, 467
Node repository box, 467
Nodes, 29, 38, 385, 442
Nodes x-partitioner, svm learner, svm predictor, x-aggregator, 448
Noise handling, 32
Nominal and ordinal clinical data, 77
Nominal clinical data, 61–65
Nominal data, 53, 59, 67
Nominal variable, 55–56
Nominal x nominal crosstabs, 69
Non-algorithmic methods, 327
Non-linear modeling, 46
Nonlinear Regression Calculator of Xuru's website, 418
Non-metric method, 327, 353
Nonnegative data, 497
Non-normal data, 196–200
Nonparametric tests, 94, 432
Non-proportional hazards, 372
Normal curve on histogram, 57, 59
Normal distributions, 177
Normality test, 253
Normalized stress, 340
Novel variables, 192
Nucleic acids sequences, 460
Numeric expression, 59

O
Observed counts, 312
Observed proportion, 476
Odds of being unhealthy, 73
Odds of disease, 245
Odds of event, 261
Odds of having had a particular prior diagnosis, 150
Odds ratio, 72, 249, 279
  (Exp (B)), 235
  and multiple regression, 118
OLAP. *See* Online analytical processing (OLAP)
One by one distances, 336
One way analysis of variance (ANOVA), 271, 276
Online analytical procedure cubes, 95–99
Online analytical processing (OLAP), 95
Online matrix-calculators, 345
Optimal binning, 26–28, 353–357
Optimal bins, 26–29
Optimal scaling, 143–148
  discretization, 148
  with elastic net regression, 147–148
  with lasso regression, 147
  with or without regularization, 148
  regularization including ridge, lasso, and elastic net regression, 148
  with ridge regression, 146
  of SPSS, 145
  without regularization, 145–146

Optimize Bins, 26
Ordered bar chart, 56
Ordinal clinical data, 67–70
Ordinal data, 53
Ordinal regression
with a complimentary log-log function, 225
including specific link functions, 227
Ordinal scaling, 223–227
for clinical scores with inconsistent intervals, 54, 60
Ordinal variable, 56–57
Ordinal x ordinal crosstabs, 69
Ordinary least squares (OLS) linear regression analysis, 155
Original matrix partitioned, 346
Orthogonal design, 360
Orthogonality of the two outcomes, 180
Orthogonal modeling of the outcome variables, 151
Outcome and predictor categories, 183–187
Outcome categories, 171–174, 233–239
Outcome prediction
with paired data, 123–129
with unpaired data, 113–121
Outcome (y-value) variables, 151
Outliers, 253
category, 33
data, 253
detection, 31
groups, 9–11
memberships, 31–34
trimming, 189
Output node, 390
Overall accuracy, 415
Overdispersion, 146, 257, 488
Overfitting, 416

P
Paired binary (McNemar test), 129
Paired chi-square tests, 475
Paired data, 113–121
Paired observations, 271
Pairwise comparisons, 181
Parallel coordinates, 43–44
Parallel-groups, 179
Parallel group study, 81, 87, 102
Parent node, 48
Pareto charts, 391–396
Pareto principle, 391
Parsimonious, 142
Partial correlation analysis, 161
Partial least squares (PLS), 137–142, 169
Partial regression coefficients, 493
Partitioning, 47, 310
Partitioning node, 50
Partitioning of a training and a test sample, 52
Path analysis, 295, 299
Pearson chi-square, 457
Pearson chi-square value, 268
Pearson goodness of fit test, 280
Penalty term, 340
Percentages of misclassifications, 65
Performance evaluation of novel diagnostic tests, 245–251
Performance indices, 109
Periodicity, 213, 423–428
Periodogram, 425
Periodogram's variance, 428
Pharmacokinetic parameters, 421
Phi and Cramer's V, 63
Phi value, 64
Pie charts, 53
Pivot, 87–94
figures, 107
tables, 32
Pivoting
the data, 89
tray, 87–94
trays and tables, 87–94
Placebo-controls, 241
Plot node, 387
Plot of the actual distances, 337
PLS. *See* Partial least squares (PLS)
Pocket calculator method for computing the chi-square value, 324
Poisson, 232
Poisson distributions, 230
Poisson regression, 133, 230
Polynomial grapher of David Wees, 493
Polynomial modeling, 419, 492
Polytomous regression, 174
Pooled t-test, 471
Post-hoc analyses in clinical trials, 118
Precision, 193
Predicted cluster membership, 33
Predicting factors, 27
Prediction accuracy, 147
Prediction table, 448–449
Predictive model markup language (PMML) document, 196
Predictive performance, 40
Predictor categories, 175–182
Preference scaling, 338–343
Preference scores, 335, 361
Principal components analysis, 139
Probabilistic graphical models using nodes and arrows, 439

Probability-probability (P-P) plot method, 258
Probit models, 279–287
Process capability indices, 106, 109
Process improvement, 435–438
Process stability, 109
Proportional hazard model of Cox, 289
Proportion of false positive, 248
Proportion of variance in the data due to the random cad effect, 220
Proportions, fractions, percentages, risks, hazards are synonymous, 481
Protein and DNA sequence mining, 459–464
Proximity and preference scores, 335
Proximity scaling, 336–338
P value calculator-GraphPad, 471
P-values, 83, 145, 166, 172

Q
Q-Q plots. *See* Quantile-quantile plots (Q-Q plots)
Quadratic modeling, 432
Quadratic (best fit second order, parabolic) relationship, 431
Qualitative data, 53
Qualitative diagnostic tests, 251
Quality control, 392
  of medicines, 105–110
Quantal effect histograms, 41
Quantile-quantile plots (Q-Q plots), 53, 237, 253–259
Quantitative data, 53
Quartiles, 57, 180
Query coverage = percentage of amino acids used, 460
Quest decision tree (Quest Tr..), 414
Quick Unbiased Efficient Statistical Trees (QUEST), 414
Quinlan decision trees, 389

R
Races as a categorical variable, 182
Radial basis neural networks, 397–400
Random effects, 185, 203
Random interaction effect, 203
Random intercept analysis, 183–187
Random intercept model, 183, 185, 186, 192
Randomization, 241
Random Number Generators, 14, 32, 114, 124, 133, 150, 177, 398
Random sample, 314
Ranges, 180
Rate analysis, 261–264
Ratios, 314, 485
  of the computed Pearson chi-square value and the number of observations, 64
  statistics, 485–489
  successful prediction with /without the model, 40
Receiver operated characteristic (ROC) curves, 245
Recoded linear model, 178
Recode variables into multiple binary (dummy) variables, 175
Regression, 94
Regression coefficient, 248
Regression equation, 177, 248
Regression lines of the 4th to 7th order, 491
Regression modeling for improved precision, 194
Regularization, 147
  procedure, 146
Regularized optimal scaling, 148
Relative health risks, 71–75, 77
Relative risk, 72, 251
  assessments, 75
Reliability, 77, 138, 139, 491
Reliability analysis, 138
Reliability assessment of qualitative diagnostic tests, 77
Repeated measures ANOVA, 271
Reports, 96
Reproducibility, 77
  of mean values, 491
  measures, 365
Rescaled distance, 5
Rescaled phi values, 64
Rescaling, 189
Residual effect, 219
Residual error of a study, 219
Residual methods of validation, 465
Residuals, 157
  sum of squares, 419
Residues, 431
Response rates, 279
Restructure, 103, 104
  data wizard, 101
  selected variables into cases, 103
Ridge regression, 146, 148
Risk analysis, 261–264
Risk and classification tables, 329
Risk of overestimating the precision, 210
Risk probabilities, 47, 52
R matrix, 347, 348
Robust Tests, 262
R partial least squares, 140
R-square values, 429

Runs test, 429–433
R value, 157, 158, 399
r-values (correlation coefficients), 141

S
Sampling plan, 314
Saved XML file, 115, 117
Scale data, 53
Scale variable, 54
Scattergram, 396, 423
Scatter plots, 42, 241, 253
Schwarz's Bayesian Criterion, 32
Scorer, 50
Scorer node, 443
Scoring Wizard, 14, 33, 115, 117, 120, 125, 128, 135, 152, 173, 311, 399
Seasonality, 211
Second derivatives, 419
Second order (parabolic) relationship, 491
SEM. *See* Structural equation modeling (SEM)
Sensitivity, 50, 146, 465, 469
  of MANOVA, 180
  of testing, 261
Sequence similarity searching, 459
Settings tab, 407, 414
Shapiro-Wikens, 253
Shareware, 186, 192
Shrinking factor, 146
Sigma, 106
Silicon Valley, 35
Simple probit regression, 279
Simple random sampling (srs) method, 317
Simulation, 195
Simulation models, 195–201
Simulation plan "splan," 197, 198
Skewed curves, 248
Skewness, 57, 58, 253, 254, 257
Skewness to the right, 58
Somer's d, 68, 69
Spearman, 339
Specification limits, 106
Spectral analysis, 425
Spectral density analysis, 426
Spectral density curve, 427
Spectral plot methodology, 423
Spectral plots, 423
Splan, 198
Splines, 43, 46, 145
Splitting methodology, 47
Spreadsheets programs like Excel, 94
Springer Heidelberg Germany, 8, 11, 15, 24, 29, 33, 34, 46, 47, 52, 53, 65, 70, 75, 77, 79, 85, 102, 104, 105, 110, 116, 118, 121, 129, 135, 142, 148, 153, 158, 163, 169, 174, 180, 182, 194, 200, 201, 206, 210, 217, 222, 230, 232, 244, 245, 248, 251, 253, 259, 261, 264–266, 269, 271, 276, 277, 279, 287, 289, 293–296, 300–302, 306, 312, 319, 325, 334, 344, 351, 353, 357, 364, 369, 375, 381, 400, 406, 407, 414, 422, 428, 433, 435, 438, 439, 444, 445, 449, 457, 464, 469, 473, 479, 482, 484, 485, 489, 491, 496
Sps file, 29
SPSS 19.0, 4, 26, 114, 117, 119, 124, 126, 132, 138, 144, 150, 310
SPSS data files, 37, 152
SPSS for starters part one, 77, 129, 206, 265, 266, 406
SPSS for starters part two, 135, 182, 261, 264, 295, 296, 300–302
SPSS modeler, 37, 300, 383, 390, 441, 447, 466
SPSS Modeler Stream file, 408
SPSS module Correlations, 161
SPSS statistical software, 87, 262, 290, 295, 378, 390, 440, 451, 486
SPSS' syntax program, 258
SPSS tutorial case studies, 271
SQL Express, 95
Square boolean matrix, 141
Squared correlation coefficient, 167, 429
Squared Euclidean Distance, 4
Square matrix Q, 347
SSCP matrices, 272
S-shape dose-cumulative response curves, 378
Standard deviation, 107, 108
Standard errors, 248
  of proportions, 482
Standardized (z transformed) canonical coefficients, 168
Standardized covariances, 305
Standardized mean preference values, 343
Standardized regression coefficients, 299
Standardized x-and y-axes, 338
Standard multiple linear regression, 190
Stationary Markov chains, 351
Stationary R square, 214
Statistical data analysis, 35
Statistical power, 158
Statistics applied to clinical studies 5th edition, 53, 65, 79, 85, 110, 116, 118, 121, 182, 194, 200, 201, 230, 232, 244, 253, 259, 269, 289, 469, 473, 482, 484, 485, 489, 491, 496

Statistics Base add-on module SPSS, 189
Statistics file node, 385, 403, 411
Statistics on a Pocket Calculator part 2, 248
Std.deviations, 57
Stepping functions, 175
Stepping pattern, 53, 67
Stochastic processes, 345–351
Stream of nodes, 403, 411, 447, 466
  called workflow in knime, 441
Stress (standard error), 340
String variable, 6
Structural equation modeling (SEM), 295–296, 300
Subgroup memberships, 13–15
Subgroup property, 219
Submatrices, 346
Subsummaries, 95
Summary tables, 53
Supervised data, 383
Support rule, 476
Support vector machine (SVM), 406, 408, 414, 445–449
SUR_1, 119
Survey data, 13
Surveys, 3–8
Survival studies with varying risks, 371–375
SVM. *See* Support vector machine (SVM)
svm, 448
Symbol ∩, 473 (COMP: Please insert correct symbol)
Synaptic weights estimates, 398
Syntax, 167
Syntax Editor dialog box, 167
Syntax file, 28, 360
Syntax text, 425

T
Tablet desintegration times, 105–110
Terminal node, 328, 330, 332
Testing parallel-groups with different sample sizes and variances, 471–473
Testing reproducibility, 79
Test-retest reliability, 138, 139
Test sample, 47
Third order (hyperbolic) relationship, 491
Three-dimensional scaling model, 343
Threshold for a positive test, 248
Ties, 69
Time-concentration studies, 418
Time-dependent covariate (called " T_" in SPSS), 373, 374
Time-dependent Cox regression, 371, 373
Time-dependent factor analysis, 121
Time series, 211
Total score = best bit score if some amino acid pairs, 460
Traditional multivariate analysis of variance (MANOVA), 165
Traditional multivariate methods, 150
Trained Decision Trees, 47–52
Training, 396, 398
  and outcome prediction, 310
  sample, 47, 310, 311, 327, 328, 334
Transform, 32, 124, 126, 133, 150, 177
Transient state, 347–350
Transition matrix, 345, 349
Trends, 211
  to significance, 85
Trend test, 265–269
  for binary data, 265
  for continuous data, 265
T-tests, 94, 146
Two by two interaction matrix, 77, 79
Two-dimensional clustering, 8, 11, 15
Two-stage least squares, 207–210
Two Step Cluster Analysis, 32
Two step clustering, 13–15
Type and c5.0 nodes, 388, 389
Type I errors, 276, 363
Type node, 403, 404, 411, 412
Typology of medical data, 53–61, 67

U
UCL. *See* Upper confidence limits (UCL)
Uebersax J. Free Software LTA (latent trait analysis)-2, 367, 369
Unadjusted p-values, 472
Uncertainty coefficient, 63–65
Univariate, 492
Univariate analyses, 277
Univariate multinomial logistic regression, 36
Univariate multiple linear regression, 140
Universal space of the imput variable, 379
Unpaired data, 123
Unpaired observations, 271
Unpaired t-tests, 471, 472
Unregularized, 146
Unrotated factor solution, 139
Unstandardized covariances, 304, 305
Upper and lower specification limits, 107
Upper confidence limits (UCL), 108, 215
US National Center of Biotechnology Information (NCBI), 459
Utilities, 14, 33, 115, 117, 120, 125, 128, 135, 152, 173, 178, 311, 316, 330, 399
Utility scores, 362

V
Variance components, 219–222
Variance estimate, 220–222
Variance stabilization with Fisher transformation, 408
Varimax, 139
Varying incident risks, 229–232
Varying predictors, 195–201
Vassarstats calculator, 483
View space, 181
Violations of the set control rules, 108
Visualization of health processes, 35–46

W
Web node, 387, 388
Weighted least squares (WLS), 155–158
  modeling, 158
  regression, 133
Weighted likelihood methodology, 439
Weighted population estimates, 313
Weka, 300
Weka Predictor node, 442
Weka software 3.6 for windows, 441
Welch's test, 471, 473
winRAR ZIP files, 186, 192
Within-Subject Factor Name, 272
WLS. *See* Weighted least squares (WLS)
Workflow, 441, 442, 466, 467
Workflow editor, 37, 441, 442, 466, 467
Workflow in knime, 441, 447, 466
WPP superfamily, 462, 463
www.john-uebersax.com/stat/Ital.htm 358, 367, 369
www.mccallum-layton.co.uk/, 477
www.wessa.net/rwasp, 140–141

X
X-aggregator, 467, 468
XML. *See* eXtended Markup Language (XML)
X-partitioner, 467
$XR-outcome, 408, 416
Xuru, the world largest business network based in Auckland CA, USA, 418

Z
Zero (0) matrix, 347
ZIP (compressed file that can be unzipped) file, 204
z-test, 248, 482
z-values, 279
  of a normal Gaussian curve, 367